# CHANGING THE U.S. HEALTH CARE SYSTEM

# CHANGING THE U.S. HEALTH CARE SYSTEM

## Key Issues in Health Services, Policy, and Management

Ronald M. Andersen
Thomas H. Rice
Gerald F. Kominski
Editors

Foreword by Abdelmonem A. Afifi

 **Jossey-Bass Publishers**
San Francisco

Substantial discounts on bulk quantities of Jossey-Bass books are available to corporations, professional associations, and other organizations. For details and discount information, contact the special sales department at Jossey-Bass Inc., Publishers (415) 433–1740; Fax (800) 605–2665.

For sales outside the United States, please contact your local Simon & Schuster International Office.

Manufactured in the United States of America

Tables 3.5, 3.7, and 4.2 are reprinted by permission of Project Hope, The People-to-People Health Foundation, *Health Affairs,* 7500 Old Georgetown Rd., Suite 600, Bethesda, MD 20814, (301) 656–7401.

Figure 10.1 is reprinted from *Visions of Entitlement: The Care and Education of America's Children,* edited by M. A. Jensen and S. G. Goffin, 1993, by permission of the State University of New York Press, Albany, NY.

Table 17.1 is reprinted from the *Journal of the American Medical Association,* 270, 1993, by permission of the American Medical Association.

**Library of Congress Cataloging-in-Publication Data**

Changing the U.S. health care system : key issues in health services,
  policy, and management / Ronald M. Andersen, Thomas H. Rice, Gerald
  F. Kominski, editors.
      p.    cm.
  Includes bibliographical references and index.
  ISBN 0–7879–0224–1
  1. Health care reform—United States.   2. Medical policy—United States.
 3. Medical care—United States.    I. Andersen, Ronald.
 II. Rice, Thomas H.   III. Kominski, Gerald F.
 RA395.AC478   1996
 362.1′0973—dc20                  95-51416

FIRST EDITION
*HB Printing*  10 9 8 7 6 5 4 3 2

# CONTENTS

## PART TWO: COSTS OF HEALTH CARE

## PART THREE: QUALITY OF CARE

## PART FOUR: SPECIAL POPULATIONS

# FIGURES AND TABLES

## Figures

# Tables

To the late Samuel J. Tibbitts and to Audrey Tibbitts, whose generosity made this work possible, we dedicate *Changing the U.S. Health Care System.*

# FOREWORD

The book you hold in your hand is a gift.

With his wife, Audrey, the late Samuel J. Tibbitts gave a generous gift to the Department of Health Services in the UCLA School of Public Health to commission a study of key issues in health policy and management challenging the American health care system. The leadership, scholarship, and charity exhibited by Sam in making this gift typified Sam's life in a number of ways.

Sam changed the health care system in California and the nation, perhaps in more ways than anyone else of his generation. After receiving a B.S. degree in Public Health from the University of California, Los Angeles in 1949 and an M.S. degree in Public Health/Hospital Administration from the University of California, Berkeley in 1950, Sam pioneered the development of integrated health care delivery and financing systems, a career course which culminated in the 1988 creation of the nonprofit UniHealth America, where he was chairman of the board until his death in 1994. Along the way, Sam founded and chaired both PacifiCare Health Systems, one of the first major health maintenance organizations, and American Health Care Systems, a group of thirty-two hospital systems across the country that organized the nation's first preferred provider system, PPO Alliance. Both a leader and a scholar, Sam served as chairman of the board of trustees of the American Hospital Association and published more than one hundred articles. Sensing the need to establish a corporate conscience in a changing health care environment, Sam became founding chairman of the Guiding Principles for Hospitals, the first program to delineate ethical and quality principles in the industry.

Even while entering the twilight of a long and storied career, Sam's concern for the future of health care remained. For that reason, he invested in the school that had nurtured him and asked the faculty to address afresh the crucial issues of cost, quality, and access to health care which now challenge the future of the United States.

The authors of this book, commissioned to guide us into an uncertain future, are gifted scholars. As dean of the UCLA School of Public Health, I have known them well and followed their research closely. Also, as a public health educator, I am keenly aware of the multidisciplinary nature of our field. To understand public health as a whole, one must have a basic level of knowledge of each of its core disciplines. But to gain a deeper understanding of public health in the United States, one needs a firm grasp of the issues facing the country in health care policy and management. Due to their complexity, discussions of these issues have been scattered in a multitude of references. To achieve Sam Tibbitts's vision, the authors sought to gather, in a single book, "a comprehensive, yet readable" account of these issues. And I believe that they have succeeded remarkably.

This book also accomplishes its self-prescribed task: "to examine where we are in achieving our country's health care goals" following the defeat by Congress in 1994 of President Clinton's comprehensive health care reform. As anticipated by Sam, the book begins by addressing three key components of health care policy: improving access, controlling costs, and ensuring quality. An early chapter notes that access to health care has always been a focus in the health care reform debate, and concludes that "the United States cannot escape the need for fundamental reforms that will extend coverage to its entire population." Cost, an element in the "trade-off" against adequate access and better quality, not only is the center of the ensuing debate in Congress but will continue to be a focus in health care policy making for the foreseeable future. In a separate chapter, the authors explore various ways of containing health care costs and emphasize the need for better data in order to make sensible policy decisions about alternative types of health care reform. Another chapter examines the measurement of health outcomes and health-related quality of life (HRQL), concluding that we need "careful and appropriate inclusion of HRQL outcomes in traditional health services research."

A number of subsequent chapters are devoted to segments of the population with special needs for health care. Subjects include long-term care for the elderly, provision of services for the growing HIV/AIDS community, multidisciplinary coordination of the fragmented child health care system, improvement of access to primary health care for low-income women, and the increase of services to the growing homeless population. Various authors advance proposals that might improve the prognosis for these vulnerable populations.

The last portion of the volume contains discussions of the fundamental challenges facing health care researchers, policy makers, and managers at the turn of the century. A very basic challenge addressed in this area is determining the appropriate role of competitive markets versus the regulatory role of government. Based on the experience of the managed care market in California, it is noted that increased price competition leads to a reduction in access for the uninsured. Despite some instances in which governmental regulation appeared to be successful in controlling expenditures and improving or maintaining access, no conclusion is drawn as to which approach should be adopted. Rather, we are presented with several research questions that require further investigation, an indication of the high degree of complexity of this topic.

After examining and comparing the experiences of health care services in other nations, the last section proceeds to deal with a variety of issues ranging from the role of preventive health care to the role of public health agencies in delivering personal health services, and from the continuing issue of medical malpractice liability to the ethics of public health and health care services. The collective message sent to the reader is clear: the time for health care reform is ripe and effective research in this area is urgently needed to support this fundamental change.

This comprehensive account of important issues facing the nation in health policy and management will be a valuable asset for health care policy researchers and analysts, as well as health care services managers, health care providers, and practitioners. Moreover, students in health care policy and management or related fields will appreciate it as a guideline to many subject areas in health care today. Finally, I believe that this book can serve as a readable guide for health care professionals and policy makers to health care reform during the next decade.

In the final analysis, health itself is a gift. I commend this volume to you, sharing the hope of Sam and Audrey Tibbitts that training and discourse will result, leading to innovations in policy and management that will enable the blessings of health to be shared by all.

*April 1996*                                                                  Abdelmonem A. Afifi
                                                           dean, and professor of biostatistics
                                                                   UCLA School of Public Health

# ACKNOWLEDGMENTS

Two people have been responsible for keeping the many authors (and the editors) coherent, organized, and more or less on schedule. They are Pamela L. Davidson, who in addition to coauthoring one chapter oversaw the entire process of developing the manuscript, and Charles Doran, who coordinated the efforts of the authors and facilitated communication with our editors at Jossey-Bass.

We also wish to thank Pat Ritter for handling the contractual arrangements so efficiently, the authors for meeting their obligations so effectively and considerably more expediently than we had expected, and the editorial staff at Jossey-Bass, who have been creative, supportive, and committed to a quality product.

*April 1996*
*Los Angeles*

Ronald M. Andersen
Thomas H. Rice
Gerald F. Kominski

# THE AUTHORS

RONALD M. ANDERSEN is the Fred W. and Pamela K. Wasserman Professor and chair, Department of Health Services, UCLA School of Public Health, and professor, UCLA Department of Sociology. Previously he was professor at the University of Chicago, serving for ten years as director of the Center for Health Administration Studies and the graduate program in health administration. He holds a B.S. degree (1960) in sociology from the University of Santa Clara and an M.S. degree (1962) and a Ph.D. degree (1968), also in sociology, from Purdue University. Andersen has studied access to medical care for his entire professional career of thirty years. He developed the Behavioral Model of Health Services Use that has been used extensively nationally and internationally as a framework for utilization and cost studies of general populations as well as special studies of minorities, low-income persons, children, women, the elderly, the homeless, and oral health among ethnic populations. He has directed three national surveys of access to care and has led numerous evaluations of local and regional populations and programs designed to promote access to medical care. Andersen's other research interests include international comparisons of health services systems, graduate medical education curriculum, physician health services organization integration, and evaluations of geriatric and primary care delivery. He is a member of the Institute of Medicine and was on the founding board of Association for Health Services Research. He has been chair of the medical sociology section of the American Sociological Association and in 1994 received the association's Leo G. Reeder award for distinguished service to medical sociology.

THOMAS H. RICE is a professor in the Department of Health Services at the UCLA School of Public Health. He is a health economist with particular interest in the health care cost containment, health insurance, and provider payment issues and in the Medicare program. Rice received his Ph.D. degree in economics at the University of California, Berkeley, in 1982. From 1979 to 1983, he was a senior health economist at the Stanford Research Institute. Between 1983 and 1991, Rice was on the faculty at the University of North Carolina School of Public Health. He spent the 1989–1990 academic year as a visiting senior analyst at the Physician Payment Review Commission. In 1988, he received the Association for Health Services Research Young Investigator Award, which is given to the outstanding health services researcher in the United States aged thirty-five or under. In 1992, he received the Thompson Prize from the Association of University Programs in Health Administration, awarded annually to the outstanding health services researcher in the country aged forty or under. Rice is currently editor of the journal *Medical Care Research and Review.*

GERALD F. KOMINSKI is an associate professor in the Department of Health Services at the UCLA School of Public Health and associate director of the UCLA Center for Health Policy Research. He also serves as a consultant at RAND and is deputy director at UCLA of the RAND/UCLA/Harvard Center for Health Care Financing Policy Research and director of training programs for the UCLA MEDTEP Outcomes Research Center for the Study of Asians and Pacific Islanders. Kominski graduated with a bachelor's degree in chemistry from the University of Chicago in 1978 and received his doctorate in public policy analysis from the University of Pennsylvania in 1985. Prior to joining the faculty at UCLA in 1989, he served for three and one-half years as a staff member at the Prospective Payment Assessment Commission (ProPAC) in Washington, D.C. He is currently principal investigator of the California Hospital Outcomes Project, a state-funded effort to develop and report risk-adjusted outcome measures for selected inpatient conditions.

◆ ◆ ◆

EMILY K. ABEL is an associate professor in the Department of Health Services at the UCLA School of Public Health, where she teaches courses entitled "Aging and Long-Term Care," "Women, Health, and Aging: Policy Issues," and "History of Public Health." She received a B.A. degree from Swarthmore College, an M.A. degree from Columbia University, a Ph.D. degree in history from the University of London, and an M.P.H. degree from UCLA. Her publications on family care for frail elderly people include *Love Is Not Enough: Family Care for the Frail Elderly; Who Cares for the Elderly? Public Policy and the Experiences of Adult Daughters;* and several articles in *The Gerontologist, Research on Aging,* and the *Journal of Aging Studies.*

CHRISTY L. BEAUDIN is a doctoral candidate in the Department of Health Services, UCLA School of Public Health. She has worked extensively in the clinical, operations, and marketing areas of health care for the past fourteen years with Loma Linda Medical Center, Mercy Hospital in San Diego, Brotman Medical Center in Los Angeles, and National Medical Management Services in Washington, D.C. She currently serves as a health care consultant in the areas of evaluation research and quality assessment and improvement programs.

LESTER BRESLOW was dean of the UCLA School of Public Health from 1972 to 1980 and is currently professor emeritus. Breslow received his M.D. and M.P.H. degrees from the University of Minnesota. He has been a member of the Institute of Medicine, National Academy of Sciences, since 1975 and was founding editor of the *Annual Review of Public Health,* from 1978 to 1990.

ROBERT H. BROOK is a corporate fellow at RAND and director of RAND's Health Sciences Program. He is professor of medicine and health services, UCLA Schools of Medicine and Public Health. Brook was head of the Health and Quality Group on the RAND Health Insurance Experiment, co-principal investigator of the Health Services Utilization Study, which developed a method for assessing appropriateness, and co-principal investigator of the national study assessing the impact of DRGs (diagnosis-related groups) on the quality and outcomes of acute hospital care. Brook received his M.D. degree from the Johns Hopkins Medical School in 1968 and his Sc.D. degree from the Johns Hopkins School of Hygiene and Public Health in 1972.

E. RICHARD BROWN is founding director of the UCLA Center for Health Policy Research and professor in the Departments of Community Health Sciences and Health Services, UCLA School of Public Health. In 1975 he received his Ph.D. degree in sociology of education from the University of California, Berkeley. He became president-elect of the American Public Health Association in November 1994 and began serving as APHA president in October 1995. He served as a senior consultant to the President's Task Force on National Health Care Reform in 1993, and was the main author of Senator Robert Kerrey's national health insurance proposal, which was introduced before the U.S. Senate in 1991.

WILLIAM S. COMANOR is professor and director of the Research Program in Pharmaceutical Economics and Policy, Department of Health Services, UCLA School of Public Health. He is also professor of economics at the University of California, Santa Barbara. Between 1978 and 1980, he served as chief economist and director at the Bureau of Economics at the Federal Trade Commission in Washington, D.C. Comanor also served as a member of the advisory board for the recent Office of Technology Assessment study of pharmaceutical research and development. He received his Ph.D. degree (1964) in economics from Harvard University

WILLIAM E. CUNNINGHAM is an assistant professor in the Department of Health Services, UCLA School of Public Health, and the Division of General Internal Medicine, Department of Medicine, UCLA School of Medicine. He received his training in health services research through the Robert Wood Johnson Clinical Scholars Program, and received his M.P.H. degree in epidemiology. Cunningham is author of several recent manuscripts on access to medical care and quality of life for persons with AIDS. He is also an investigator at RAND, and a collaborator on a new national study of AIDS costs and AIDS patients' access to and quality of care.

PAMELA L. DAVIDSON is study director for the International Collaborative Study of Oral Health Outcomes (ICS-II) USA Ethnicity and Aging Project, UCLA School of Public Health. She has been a health services researcher for more than a decade. Prior to her appointment at UCLA, she was employed as a director for California Health Decisions, Inc., and as research coordinator for the Orange County Community Consortium. In addition to health services research and policy analysis, Davidson's professional activities include strategic programming and evaluation, health promotion, and management and organization development. She received her Ph.D. degree from UCLA in health services in 1995.

JONATHAN E. FIELDING is a professor of health services and pediatrics in the UCLA Schools of Public Health and Medicine. He has served as vice president and health director of Johnson & Johnson Health Management Inc., and as vice president, health policy analysis and planning, for Johnson & Johnson. Fielding holds graduate degrees in medicine and public health from Harvard University and an M.B.A. degree in finance from the Wharton School of Business. He was founding co-director of the UCLA Center for Health Enhancement, Education and Research, a founding member of the U.S. Preventive Services Task Force, and Commissioner of Public Health for the Commonwealth of Massachusetts from 1975 through 1979.

PATRICIA A. GANZ is professor in the UCLA Schools of Public Health and Medicine. She also serves as director of the division of cancer prevention and control research in the UCLA Jonsson Comprehensive Cancer Center. She has been instrumental in incorporating quality-of-life assessment into cancer clinical trials and chaired a National Cancer Institute workshop on this topic in 1990. She serves as associate editor of the journal *Quality of Life Research*. Ganz received her M.D. degree from the UCLA School of Medicine in 1973.

LILLIAN GELBERG is an assistant professor in the division of family medicine, UCLA School of Medicine. She is currently a member of the American Academy of Family Physicians, American Public Health Association, Society of Teachers of Family Medicine, Association for Health Services Research, and Society of General Internal Medicine. She was a fellow in the Robert Wood Johnson Clinical Scholars Program; was a recipient of the National Research Service Award for Individual Fellowship, Agency for Health Care Policy and Research; received the 1995 Young Investigator Award of the Association for Health Services Research; and received the Robert Wood Johnson Foundation Generalist Physician Faculty Scholars Program Award. She has conducted research on the health status and access to care of the homeless and other vulnerable populations since 1984. Gelberg received her M.D. degree from Harvard Medical School in 1981 and her M.S.P.H. degree from UCLA in 1987.

NEAL HALFON is an associate professor of pediatrics, UCLA School of Medicine; associate professor, Department of Community Health Sciences, UCLA School of Public Health; and a consultant at RAND. Halfon received his B.S. degree in psychobiology and chemistry at the University of California, Santa Cruz, and his M.D. degree (1978) at the University of California, Davis, where he was a Regents Scholar. He is director of the Child and Family Health Program at UCLA, co-director of the National Maternal and Child Health Policy Research Center, and a member of the Child Health Consortium. He co-chairs the committee on serving underserved children for the Ambulatory Pediatric Association, and is a member of the committee on child health financing for the American Academy of Pediatrics.

MOIRA INKELAS is a research associate in the UCLA School of Public Health, and a doctoral fellow in health policy analysis at the RAND Graduate School. She is a member of the Ambulatory Pediatric Association and the American Public Health Association. She has conducted research on intake and case disposition in child welfare, and on access to care of other vulnerable populations. Her current research activities include access to health services under Medicaid managed care, systems of care for children with special health needs, and the child welfare system. She received her M.P.H. degree from UCLA in 1993.

CHARLES E. LEWIS is a professor in the UCLA Schools of Medicine and Public Health and Nursing and director of the UCLA Center for Health Promotion and Disease Prevention. He is a member of the Institute of Medicine of the National Academy of Science. He became a regent of the American College of Physicians in 1988 and served in that capacity until 1994. Since 1990, Lewis has served as a commissioner for the Joint Commission on Accreditation of Healthcare Organizations. He received his M.D. degree from Harvard Medical School and his Sc.D. degree in environmental health from the University of Cincinnati.

MARK S. LITWIN is an assistant professor in the UCLA Schools of Public Health and Medicine. Litwin received a bachelor's degree in economics from Duke University (1981) and his M.D. degree from Emory University (1985). He completed his residency training in urological surgery at Harvard Medical School's Brigham and Women's Hospital and spent two years as a Robert Wood Johnson Clinical Scholar at UCLA. Litwin's research activities include medical outcomes assessment, health-related quality of life, urologic oncology, cost-efficacy in urological care, physician payment systems, and patient preferences.

ELIZABETH A. MCGLYNN is a health policy analyst at RAND. She was a senior investigator on the HMO Quality of Care Consortium, a collaborative effort between RAND and eleven managed care organizations to design and test a clinically based approach to measuring the quality of care. She was principal investigator on a project to develop criteria for assessing the quality of inpatient care for persons with schizophrenia and is a coinvestigator on the AHCPR-funded Schizophrenia PORT. She is currently principal investigator on an HCFA-funded project to develop a more comprehensive approach to monitoring the quality of care for women and children in managed care systems. McGlynn received her Ph.D. degree in policy analysis from the RAND Graduate School in 1988.

GLENN MELNICK is an associate professor, Department of Health Services, UCLA School of Public Health, and a consultant with RAND. He was principal investigator of a project funded by the Bureau of Health Facilities that involved the development of one of the first hospital market-level databases in the United States necessary for the evaluation of the effects of market-based procompetition policies on the health care sector. Melnick has numerous publications on the effects of competition in the market for hospital services and is frequently called upon to provide expert advice to policy makers in the area of health care competition. He received his Ph.D. degree in urban and regional planning, with an emphasis on health, from the University of Michigan in 1983.

CHRISTOPHER J. PANARITES is a senior associate at Health Technology Associates, Inc. He recently received his Ph.D. from the Department of Health Services, UCLA School of Public Health. He wrote his dissertation based on data from the UCLA Homeless Health study, which explored physical health problems and service use among homeless adults in Los Angeles County. Panarites was a recipient of a University of California AIDS Research Program (UARP) fellowship and a training fellowship from the Agency for Health Care Policy and Research.

MILTON I. ROEMER is professor emeritus in the Department of Health Services, UCLA School of Public Health. He earned his M.D. degree in 1940 from New York University and also holds master's degrees in sociology from Cornell and in public health from the University of Michigan. Roemer has served at all levels of health administration—as a county health officer, a state health official, an officer of the U.S. Public Health Service, and a section chief of the World Health Organization. He has been a member of the Institute of Medicine of the National Academy of Sciences since 1974. In 1977, he received the American Public Health Association International Award for Excellence in Promoting and Protecting the Health of People. In 1983, the APHA awarded Roemer its highest honor, the Sedgwick Memorial Medal for Distinguished Service in Public Health.

RUTH ROEMER is adjunct professor emerita, Department of Health Services, UCLA School of Public Health, and past president (1987) of the American Public Health Association. As consultant to the World Health Organization on health legislation, she has worked on nursing education and regulation, legislation on human resources for health, uses of fluorides for dental health, ethical aspects of maternal and child health, and tobacco control. She is author of a monograph published by WHO in 1982, with a second edition in 1993, *Legislative Action to Combat the World Tobacco Epidemic.* Among her honors are the WHO Medal on Tobacco or Health and the American Public Health Association Sedgwick Memorial Medal for Distinguished Service and Advancement of Public Health. She received her J.D. degree (1939) from Cornell Law School.

PAULINE VAILLANCOURT ROSENAU is an associate professor at the School of Public Health, University of Texas Health Science Center at Houston, where she is affiliated with the Department of Management and Policy Sciences, the Department of Health Services Organization, and the Health Policy Institute.

She was a professor at the University of Quebec in Montreal for two decades before joining the School of Public Health in 1993. Her edited book, *Health Reform in the Nineties,* appeared in June 1994. Her last two books received Choice Magazine's Annual Outstanding Academic Books Awards. She received her Ph.D. degree (1972) in political science from the University of California, Berkeley, and her M.P.H. degree (1992) from UCLA.

MARK A. SCHUSTER is an assistant professor in the Department of Pediatrics, UCLA School of Medicine, and a senior natural scientist at RAND. Schuster received a B.A. degree in history from Yale in 1981, M.D. and M.P.P. degrees from Harvard in 1988, and a Ph.D. in Public Policy Analysis from the RAND Graduate School in 1994. His research focuses on child and adolescent quality of care, adolescent sexuality and risk prevention, and access to and cost of care for children with HIV infection. He completed his residency in pediatrics at the Children's Hospital of Boston in 1991 and his fellowship with the Robert Wood Johnson Clinical Scholars Program at UCLA/RAND in 1993.

STUART O. SCHWEITZER is a professor in the Department of Health Services, UCLA School of Public Health. He earned his Ph.D. degree (1966) in economics from UCB. He has been on the research staff of the Urban Institute, in Washington, and at the National Institutes of Health. In 1980, Schweitzer was in charge of health policy development for President Carter's Commission for a National Agenda for the Eighties. He has held visiting appointments at Nuffield College, Oxford; the School of Public Health at the Shanghai Medical University; and the Centre de recherche, d'étude, et de documentation en économie de la santé (CREDES) and the École supérieure des sciences économiques et commerciales (ESSEC) in Paris.

PAMELA STEFANOWICZ is a doctoral candidate in the Department of Health Services, UCLA School of Public Health. She is currently conducting research for her dissertation, "Home Care for the Frail Elderly: The Process of Delivering and Receiving Care." She was the recipient of a National Center for Health Services Research fellowship and is a member of Delta Omega, the national scholarly honor society in public health.

STEVEN P. WALLACE is associate professor of public health in the Department of Community Health Sciences at UCLA. He is also co-director of the California Geriatric Education Center's Health and Aging Faculty Development Program and is chair of the Association of Schools of Public Health Task Force on

Health and Aging. He has published widely on his research in long-term care, minority aging, and health policy in journals such as the *Gerontologist, Journal of Gerontology: Social Sciences, American Journal of Public Health,* and *Journal of Aging Studies.* His current research focuses on access to long-term care by minority elderly. Wallace received his Ph.D. degree in sociology from the University of California, San Francisco, in 1987.

DAVID L. WOOD is a faculty member of the UCLA School of Medicine. Wood received combined M.D. and M.P.H. degrees from UCLA in 1982. He is currently the principal investigator of a CDC-funded study examining the delivery immunizations for African American and Latino families. Wood has also analyzed data on access to care for poor children from the Robert Wood Johnson Access to Care Survey and the National Health Interview Survey. His clinical practice has been among poor and disadvantaged populations.

ROBERTA WYN is associate director for research at the UCLA Center for Health Policy Research. She received her Ph.D. degree (1995) in public health from UCLA. Wyn has conducted research in several health care policy areas, with a particular focus on access to health insurance coverage and health care for women, ethnic populations, and low-income populations. She has also conducted analysis of the effects of alternative health care reform proposals on disadvantaged subgroups of the population. Her most recent research has focused on access to clinical preventive services for women.

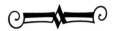

# INTRODUCTION AND OVERVIEW

Ronald M. Andersen, Thomas H. Rice,
and Gerald F. Kominski

The early 1990s were heady times for advocates of health care reform. The central role played by health care in the 1992 presidential election, the workings of the White House Task Force on Health Care Reform, and the debate in Congress that followed the airing of the Clinton proposal all signaled that the United States was finally ready to make fundamental changes in health care reform—although the exact nature of this reform was not yet clear. This optimism quickly subsided, however, as the 103rd Congress did not approve any major health care reform legislation. This was soon followed by the election of a Republican Congress that believed it had received a strong mandate from the voters *not* to substantially alter the health care delivery and financing system. In fact, the legacy of this Congress has been substantial reductions in Medicare and other federally supported health care programs.

The defeat of comprehensive health care reform did not, of course, make our problems go away. Rather, it clarified that:

- Many, if not most, of the problems we face in ensuring access to affordable, high-quality health care would have to be dealt with incrementally rather than through comprehensive reform.
- Greater reliance would be placed on the workings of the market rather than on additional governmental regulations.

The defeat of comprehensive reform efforts makes the work performed by the entire health care policy and management community more critical than ever. The mechanisms necessary to improve access, ensure quality, and control costs were not put into place. Rather, these goals will have to be achieved more circuitously, either through the market or through the subsequent enactment of piecemeal legislation. It is therefore an unusually opportune time to examine where we are in achieving our country's health care goals.

In this volume, we attempt to accomplish this task by taking a comprehensive and careful look at current issues in health care policy and management. To carry this out, we have assembled a large group of very talented and experienced researchers, and asked them to take stock of the past, present, and future in their particular areas of expertise. For a specific topic, each author or group of coauthors was asked to present the primary research and policy issues facing that topic, summarize existing empirical research on the topic, and discuss research and management strategies that can be used to address current problems.

The book is aimed at providing, in a single source, a comprehensive yet readable account of the issues facing the United States in health care policy and management. We hope that it will be of benefit to a variety of audiences, including:

- *Students.* Both those specializing in health care policy and management and those in other fields will benefit from having a thorough and up-to-date review of the literature in many subject areas in the health care field.
- *Health services researchers and policy analysts.* Those responsible for coming up with ideas will find it useful to have ready access to the state of the art in research, as well as an analysis of policy options relevant to many aspects of the health care market.
- *Health care managers.* Those responsible for organizing services will benefit from having a single source of information on how to promote quality and better health outcomes while controlling expenditures.
- *Practitioners and providers.* Those responsible for direct care, especially doctors and nurses, will find special issues of interest addressed in various chapters.

## Organization and Summary of the Volume

The volume is divided into five sections. Each of these sections contains two or more chapters relevant to that particular topic. The first three sections are on the three key components of health care policy: access, costs, and quality. In each of these sections, there are chapters on measurement and trends as well as chapters on policy options. The fourth section addresses special populations, with individual chapters on long-term care and the elderly, AIDS, children's and families' health, women's health, and the homeless. The fifth and final section concerns directions for change, with chapters on hospital price competition, regulation, lessons from other countries, the role of prevention, public and personal health, medical malpractice, and ethical issues in public health and health services management.

Here are brief summaries of some of the key material contained in these chapters.

## Access to Health Care

It is particularly appropriate to start with this topic, as concerns about access were largely responsible for instigating the health care reform debate. Consequently, access was also the major casualty. The United States holds the dubious distinction of being the only developed country that does not ensure access to health care through guaranteed coverage. Furthermore, many analysts—ourselves included—believe that one of the major barriers to controlling health care costs is exactly this lack of universal coverage. This is not only because it makes it difficult for poor and sick people to seek preventive care, but also because it fragments the financing system, requiring the existence of an expensive safety net as well as aggravating the problem of cost shifting.

Chapter One, by Ronald M. Andersen and Pamela L. Davidson, provides a comprehensive examination of access to health care. The authors argue that understanding access is the key to understanding health policy because the access framework predicts and measures health service use, can be used to promote social justice, and can be used to promote health outcomes. The chapter uses a behavioral model to explain the many aspects of access, defines exactly how access can be measured, and presents data on the levels of access and trends in the United States. Trends that emerge from this analysis include a substantial decline since 1980 in the ownership of private insurance (and a concomitant rise in the proportion of the population uninsured), which cuts across demographic groups. There has also been a gradual movement over the last sixty-five years toward equity of access by income and by race for hospital and physician services, but substantial inequalities remain in the area of dental services. The chapter also presents data on the adequacy of prenatal care and vaccine-preventable childhood diseases, which indicate that substantial racial inequalities still exist.

Chapter Two, by E. Richard Brown and Roberta Wyn, follows this tack by examining alternative public policies for achieving greater health care coverage in the United States. After providing a historical perspective on why so much of the population remains uninsured, the authors discuss the successes and failures of the Medicare and Medicaid programs, with regard to providing access to affordable high-quality coverage. The remainder of the chapter focuses on the pros and cons of alternative public and private policy options for extending coverage, including consideration of Medicaid expansions, employer mandates, risk-pooling, purchasing cooperatives, and subsidies for small-group and individual coverage. Special attention is given to managed care coverage (through both the public and private sectors), as this approach is currently favored by many policy makers. In spite of the plethora of options examined, the authors conclude that the United States cannot escape the need for fundamental reforms that will extend coverage to its entire population.

## Costs

Even though concerns about access to care provided the primary impetus behind the reform movement, it was clearly the cost issue that dictated the ensuing debate in Congress. (In fact, a case can be made that the viability of any proposal was—and still is—determined to a great degree by how the Congressional Budget Office scores its costs.) Health care costs in the United States far exceed those of other developed countries, but these costs are still not sufficient to provide universal coverage of the population. Perhaps the major reasons that policy makers and managers are concerned about the quality of care delivered is not a lack of technical expertise and equipment, but the inability to *afford* high-quality care. It is the trade-offs between costs on the one hand and access and quality on the other that will continue to provide the major tension in health care policy for the foreseeable future. Thus, the ability to control costs will have the fortuitous effect of allowing for increased access and better quality.

Chapter Three, by Thomas H. Rice, focuses on measuring health care costs and presenting their trends. With regard to measurement, the chapter distinguishes between expenditures and costs, focusing thereafter on the more easily measured concept of expenditures. It also discusses the advantages and disadvantages of various measures of alternative health care prices and expenditures, and the reliability of the data sources used to measure expenditures in the United States and throughout the world. A number of tables are used to present trends in actual expenditures; some of the more noteworthy ones include a recent decline in the rate of growth of expenditures in the United States and yet a growing disparity between how much of national income is devoted to health care in the United States versus other countries. In 1985, for example, the proportion of national income spent on health was 24 percent higher in the United States than in the next highest country; by 1992, the figure had risen to 32 percent. The chapter ends with a discussion of the need for better data in the United States, concluding that requiring private insurers to collect and release data on expenditures is essential for making sensible policy decisions about alternative types of health care reform.

Chapter Four, also by Thomas H. Rice, focuses on alternative ways of containing health care costs. It begins by developing a conceptual framework that allows cost containment methods to be divided into two different categories: those based on fee-for-service, and those based on capitation. Within fee-for-service, strategies fall into one of three groups: price controls, volume controls, and expenditure controls. Most of the remainder of the chapter reviews the literature and experiences, both in the United States and in other developed countries, on the success and failures of the many strategies that have been employed to contain costs, including hospital rate-setting programs, diagnosis-related groups, certificate-of-need programs, utilization review, technology controls, physician fee controls, practice guidelines, expenditure controls, health maintenance organizations, and managed competition (with and without premium controls). Although no conclusions are warranted concerning what is the best way to control costs, the chapter indicates the basic trade-offs involved for whatever options are chosen.

Chapter Five, by Stuart O. Schweitzer and William S. Comanor, examines a particular aspect of health care costs: pharmaceuticals. The cost of pharmaceuticals has been an important policy issue for decades, with a concern among many consumer advocates that it is too high and should be controlled—an interesting phenomenon analyzed by the authors because pharmaceutical costs have increased *less quickly* than most other components of health care costs. The authors analyze the causes of increasing pharmaceutical costs, first by critiquing studies conducted by others and then by conducting their own review of drug prices and expenditures over time in the United States and in other countries, adjusting for improvements in quality. They also review the many public policies that have been employed to control these costs, which have been aimed at consumers, physicians, and manufacturers. Although the authors do not reach any definitive conclusion about which policy levers are best, they are particularly concerned whether success can be achieved without sacrificing the vitality and viability of the industry, whose hallmark is a large investment in R&D for new products.

## Quality

There is little question that establishing and preserving quality in health care has become the leading issue for health care managers. With tremendous competitive pressures to control health care costs, managers are faced with the task of formulating financial incentives and other mechanisms that will help ensure that a high-quality, cost-effective product is provided to patients. The advent of health care report cards symbolizes consumers' need for easily digestible information on the relative quality of their alternative insurance choices. This interest is paralleled on the research front, where a great deal of effort is being expended to produce reliable measures of health care outcomes.

Chapter Six, by Patricia A. Ganz and Mark S. Litwin, examines the measurement of health outcomes and quality of life. After providing a historical perspective on the health outcomes movement, the authors present an overview of the concept of health-related quality of life (HRQL), which focuses on the patient's own perception of health and the ability to function as a result of health status or disease experience. Much of the remainder of the chapter is devoted to the challenging goal of measuring HRQL and to presenting health services research studies that have attempted to measure HRQL. An important conclusion is that patients are most concerned not with prolonging their lives per se but rather with improving the quality of their remaining years. Therefore, the authors argue, consumers are anxious to have information about the HRQL impact of new treatments. What is needed is the careful and appropriate inclusion of HRQL outcomes in traditional health services.

Chapter Seven, by Elizabeth A. McGlynn and Robert H. Brook, focuses on ensuring quality of care. It reviews various methods for assessing quality and presents data on what is known about the current level of quality in the United States. As the longest chapter in this volume, it covers a number of topics, including how to select the health conditions or problems to be examined; definitions and determinants of quality; what is known—and perhaps more significantly, not known—about structural, process-oriented, and outcomes-related quality of care; and finally, how information about quality can be used by the many actors in the health care arena. The authors conclude that over the next decade, the need to measure, monitor, and report on the quality of care will only become more important. Nevertheless, much work remains to be done, in part because of the difficulty of adjusting the results of quality assessment for differences in the severity and other characteristics of the populations whose care is being evaluated. Paramount in doing so is obtaining the necessary data from administrative, clinical, and survey sources.

## Special Populations

The problems of access, cost, and quality have varied historically for segments of the U.S. population due to their special needs and the way the health care system has responded to those needs. It is likely that the nature of the problems faced by different groups will continue to change in the face of major alterations in the way health services are organized and financed. All of the authors in this section have suggestions for health services research and policy implementation that might improve the prognosis for these vulnerable populations.

Chapter Eight, by Steven P. Wallace, Emily K. Abel, and Pamela Stefanowicz, provides a comprehensive overview of the long-term care system as a response to the rapidly increasing number of elderly in the United States and their needs for treatment of chronic and disabling illness. They provide up-to-date information on nursing homes, the range of community-based care, informal long-term care, and workers in the long-term care system. They emphasize that long-term care includes social as well as medical services, is provided overwhelmingly by family and friends, and is financed primarily by Medicaid and out-of-pocket payments. After documenting that the driving force in policy and research in long-term care for the past twenty years has been cost containment and efficiency, they identify as the most critical policy and research question, how to provide adequate high-quality long-term services to a growing and diverse older population. They conclude that the limited financial resources of many older persons, especially among racial/ethnic minorities, widows, and the working class, create a need for a universal Medicare type of social insurance.

William E. Cunningham, Christy L. Beaudin, and Christopher J. Panarites argue in Chapter Nine that the characteristics of HIV/AIDS—contagious, chronically disabling, fatal, and of emerging epidemic proportions—will increasingly force health care policy makers and managers to reevaluate the organization, delivery, and financing of health services for the HIV population. To assist in this task, they review current knowledge and research needs concerning the changing epidemiology and treatment of AIDS; measures of access, costs, and quality; and the range of services needed to treat AIDS, including not only formal medical services but also prevention, psychosocial services, and community-based health and social services. They discuss the increasing challenges to provide and pay for services as the HIV/AIDS epidemic moves from its initial epicenters of Caucasian homosexual men to much broader communities of socially and economically disadvantaged populations including women, children, adolescents, and minority groups.

Chapter Ten, by Neal Halfon, Moira Inkelas, David L. Wood, and Mark A. Schuster, examines the key issues underlying the incongruities between the needs of children and families and the current and evolving structure of the health services organization in the United States. The authors review the health needs of children and families by examining children's unique vulnerabilities, current health risks and conditions, and service needs. Next, they describe the characteristics of the health care system that influence children's access to care and the overall efficiency of health care for children. They find the organization of services to be disjointed, with multiple financial and structural barriers to children's receipt of care. They note that the movement to manage care so as to rationalize the delivery of personal medical services may substantially improve children's access to basic medical care, but many of their health needs—especially for complex medical or socially based health problems—may not be adequately addressed. The authors conclude that adequate response to the health care needs of at-risk children requires coverage for the uninsured and also the development of multi-disciplinary coordination to integrate the fragmented child health system.

Chapter Eleven, by Roberta Wyn and E. Richard Brown, examines how women's health status, socioeconomic status, and multiple role responsibilities interface with their access to and use of services. While women have lower uninsured rates and higher utilization rates than men, the authors call attention to women's more limited health insurance options and large discrepancies among women in coverage rates and health care use according to income, education, and ethnicity. They also document women's differential access to procedures and outcomes after they gain access to the system. They find that financial barriers have a profound effect on women's access to health care and health status—especially among low-income women, who have the lowest rates of screening for certain clinical services, the poorest health status, and the greatest vulnerability to the effects of increasing medical care costs. However, they note that providing financial access is not sufficient to improve women's use of health services. Services need to be organized to provide a regular source of care and incentives to physicians to promote primary and preventive services. More research is needed on the benefit to women from having a women's health specialist as a primary care provider and what this would do to their overall access to non-reproductive-related primary care services. While the authors observe that managed care plans are well positioned to promote integrated preventive and primary care for women, they also caution about the need to monitor the incentive for managed care to underserve, which might be particularly detrimental to women with chronic conditions or who require specialty care.

In Chapter Twelve, Lillian Gelberg describes the sociodemographic characteristics of homeless adults and children as well as their health status, risk factors for illness, barriers to care, quality of care, and current access to medical programs. She notes that homelessness has reached crisis proportions with estimates of up to three million currently homeless heterogeneous persons including families, runaway youth, the physically and mentally ill, and substance abusers. They experience high rates of acute and chronic illness but have limited access to medical care as reflected by high inpatient utilization and low ambulatory service use relative to their high level of need. The medical care they do receive is limited in terms of availability, continuity, and comprehensiveness. The author also details the special requirement for providers to address the housing and social service needs of the homeless at the same time their medical care needs are addressed. She finds the homeless particularly vulnerable in the policy arena because of the absence of strong advocates, tendencies by the public to accept large-scale homelessness as inevitable, and commonly held beliefs that the homeless are responsible for their status. Still, she notes that their plight could be improved by stabilizing funding for health care for the homeless, funding respite care, and medical education reform. She concludes that typical managed care models of health service delivery may not be effective for the homeless and a parallel system of care will need to be developed to address their unique needs.

## Directions for Change

As previously stated, the defeat of comprehensive health care reform at the national level provides a unique opportunity to reexamine the goals of health care reform and the methods for achieving those goals in a political environment strongly polarized over the need for such reform. Health services research has clearly played an influential role in the development of policy options at the local, state, and national levels during the past two decades. What significant contributions will health services researchers make during the next decade? The remainder of the volume addresses some of the fundamental challenges facing health care researchers, policy makers, and managers as we enter the twenty-first century.

Perhaps the most basic challenge involves determining the appropriate role of markets versus the role of governments in addressing issues of access, cost, and quality. Chapters Thirteen and Fourteen deal directly with the research evidence and policy issues related to competitive versus regulatory approaches.

Chapter Thirteen, by Glenn Melnick, evaluates the role of market forces and managed care in the control of health care costs. Drawing largely on his own research on this topic, the author argues that because California is considered to be the most mature managed care market in the country, it can serve as a laboratory to inform policy makers on what might be expected in other parts of the country as managed care expands nationally. The introduction of price competition among California hospitals, beginning in 1982, had a dramatic effect on hospitals in highly competitive markets by the end of the 1980s. Hospitals in the most competitive markets had significantly lower revenue growth compared to hospitals in the least competitive markets. As managed care continues to grow rapidly in private markets and in the Medicare and Medicaid programs, important issues require further investigation. These include how hospitals achieve their cost savings in response to increased competition and the implications of a competitive system on quality and access. The author notes that recent findings from California indicate that increased price competition leads to a reduction in access for the uninsured.

Chapter Fourteen, by Gerald F. Kominski, examines the role of regulatory approaches at both the state and national level in controlling costs and improving access. State all-payer rate-setting programs for hospital care and federal reforms in hospital and physician payment have been successful, according to the author, in controlling expenditures and in improving or maintaining access. Despite this evidence, policy makers and analysts still do not agree on what are the best mechanisms for controlling costs and expanding access, and whether regulatory controls will be more effective than market-based approaches in achieving these goals in the future. The author identifies five major research questions that will require further investigation as governments abandon regulatory approaches in favor of market-based reforms. He concludes that health services research can make a valuable contribution to future debates concerning regulatory versus competitive strategies by focusing on the distributional consequences of different approaches.

In Chapter Fifteen, Milton I. Roemer examines the experience from other nations concerning the financing, organization, and delivery of health care services. This experience, often dismissed in the debate over national reform in the United States, has shaped the nation's health care system in the past and continues to provide possible models for future improvement. The author points out that the broad thrust of health policy in the major industrialized countries of the world has been the development of health protection. There are many new lessons that could be learned to improve the effectiveness of the U.S. health system, including innovations in health personnel, such as midwives and dental nurses; the expansion of ambulatory care; regulation of hospital beds and budgets; and general revenue financing of social insurance.

Chapter Sixteen, by Charles E. Lewis, discusses the role of preventive health services and reasserts the continuing value of these services in maintaining individual and population health. The author focuses on three major questions: What is preventible? How can barriers to the application of effective treatments be overcome? and What value does society place on prevention? After discussing the recent history of prevention, the author applies these questions to case studies dealing with infectious diseases in children, cardiopulmonary diseases attributable to cigarette smoking, and deaths due to gunshot wounds. Although there are scientifically valid preventive interventions in each of these cases, values (confounded with economic interests) are the primary obstacles to successful prevention of tobacco- and firearm-related deaths.

In Chapter Seventeen, Lester Breslow and Jonathan E. Fielding reexamine the significant role of public health agencies in the delivery of personal health services in the United States. They find that these agencies have a vital interest in health care delivery because a substantial portion of the population has inadequate access to services or unstable health benefits. Public health has traditionally been directed at assuring a safe environment and at addressing the behavioral influences on health. Access to quality personal health services provided by the public health system, they argue, is also an important determinant of health. The ability of public health agencies to perform all their core public health functions, however, requires greater commitment to public health and health promotion.

Chapter Eighteen, by Ruth Roemer, deals with the continuing issue of medical malpractice liability. The author first explores the history of malpractice insurance crises of the 1970s and 1980s, state legislative responses, and the impact of those responses. She then discusses major potential reforms to the tort system, including alternative dispute resolution, enterprise liability, no-fault insurance, and medical accident compensation. Reviewing U.S. and international experience with these options, the author concludes that despite the soundness of the no-fault approach, political realities seem to militate against adoption of this alternative. Instead, the climate may be favorable for rationalizing our handling of medical injury compensation by adopting an administrative system that is more equitable and less costly than the tort system.

Chapter Nineteen, by Pauline Vaillancourt Rosenau and Ruth Roemer, deals with the ethics of public health and health care services. They argue that the cardinal principles of medical ethics—autonomy, beneficence, and justice—apply in public health ethics, but in a somewhat altered form. The authors contrast these principles as usually applied in medical ethics, where individual rights and autonomy prevail, with a broader social perspective in which individual rights may be subsumed by considerations of social welfare. At a time when we continue moving toward market-based solutions, the authors provide a framework for reexamining some of the ethical and social issues related to resource development, economic support, organization, management, delivery, and quality of care. Ethical issues in public health and health services management are likely to become increasingly complex in the future. The authors conclude, however, that even in the absence of agreement on ethical assumptions and in the face of diversity and complexity that prohibit easy compromise, mechanisms for resolving ethical dilemmas in public health do exist.

## Conclusion

When we initially planned this monograph, we expected the passage of comprehensive national health care reform to make fundamental changes in the health care system. We wished to explore the lessons to be learned from health services research for implementing these approved policies. However, the failure to pass comprehensive reform now makes the role of health services research and its lessons even more important. We have asked the authors of this volume to explore what health services research has to tell us about making fundamental changes to ensure access to affordable high-quality health care. We think that as an informed reader, you will find the authors rose to the challenge of providing comprehensive reviews of key policy and management issues regarding problems of access, cost, and quality as well as of serving special populations and assessing various strategies for reform. Unfortunately, neither the authors of this volume (nor any other possible set of authors for that matter) have answers for all the major challenges facing our health care system, but you will find that they delineate the critical set of questions and propose a number of informed, innovative solutions.

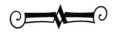

CHAPTER ONE

# MEASURING ACCESS AND TRENDS

Ronald M. Andersen and Pamela L. Davidson

The purpose of this chapter is to present basic trends as well as research and policy issues related to health care access. We define *access* as the actual use of personal health services and everything that facilitates or impedes the use of personal health services. It is the link between health services systems and the populations they serve. The conceptualization and measurement of access is key to the understanding and formulating of health policy because it predicts health services use, can be used to promote social justice, and can be used to promote health outcomes.

The chapter presents a conceptual framework for understanding access to medical care. The various types of access are considered and related to their policy purposes. Examples of key access measures are provided and trend data are used to track changes that have occurred over time in these access indicators. Findings from various national studies are synthesized to determine whether access is improving or declining in the United States—for whom and according to what measures. The chapter concludes by discussing future access indicators and research directions.

## Understanding Access to Health Care

This section provides a conceptual framework for understanding access to medical care based on a systems perspective. The framework is a potentially powerful analytical tool that can be applied by policy analysts and health services managers to describe, predict, and explain population-based health services utilization and health outcomes. Also reviewed are the types of access measures and their definitions according to components of the framework.

## Conceptual Framework

Figure 1.1 presents a behavioral model of health services use, which is helpful in understanding access to medical care. The conceptual framework presents a systems approach to understanding a population's access to health care and consists of four major components: environmental factors, population characteristics, health behaviors, and health outcomes.

External environmental factors affect the health status of individuals within the community. Environmental factors reflect the economic climate, relative wealth, politics, level of stress and violence, and prevailing norms of the society that may affect the way society views health and whether access to health care is considered the responsibility of the individual or the state.

Health care system characteristics are the policies, resources, organization, and financial arrangements influencing the accessibility, availability, and acceptability of medical care services.

Personal characteristics of the population at risk—conceptualized as predisposing characteristics, enabling resources, and need—influence personal health practices and utilization of health services, which in turn influence health status and consumer satisfaction. Among the predisposing characteristics, demographic factors such as age and gender represent biological imperatives suggesting the like-

## FIGURE 1.1. A BEHAVIORAL MODEL OF HEALTH SERVICES USE.

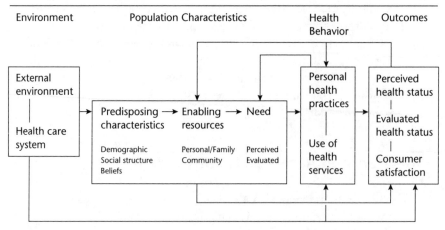

lihood that people will need health services.[1] Social structure is measured by a broad array of factors that determine the status of a person in the community, his or her ability to cope with presenting problems and command resources to deal with these problems, and how healthy or unhealthy the physical environment is likely to be. Traditional measures used to represent social structure include education, occupation, and ethnicity. Expanded measures of social structure might include social networks, social interactions, and culture.[2]

Health beliefs are attitudes, values, and knowledge people have about health and health services that influence their subsequent perceptions of need and use of health services. Health beliefs provide one means of explaining how social structure might influence enabling resources, perceived need, and subsequent use.

Both community and personal enabling resources must be present for use to take place. Community resources include supply factors, such as physician and hospital bed population ratios. Health personnel and facilities must be available where people live and work. Then people must have the personal means and know-how to obtain those services. Income, health insurance, a regular source of care, transportation, and acceptable travel and waiting times are some of the important measures of enabling resources. More detailed organizational measures, such as utilization control mechanisms, managed care gatekeepers, certification for emergency room use, second opinions for surgery, and coordination of services can also be included as enabling factors.

Any comprehensive effort to model access to health care must consider how people view their own general health and functional state, as well as how they experience symptoms of illness, pain, and worries about their health. This assessment leads to judgments about their health condition and whether it is of sufficient importance and magnitude to seek professional help. Perceived need is largely a social phenomenon that, when appropriately modeled, should itself be largely explained by social factors (such as ethnicity and education) and health beliefs (such as health attitudes and knowledge about health care).

However, within rather broad limits established by predisposing and enabling factors, a biological imperative accounts for some people's help seeking and consumption of health services.[3] This imperative is better represented by the evaluated component of need.[4] Evaluated need represents professional judgment and objective measurement about a patient's physical status and need for medical care (for example, blood pressure readings, temperature, blood cell count). Of course, evaluated need is not simply—or even primarily—a valid and reliable measure from biological science. It also has a social component and varies with the changing state of the art and science of medicine as well as the training and competency of the professional expert doing the assessment. Logical expectations of the model are that *perceived need* will help us to better understand the care-seeking process and adherence to a medical regimen, while *evaluated need* will be more closely related to the kind and amount of treatment that will be provided after a patient has presented to a medical care provider.

The environment and population characteristics may have direct effects but also work through health behaviors to influence outcomes. Health behavior includes personal health practices as well as use of formal health services. Personal health practices performed by the individual to maintain or improve health can include appropriate diet and nutrition, exercise, stress reduction, control of alcohol and tobacco use, self-care, and compliance with medical regimens.

The purpose of the original behavioral model was to predict health services use measured rather broadly as units of physician ambulatory care, hospital inpatient services, and dental care consumed during a given year. We hypothesized that predisposing, enabling, and need factors would have differential ability to explain use depending on what type of service was examined.[5] Hospital services utilized in response to more serious problems and conditions would be primarily explained by need and demographic characteristics, while dental services, considered more discretionary, would likely be explained by social structure, health beliefs, and enabling resources. We expected all the components of the model to explain ambulatory physician use because the conditions stimulating care seeking would generally be viewed as less serious and demanding than those resulting in inpatient care, but more serious than those leading to dental care.

More specific measures of health services use could be used to describe a particular medical condition or type of service or practitioner or could be linked to an episode of illness. For example, a longitudinal study of rheumatoid arthritis patients could measure visits to different types of providers, treatment provided, level of patient compliance to treatment, and associated changes in functional status and pain over time. While such linked analyses are in many ways likely to be more informative—the more global ones (for example, number of physician visits, self-rated general health status) still have a role to play. Global measures provide needed comprehensive indicators of the overall effects of policy changes over time.

Outcomes include people's perception of their health status and clinical assessment by health care professionals as well as their general satisfaction with the care they receive. Perceived health status relies on the judgment and values of the individual or others responsible for the individual's welfare. It indicates the extent to which a person can live a functional, comfortable, and pain-free existence within society. Evaluated outcomes are dependent on the judgment of the professional, based on established clinical standards and state-of-the-art practices. Consumer satisfaction describes how individuals feel about the health care they receive and can be judged by ratings of waiting time, travel time, communications with providers, and technical care received.

The model also includes feedback. We expect health behavior to alter people's need for services. Outcomes (health status and satisfaction) might also result in changes—in both health behavior and population characteristics (such as predisposing beliefs or perceived need).

## Types of Access

A major goal of the behavioral model is to provide measures of access to medical care. Access is a relatively complex health policy measure and can be reasonably defined in multidimensional terms. Figure 1.2 presents the types of access to health care and their definitions according to components of the Behavioral Model.

*Potential.* Potential access may be described in terms of structural indicators such as characteristics of the health care delivery system and enabling resources that influence potential care seekers' use of health services. More enabling resources provide the means for, and increase the likelihood that, use will take place.

### FIGURE 1.2. TYPES OF ACCESS TO HEALTH SERVICES.

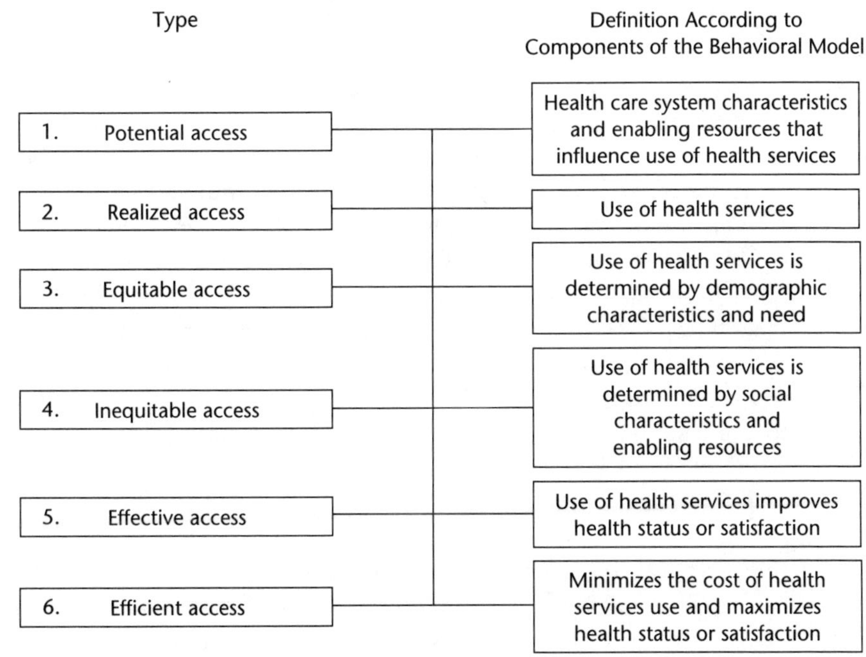

| Type | Definition According to Components of the Behavioral Model |
| --- | --- |
| 1. Potential access | Health care system characteristics and enabling resources that influence use of health services |
| 2. Realized access | Use of health services |
| 3. Equitable access | Use of health services is determined by demographic characteristics and need |
| 4. Inequitable access | Use of health services is determined by social characteristics and enabling resources |
| 5. Effective access | Use of health services improves health status or satisfaction |
| 6. Efficient access | Minimizes the cost of health services use and maximizes health status or satisfaction |

*Realized.*  Realized access is the actual use of services. Realized access indicators include actual utilization of physician, hospital, and other health services.

*Equitable and Inequitable.*  Access is defined as equitable or inequitable according to what determinants (for example, age, ethnicity, insurance status, or symptoms) of realized access are dominant in predicting utilization. Equity is in the eyes of the beholder. Value judgments about which components of the model should explain utilization in an equitable health care system are crucial to the definition. Traditionally, equitable access has been defined as occurring when demographic and need variables account for most of the variance in utilization.[6] Demographic characteristics (such as age or gender differences) are indicators of equitable access to the extent that they are precursors of need. Inequitable access occurs when social characteristics and enabling resources (such as ethnicity or income) determine who gets medical care.

*Effective.*  Effective access is the link between realized access (utilization of health services) and health outcomes (health status, consumer satisfaction). It assesses the benefit of medical care as measured by improvements in health outcomes.[7] Measures of effectiveness examine the relative impact of health services utilization within the context of other predisposing, enabling, need, and health behavior variables. Predisposing variables, such as age, gender, and social support, can influence the patient's health status following treatment. Access to personal enabling resources (health insurance, income, regular source of care) can result in expeditious medical treatment with highly trained practitioners using state-of-the-art medical technology. Conversely, lack of enabling resources can lead to delays in seeking medical advice and episodic, fragmented treatment with a potential negative impact on health outcomes and satisfaction with medical care. Researchers conducting effectiveness and outcomes research have developed strategies for risk adjustment to control for the effects of medical need (for example, severity of illness, number of symptoms, and co-morbidities) before intervention. Personal health practices (diet, exercise, stress management) and compliance with medical regimens prior and subsequent to treatment can also influence health outcomes. Analytical models used to determine the effectiveness of alternative medical treatments on health outcomes must consider the influence of these varying personal and behavioral factors as well as differences in health care delivery systems and external environment.

*Efficient.*  Efficient access links resources consumed to health services and associated health outcomes. Efficient access minimizes the cost of health services and maximizes health status or consumer satisfaction. Aday and her colleagues describe efficiency as producing the combination of goods and services with the highest attainable total value, given limited resources and technology.[8] Efficiency consists of two components, allocative and productive. Allocative efficiency requires the attainment of the most valued mix of outputs. Productive efficiency means producing a given level of output at minimum cost. Efficiency attempts to quantify the cost-effectiveness or cost-benefit of health services in assessing the extent to which finite private, public, or personal resources should be invested in assuring access to those services.[9]

## Policy Purposes of Access Measures

Earlier policies were designed to increase health services use and promote social justice. The cost containment movement resulted in the design of strategies to control utilization. Eventually, policy analysts linked medical services use to health outcomes to measure the actual benefit of medical care. Resource management efforts now identify the most cost-effective interventions to promote health outcomes and minimize cost. Figure 1.3 summarizes the major policy uses of access

### FIGURE 1.3. POLICY PURPOSES OF ACCESS MEASURES.

| Type | Policy Purpose |
|---|---|
| 1. Potential access | To increase or decrease health services use |
| 2. Realized access | To monitor and evaluate policies to influence health services use |
| 3. Equitable access | To ensure health services distribution is determined by need |
| 4. Inequitable access | To reduce the influence of social characteristics and enabling resources on health services distribution |
| 5. Effective access | To improve the outcomes (health status, satisfaction) from health services use |
| 6. Efficient access | To minimize the costs of improving outcomes from health services use |

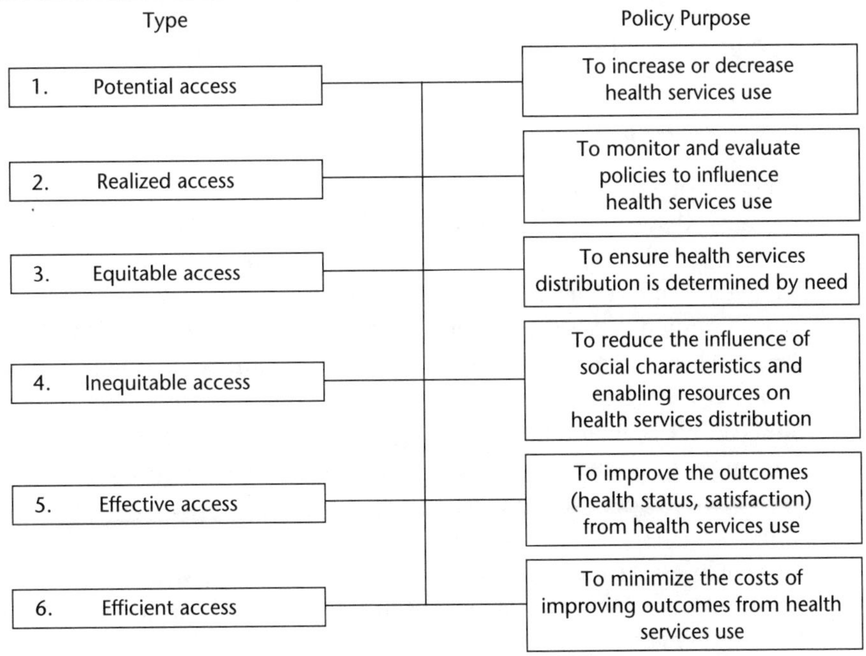

measures and how the emphasis has changed from one policy goal to another with the passage of time.

## To Change or Monitor Utilization

Historically, the United States experienced improving trends in access to health care as measured by increasing health services utilization rates. Access to health services was considered an end goal of policy change. Potential access measures were used as indicators of increasing access to medical care services. Realized access measures were used to monitor and evaluate policies to influence health services use. Policies were implemented in the 1950s and 1960s to increase the numbers of physicians, to supply hospital beds in rural communities, and to create federal programs to increase access including Medicare and Medicaid legislation.

The U.S. health care system evolved from decision making grounded in altruism through increasing the access and supply of resources to a position of caution and financial prudence.[10] The predominant focus on increasing medical care utilization shifted in the 1970s to concern for health care cost containment and creation of mechanisms to limit access to health care, including HMO legislation, coinsurance, deductibles, utilization review, and the genesis of managed care. In the 1980s and 1990s, HMOs competing with fee-for-service organizations enjoyed double-digit growth in profit margins.[11] HMO growth, however, may be slowing as the managed care market becomes saturated.

## To Promote Social Justice

The social justice movement, dominant in the 1960s and early 1970s with the passage of Medicare and Medicaid, sought to ensure that health services distribution was determined by need and to reduce the influence of social characteristics and enabling resources on health services distribution.

Equity of access to medical care is the value judgment that the system is deemed fair or equitable if need-based criteria rather than enabling resources (insurance coverage or income) are the main determinants of whether or not, or how much, care is sought. Subgroup disparities in the utilization of health services (for example, according to race/ethnicity or health insurance coverage) would be minimized in a fair and equitable system, while underlying need for preventive or illness-related health care would be the principal factor determining utilization. In reality, social and economic factors are related in varying degrees to health risk and health outcomes in countries with all types of political, economic, and health care systems.[12]

This dominant emphasis on social justice declined in the 1970s and 1980s with increasing concern for cost containment. The 1990s are turbulent times in health care and significant portions of high-risk vulnerable subgroups in the nation are uninsured and unable to pay for health care services.[13]

## To Promote Health Outcomes

The cost containment movement became more sophisticated in the late 1980s and 1990s. The next generation of health services research began to measure the impact of health services utilization on health outcomes. Accordingly, the Institute of Medicine Committee on Monitoring Access to Personal Health Care Services defined *access* as "the timely use of personal health services to achieve the best possible health outcomes."[14] This definition relies both on the use of health services and health outcomes as yardsticks for judging whether access has been achieved. The resulting measures are referred to as effective access.

While improving health status is an essential goal of medical care, it is often challenging to link differential outcomes to specific components of the health care system. Weissman and Epstein[15] provide this example of our limited ability to link access to health care to health status outcomes. One group of patients suffers higher rates of complications several weeks after discharge from the hospital. It is difficult to determine whether the causes of the poor outcomes were initiated during the hospital stay or postdischarge in the ambulatory setting, by differences in the home environment or individual health behaviors, or by measured differences between the groups in severity of illness. In spite of these measurement challenges, health outcomes are important ultimate indicators of access to health care.

## To Promote Health Outcomes and Minimize Cost

Most recently concerns about cost containment have been combined with those directed to improving health outcomes. The results are measures of efficient access. These measures are similar to measures of effective access with the added emphasis on measuring resources used to influence outcome. The policy purpose is to promote health outcomes while minimizing the resources required to attain improved outcomes.

# Examples of Key Access Measures

This section discusses the kinds of measures used to describe the various types of access. Data are collected and analyzed from multiple sources to measure access to health care, including hospitals and other health organizations at the national, state, or regional level, or within a single health services organization or community clinic. Tables 1.1 and 1.2 provide visual summaries of the material.

## Potential

Potential access measures are the structural characteristics of the health care delivery system and enabling resources. The first section of Table 1.1 presents these measures. Structural characteristics include measures of capacity (for example, physician/population ratio or hospital bed/population ratio), organization (percentage of the population enrolled in managed care programs), and financing (per capita expenditures for health services or percentage of population with health insurance). Enabling characteristics are personal resources (regular source of care, income, health insurance coverage) and community resources (urban or rural community, region of residence) that may be associated with potential access.

## Realized

Realized access is measured by number, type, site, and purpose of services, as shown in Table 1.1. Type of services utilized can be ambulatory, inpatient, prescriptions, or dental care services. The site of service utilization can be the physician's office, hospital, or community clinic. Service purpose can be primary (preventive or early treatment), secondary (more complex treatment for acute or chronic conditions), or tertiary (rehabilitative or custodial) care.

## Equitable

The test of equity of access involves determining whether there are systematic differences in use and outcomes among groups in U.S. society and whether these differences are associated with financial or other barriers to care.[16] Equitable access is indicated when services are distributed according to need for care, as shown in the third section of Table 1.1. Perceived need is captured by patient self-reporting of symptoms, pain, and general health status. Evaluated need is documented in medical records and test results recorded by medical professionals. Inequitable access (the fourth section of Table 1.1) is indicated when services are distributed according to predisposing social characteristics (such as race/ethnicity, education, or occupation) and enabling resources (such as regular source of care, income, or health insurance coverage).

### TABLE 1.1. POTENTIAL, REALIZED, AND
### EQUITABLE ACCESS MEASURES.

| Type | Measures | Examples |
|---|---|---|
| *Potential Access* | | |
| Health Care System Characteristics | Capacity | Physician/population ratio<br>Hospital bed/population ratio |
| | Organization | Percentage of population in managed care |
| | Financing | Per capita expeditures for health services<br>Percentage of population with health insurance |
| Enabling Characteristics | Personal Resources | Regular source of care<br>Income<br>Health Insurance coverage |
| | Community Resources | Urban or rural community<br>Region of residence |
| *Realized Access* | Type of Service | Ambulatory<br>Inpatient<br>Prescription<br>Dental |
| | Site of Service | Physician office<br>Hospital<br>Community clinic |
| | Purpose of Service | Primary care<br>Secondary care<br>Tertiary care |
| *Equitable Access* | Services distributed according to perceived patient need | Symptoms<br>Pain<br>General health status<br>Functional status |
| | Services distributed according to evaluated need | Medical history<br>Test results |
| *Inequitable Access* | Services distributed according to predisposing social characteristices | Race/Ethnicity<br>Education<br>Occupation |
| | Services distributed according to enabling characteristics | Regular source of care<br>Income<br>Health insurance coverage |

## Effective and Efficient

Table 1.2 presents examples of objectives for primary prevention and illness-related care linked to measures of realized access (use of services) and health outcomes.

### TABLE 1.2. EFFECTIVENESS AND EFFICIENCY ACCESS MEASURES.

| Objective | Realized Access Measures (Use of Services) | Outcome Measures |
|---|---|---|
| *Primary Prevention* | | |
| 1. Promoting successful birth outcomes | Percentage of women obtaining adequate care based on Kessner index (trimester in which care first sought, number of visits, gestational age) | Infant mortality rate<br>Low birthweight<br>Congenital syphilis |
| 2. Reducing the incidence of vaccine-preventable childhood diseases | Percentage of preschool-age-children (age one to four years) who have been vaccinated | Incidence of preventable childhood communicable diseases (diphtheria, measles, mumps, pertussis, polio, rubella, and tetanus)—cases per 1,000 population |
| 3. Early detection and diagnosis of treatable diseases | Breast and cervical cancer screening—percentage of women undergoing selected procedures (clinical breast exam, mammography, Pap test in given period | Percentage of (breast, cervical cancer) tumors diagnosed at early stages |
| 4. Promoting functional dentition status | Percentage of population with a dental visit in the past year | Percentage of children with untreated decayed teeth<br>Percentage of adults with no teeth |
| *Illness-Related Care* | | |
| 1. Reducing the effects of chronic diseases and prolonging life | Average number of annual physician contacts for those in poor health<br>Use of high-cost, high-tech procedures | Avoidable hospitalization for chronic diseases<br>Number of deaths per 100,000 population estimated to be due to access problems |
| 2. Reducing morbidity and pain through timely and appropriate treatment | Percentage of individuals with acute illness who have no physician contact | Avoidable hospitalization for acute conditions |

Measures of effectiveness link utilization to health outcomes. Efficiency measures are measures of effectiveness with a valuation of resources expended (such as cost per unit of improved health) to attain effectiveness. The particular objectives listed are based on those selected by the Institute of Medicine Committee on Monitoring Access and the Robert Wood Johnson report *Key Indicators for Policy.*[17]

***Promoting Successful Birth Outcomes.***  A realized access measure expected to be associated with successful birth outcomes is the Kessner index, which is based on trimester of initiation, frequency of prenatal care, and gestational age. Outcome measures of effectiveness assumed to be affected by prenatal care include rates of infant mortality, low birthweight, and congenital syphilis. Efficiency might measure the relative impact on infant mortality of resource allocation for prenatal care services compared to neonatal intensive care services.

***Reducing Vaccine-Preventable Childhood Diseases.***  The relevant realized access measure here is percentage of children vaccinated. The outcome measures of effectiveness would be the incidence of preventable childhood communicable diseases, and related efficiency measures would be estimates of the costs of reducing incidence through vaccinations.

***Promoting Early Detection and Diagnosis.***  Examples of realized access measures are breast and cervical cancer screening rates for women. Important outcomes measures, in this case, are the stage at which tumors are diagnosed. An increased proportion of tumors diagnosed in early stages would suggest more effective and, perhaps, more efficient access. Efficiency measures would help providers determine the optimal age for allocating fixed resources to provide mammography screening in the adult female population.[18]

***Promoting Functional Dentition Status.***  A realized access measure is the proportion of people who see a dentist. Among the relevant outcome measures of effectiveness are reduced proportions of children with untreated decayed teeth and adults who experience total tooth loss. Efficiency measures might compare the relative time, cost, and personnel mix required to provide dental services in alternative practice settings.[19]

In addition to the primary prevention objectives already discussed, realized access may influence the course of a current illness. Illness-related objectives include the following.

***Reducing the Effects of Chronic Diseases and Prolonging Life.***  Realized access measures selected here include number of physician contacts for people reporting poor health. The related outcome measure is avoidable hospitalizations for chronic disease through physician contact. Another realized access measure is the use of high-cost, high-tech procedures such as open heart surgeries or transplants, with the related outcomes being reduced chronic disease or prolonged life. Efficiency measures might compare the cost for routine physician monitoring of chronic disease to the cost of avoidable hospitalizations.

***Reducing Morbidity and Pain.*** A realized access measure in response to acute illness is the proportion of individuals who do not see a physician. A related effectiveness outcome measure is an estimate of hospitalizations for acute conditions that might have been avoided with appropriate physician monitoring. Efficiency measures might compare the cost of visits for acute illness to the costs of hospitalization for acute conditions that might have been avoided.

## Trends in Access

In this section, the trends in access are examined according to different types of access measures. We consider changes over time in potential access (health insurance coverage), realized access (use of hospital, physician, and dental services) and equitable access (health insurance availability and health services use according to income and race). We will also examine some key research findings concerning effective and efficient access.

### Potential Access

Table 1.3 reports a critical potential access measure—health care coverage for persons under sixty-five years of age from 1980 to 1993. The uninsured proportion of the population increased from 13 percent to 17 percent in that time period. While Medicaid coverage increased (from 6 percent to 10 percent), the overall decline in coverage resulted from a drop in the proportion covered by private insurance from 79 percent to 71 percent.

The proportion of the uninsured population increased for adults aged fifteen to forty-four years since 1980, reaching 22 percent in 1993. The proportion covered by private insurance decreased for every age group and the decline was especially noticeable for children under fifteen, declining from 75 percent to 66 percent. However, since 1980, Medicaid has covered an increasing portion of children, reaching 19 percent in 1993. This increase reflects the expanded Medicaid income eligibility enacted by Congress in the mid 1980s (as discussed in Chapter Two). However, even for children, the proportion uninsured is greater in

1993 (15 percent) compared to 1980 (13 percent). The results overall leave little doubt that a significant decline in potential access has occurred for the U.S. population, particularly for people aged fifteen to forty-four years, because of a decline in health insurance coverage.

### TABLE 1.3. HEALTH CARE COVERAGE BY AGE, RACE/ETHNICITY, AND INCOME.

| | Private Insurance[c] | | | Medicaid[c] | | | Not Covered[c] | | |
|---|---|---|---|---|---|---|---|---|---|
| | | | | Percentage of Population | | | | | |
| | 1980 | 1989 | 1993 | 1980 | 1989 | 1993 | 1980 | 1989 | 1993 |
| *Age* | | | | | | | | | |
| Under 15 | 75 | 72 | 66 | 10 | 11 | 19 | 13 | 16 | 15 |
| 15–44 | 79 | 77 | 71 | 4 | 4 | 6 | 14 | 18 | 22 |
| 44–64 | 84 | 83 | 81 | 3 | 3 | 3 | 9 | 11 | 12 |
| *Race/Ethnicity* | | | | | | | | | |
| White | 82 | 80 | 75 | 3 | 4 | 7 | 11 | 14 | 16 |
| Black | 60 | 59 | 51 | 18 | 17 | 24 | 19 | 22 | 23 |
| Hispanic origin[a] | — | 51 | 49 | — | 10 | 16 | — | 31 | 34 |
| *Income[b]* | | | | | | | | | |
| Less than $14,000 | 39 | 35 | 26 | 28 | 27 | 37 | 38 | 37 | 35 |
| $14,000–$24,999 | 61 | 71 | 60 | 9 | 5 | 11 | 26 | 21 | 27 |
| $25,000–$34,999 | 79 | 88 | 81 | 3 | 1 | 2 | 15 | 9 | 14 |
| $35,000–$49,999 | 90 | 92 | 89 | 1 | 1 | 1 | 6 | 6 | 8 |
| $50,000 or more | 94 | 96 | 94 | 1 | * | * | 4 | 3 | 5 |
| *Total* | 79 | 77 | 71 | 6 | 6 | 10 | 13 | 16 | 17 |

—Not Available

*Less than 0.5 percent

[a]Hispanic origin based on self-report; may include persons classified as either white or black according to race.

[b]Family income categories for 1989 and 1993. Family income categories for 1980 are less than $7,000, $7,000–$9,999, $10,000–$14,999, $15,000–$24,999, $25,000 or more.

[c]The sum of the percentages for private insurance, Medicaid, and no coverage may not come to 100 percent because other types of health insurance (such as Medicare or military policies) do not appear in the table and because persons with both private insurance and Medicaid are counted in both columns.

*Source:* National Center for Health Statistics, *Health United States, 1994* (Hyattsville, Md.: Public Health Service, 1995), p. 240.

## Realized Access

Table 1.4 presents a historical perspective of personal health care use for the U.S. population from 1930 to 1993. It provides trend data on realized access for three types of services: services in response to more serious illness (hospital admissions), services provided for a combination of primary and secondary care (physician visits), and services for conditions that are rarely life threatening and generally considered discretionary but still have an important bearing on people's functional status and quality of life (dental visits).

The hospital admission rate for the U.S. population doubled between 1930 (six admissions per hundred persons per year) and the early 1950s (twelve admissions). A rising standard of living, the advent of voluntary health insurance, the increasing legitimacy of the modern hospital as a place to have babies and treat acute illness, and the requirements necessary for developing more sophisticated medical technology—all contributed to expanded use of the acute care hospital. Hospital admissions further increased in the 1960s and early 1970s (reaching fourteen admissions per hundred in 1974) reflecting continued growth in medical technology, private health insurance, and the advent of Medicare coverage for the elderly and Medicaid coverage for the low-income population in 1965.

However, beginning in the mid 1970s use of the acute care hospital began to decline, dropping to ten admissions per hundred population by 1987 and nine in 1993. Those declines accompanied increasing efforts to contain health care costs by a shift in care from the more expensive inpatient setting to less expensive outpatient settings, a shift from fee-for-service to prospective payments by Medicare, reduced coverage and benefits with increasing coinsurance and deductibles for health insurance, and a shift in certain medical technology and styles of practice reducing reliance on the inpatient settings.

Physician visits (Table 1.4) also increased substantially from the 1930s (2.6 visits per person per year) to the early 1950s (4.2 visits), for many of the same reasons that hospital admissions were increasing in this period. However, unlike hospital admissions, number of physician visits continued to increase, reaching 4.9 visits in 1974 and 6.0 visits in 1993. In part, the relative deemphasis of the inpatient setting and the shift to outpatient settings may account for the divergence in trends of these basic realized access measures.

Trends in dentist visits (Table 1.4) for the total U.S. population paralleled those for physician visits. Twenty-one percent of the population visited a dentist in 1930. The proportion increased consistently, reaching one-half of the population in 1974. Further increases in the last twenty years resulted in 61 percent of the population visiting a dentist in 1993.

## TABLE 1.4. PERSONAL HEALTH CARE USE BY INCOME.

| | 1928–1931[a] | 1952–1953[a] | 1963–1964[a] | 1974[a] | 1987[b,g] | 1993[c] |
|---|---|---|---|---|---|---|
| *Hospital Admissions* (Admissions per 100 persons per year) | | | | | | |
| Low income[d] | 6 | 12 | 14 | 19 | 14 | 14 |
| Middle income[e] | 6 | 12 | 14 | 14 | 11 | 9 |
| High income[f] | 8 | 11 | 11 | 11 | 8 | 7 |
| Total | 6 | 12 | 13 | 14 | 10 | 9 |
| *Physician Visits* (Visits per person per year) | | | | | | |
| Low income[d] | 2.2 | 3.7 | 4.3 | 5.3 | 6.8 | 7.3 |
| Middle income[e] | 2.5 | 3.8 | 4.5 | 4.8 | 5.4 | 5.9 |
| High income[f] | 4.3 | 6.5 | 5.1 | 4.9 | 5.3 | 5.9 |
| Total | 2.6 | 4.2 | 4.5 | 4.9 | 5.4 | 6.0 |
| *Dentist Visits* (Percentage seeing a dentist within year) | | | | | | |
| Below poverty[h] | | | | | 33% | 36% |
| Low income[d] | 10% | 17% | 21% | 35% | 42 | |
| At or above poverty[h] | | | | | 52 | 64 |
| Middle income[e] | 20 | 33 | 36 | 48 | 60 | |
| High income[f] | 46 | 56 | 58 | 64 | 76 | |
| Total | 21% | 34% | 38% | 49% | 58% | 61% |

[a]*Source:* Various surveys, reported in R. Andersen and O. Anderson, "Trends in the Use of Health Services," in *Handbook of Medical Sociology* (3rd ed.), eds. H. E. Freeman, S. Levine, and L. G. Reeder (Englewood Cliffs, N.J.: Prentice Hall, 1979), pp. 374, 378, 379.

[b]*Source:* National Center for Health Statistics, *Health United States, 1994* (Hyattsville, Md.: Public Health Service, 1995), pp. 171, 179, 180.

[c]*Source:* National Center for Health Statistics, *Health United States, 1994* (Hyattsville, Md.: Public Health Service, 1995), pp. 169, 177, 178.

[d]Low income = lowest 15 percent to 27 percent of family income distribution.

[e]Middle income = middle 51 percent to 73 percent of family income distribution.

[f]High income = highest 12 percent to 32 percent of family income distribution.

[g]1989 for dental visits

[h]Dental visit data from National Center for Health Statistics, unpublished data from the National Health Interview Survey, persons aged twenty-five years or older.

## Equitable Access

Table 1.5 completes the picture begun in Tables 1.3 and 1.4 of health insurance coverage and personal health care use among the U.S. population. Equitable access is indicated by similar levels of insurance coverage and use by different income and ethnic groups. Inequitable access is suggested by discrepancies in coverage and use for these groups.

### TABLE 1.5. PERSONAL HEALTH CARE USE BY RACE.

|  | 1964[a] | 1981–1983[b] | 1987–1989[a,c] | 1993[d] |
|---|---|---|---|---|
| *Hospital Admissions* (Admissions per 100 persons per year) |  |  |  |  |
| Black[e] | 8 | 14 | 12 | 11 |
| White | 11 | 12 | 10 | 9 |
| Total | 11 | 12 | 10 | 9 |
| *Physician Visits* (Percentage with physician visit within year) |  |  |  |  |
| Black[e] | 58% | 75% | 75% | 79% |
| White | 68 | 76 | 77 | 79 |
| Total | 67% | 76% | 77% | 79% |
| *Dental Visits* (Percentage seeing a dentist within year) |  |  |  |  |
| Black[e] | 22% | 36% | 44% | 47% |
| White | 45 | 53 | 60 | 64 |
| Total | 43% | 50% | 58% | 61% |

[a]*Source:* National Center for Health Statistics, *Health United States, 1993* (Hyattsville, Md.: Public Health Service, 1994), pp. 174, 179, 180.

[b]*Source:* National Center for Health Statistics, *Health United States, 1988* (Hyattsville, Md.: Public Health Service, 1989), pp. 107, 111.

[c]1989 for dental visits

[d]*Source:* National Center for Health Statistics, *Health United States, 1994* (Hyattsville, Md.: Public Health Service, 1995), pp. 172, 178.

[e]For 1964, the total given as "black" actually includes all non-Caucasians.

*Health Insurance.* Table 1.3 suggests considerable inequity in insurance coverage in 1980, continuing to the present time. Minorities and low-income people are least likely to have private health insurance. Medicaid compensates for some of this inequity but still leaves high proportions of blacks (23 percent), Hispanics (34 percent), and the low-income persons (35 percent) uninsured in 1993.

The trends in Table 1.3 provide a somewhat mixed picture as to whether inequities in health insurance coverage are increasing over time. Between 1980 and 1993, coverage through private health insurance declined for all ethnic groups while the proportions covered by Medicaid or without coverage increased for all of them. While potential access as measured by insurance coverage declined for all ethnic groups and inequities existed over the entire period (whites were less likely to be uninsured than minorities), there is no clear trend toward greater or less inequity according to ethnicity.

Trends in equity according to income level are even more complex. Between 1980 and 1993, private health insurance coverage of the lowest income group declined consistently, with the rate of decline apparently increasing in recent years. For the lower-middle income groups, private insurance coverage increased during the early 1980s but then declined considerably in the early 1990s, so that by 1993 the coverage was similar to what it was in 1980. Most of the highest income groups had private health insurance coverage throughout the period. Increases in Medicaid coverage more than compensated for decline in private insurance coverage for the lowest income group, so that the proportion uninsured actually declined for the thirteen-year period. This was not the case for the lower-middle income groups, where for the last few years the proportion uninsured has been increasing (21 percent to 27 percent). Consequently, it appears that inequities in insurance coverage have been increasing for the lower-middle income groups.

*Hospital Admissions.* Tables 1.4 and 1.5 suggest increasing equity according to income and race for hospital admissions. In 1928–1931, the highest income group had the highest admission rate (Table 1.4). By the 1950s, the rates had equalized. In subsequent years the rates by income diverged. Hospitalization for the lowest income group increased relative to those with higher incomes, so that by 1993 the lowest income group had a rate (fourteen per hundred) twice that of the highest income group (seven). Does this indicate that inequity exists in favor of the low-income group? Probably not. Studies taking into account need for medical care suggest that the greater hospital use for low-income persons can be largely accounted for by their higher rates of disease and disability.[20] The hospital admission rate in 1964 for whites (eleven) was still considerably higher than the rate for blacks (eight), as shown in Table 1.5. However, by the 1980s the rate for blacks exceeded the rate for whites and the higher rate for blacks continued into the 1990s. The higher hospital admission rates for blacks, similar to the higher rates for low-income people, can be largely accounted for by higher levels of medical need.[21]

***Physician Visits.*** The trends in Tables 1.4 and 1.5 also suggest increasing equity for physician visits according to income level and ethnicity. In 1928–1931, the lowest income group averaged only one-half as many visits to the doctor (2.2 visits) as the highest income group (4.3 visits), as shown in Table 1.4. Over time the gap narrowed. By 1974, the lowest income group was actually visiting a physician more compared to the higher income groups and the difference increased in the 1980s and early 1990s. Again, research results suggest that the apparent excess for the low-income population can be accounted for by their greater levels of medical need.[22] Similar trends have taken place for the black population, as shown in Table 1.5, but parity with the white population in proportions seeing a doctor did not take place until the early 1980s and the proportions seeing doctors have remained the same for blacks and whites into the early 1990s. The physician use rate for the growing Latino population remains considerably below that for both blacks and whites.[23]

***Dental Visits.*** Tables 1.4 and 1.5 tell a story of major inequities according to income and race in dental visit rates that existed in 1928–1931 and continue to exist into the 1990s. The proportion seeing a dentist has increased considerably for all income and racial groups. Still, by 1993, only 36 percent of the below-poverty group saw a dentist compared to 64 percent of those at or above poverty, as shown in Table 1.4. Similarly, Table 1.5 shows that 47 percent of blacks saw a dentist compared to 64 percent of whites.

## Key Findings for Effective Access

The effectiveness and outcomes movement initiated in the late 1980s was in response to several major developments converging on the national scene.[24] The Health Care Financing Administration proposed a research program called the Effectiveness Initiative, stimulated by their needs to ensure quality of care for the 30 million Medicare beneficiaries; to determine which medical practices worked best; and to aid policy makers in allocating Medicare resources. At about the same time, an Outcomes Research Program was authorized by Congress, largely inspired by the work of John Wennberg and associates in small-area variations in the utilization and outcomes of medical interventions. A third major development stimulating the effectiveness movement stemmed from efforts led by Robert H. Brook and associates to determine whether medical interventions used in the normal practice setting were being used appropriately. Within the same time period, the Agency for Health Care Policy and Research was created, with a responsibility for developing medical practice guidelines. The guidelines represent the practical application of the outcomes and effectiveness research movement.

Prior to the effectiveness initiative, research was limited by weak study designs (observational and cross-sectional) that were not capable of determining the clear direction of effects and their potential causality.[25] Most studies used mortality as the outcome variable, which was shown to be more sensitive to environmental and socioeconomic factors than to medical care utilization.[26] Moreover, the appropriate risk adjustments were usually not available in mortality data sets.

The Medical Outcomes Study (MOS) was undertaken in response to these methodological limitations. The MOS sampled physicians and patients from different health care systems—including traditional fee-for-service (FFS) plans, independent practice associations (IPAs), and health maintenance organizations (HMOs)—and health care settings to investigate the relationships between structure, process, and medical outcomes. Specifically, the MOS was designed to determine whether variations in medical outcomes were explained by differences in the system of care (structure and process) and medical specialty, and to develop instruments to assess and monitor medical outcomes (such as clinical endpoints, functioning, perceived general health status and well-being, and satisfaction with treatment).[27] Results from the MOS indicated that patient mix was related to utilization, that is, increasing levels of severity were associated with decreasing levels of functional status and well-being and increasing levels of utilization (hospitalizations, physician visits, prescription drugs), and differed significantly across systems of care and medical specialties.[28] Variations in resource use, while related to patient mix, were significantly influenced by specialty training, payment system, and practice organization.[29] The MOS also compared indicators of primary care quality across the various health care systems, controlling for patient and physician characteristics.[30] Performance indicators in the three payment settings revealed notable differences in primary care quality: financial access was highest in prepaid systems; organizational access, continuity, and accountability were highest in the FFS system; and coordination was highest and comprehensiveness lowest in HMOs. Ultimately, research results demonstrated that multiple factors—patient mix, medical specialty, and system of care—influence patient outcomes, and when patient and physician characteristics are controlled, quality indicators of primary care vary across system of care.

## Key Findings for Efficient Access

Efficiency studies have been conducted at multiple levels including the macroeconomic level, the health plan system level, and the consumer behavior level. At the macroeconomic level, comprehensive data available on major, industrialized countries have been used to compare health services utilization, health resources and expenditures, and health outcomes. The Organization for Economic Cooperation and Development study comparing per capita health care expenditures in seven major industrialized countries, found that the United States spent about 40 percent more than Canada and almost three times more than the country with the lowest expenditures, the United Kingdom. The large expenditure gap for the United States was not offset by health outcome advantages, which raised concerns that resources were being misallocated to services with low benefit relative to cost.[31]

Efficiency analyses conducted at the health plan system level usually compare traditional indemnity plans with FFS providers to HMOs. Results from the randomized RAND Health Insurance Study (HIS) indicated that the HMO provided care at 25 percent less expense with no adverse health effects on the general population. The change in financial incentives and better resource management (for example, fewer hospital admissions) were seen as strategies to reduce inefficiencies.[32] Other studies have conducted production efficiency analyses concentrating on the size and personnel mix of physician practices and other medical care delivery settings, and results indicate that physicians could raise the productivity of their practices and lower the total cost per office visit by employing more aides.[33]

Efficiency analyses focusing on the consumer population have investigated whether health services were being utilized in the most efficient way. Cost sharing is portrayed as a mechanism to decrease inappropriate utilization and therefore produce more efficient health services delivery. Participants in the HIS were randomly assigned to a free-care group or to insurance plans requiring them to pay part of the cost (cost sharing). A physician panel judged whether symptoms were minor (not warranting a physician visit) or serious (warranting a physician visit). No significant differences were reported between the free-care and cost-sharing groups in visiting the physician for serious symptoms. However, utilization for minor symptoms was decreased by more than 30 percent in the cost-sharing group compared to the free-care group. These findings provided empirical evidence demonstrating that efficient utilization management could be achieved by modifying patient behavior through cost sharing, without compromising health outcomes.[34]

## Conclusion: Trends in Access

Is access improving or declining in the United States? For whom and according to what measures? While we have documented continuing increases in some realized access measures, including physician and dental visits, inpatient hospital use has been declining for twenty years. And a key potential access measure, health insurance, reveals that while increasing numbers of persons are being covered by Medicaid (although the program is currently under severe threat), there has been a decline in the numbers covered by private insurance in the last fifteen years and an overall increase in the proportion without any health insurance coverage. Low-income and black populations appear to have achieved equity of access according to gross measures of hospital and physician utilization (not adjusting for their greater need for medical care) but continue to lag considerably in receipt of dental care. Equity has certainly not been achieved according to health insurance coverage as the proportion uninsured is 50 percent higher for blacks and more than twice as high for Latinos and the low-income population as for whites.

A number of recent national investigations of access considering effectiveness and efficiency as well as potential and realized measures provide rather discouraging conclusions about trends—particularly those regarding equity of access. The Commonwealth Fund, citing "serious health problems," "shorter life spans," and "higher infant mortality" of minority Americans compared to white Americans, sponsored a national health access survey of more than 3,700 African American, Hispanic, Asian, and white adults in 1994. Two-fifths of Hispanics and Asians reported no regular doctor or provider compared to one-fifth of white adults. Waiting too long to seek care is a major problem for 27 percent of minority adults (46 percent for those of Chinese descent) compared with 16 percent of white adults. Of Americans who visited a doctor in the last year, the proportion that did *not* receive preventive care services such as blood pressure tests, Pap smears, and cholesterol readings was considerably larger for some minorities (Vietnamese, 47 percent; Mexican, 39 percent; and Puerto Rican, 38 percent) than for whites (26 percent). Karen Davis, president of the Commonwealth Fund, thus asks, "if minority Americans already face problems obtaining care . . . how will they be affected by changes in health care financing and practice, the competitive pressures under managed care, and future curbs in Medicaid and public health programs?"[35]

The Center for Health Economics Research, commissioned by the Robert Wood Johnson Foundation to investigate access to health care in the United States, notes that while "in the last few decades the United States has made notable improvements in health status attributable in part to improved access—for example, striking declines in deaths from heart attacks and strokes (linked to better control of high blood pressure and cardiovascular treatments) and greater survival among low birthweight White infants (linked to neonatal intensive care) . . . *the access picture has worsened for many, particularly the poor.*"[36] The study concludes that even though people in the United States are spending more on health care than on food and housing combined, pressures to curtail costs threaten to further erode access to care. Supporting evidence includes:

- The proportion of unintended births (associated with insufficient prenatal care and low birthweight infants) is rising.
- Neonatal death rates for blacks are twice the rates for whites.
- Rates of early prenatal care—a service that may save $3 for every dollar spent—show almost no progress.
- U.S. immunization rates are lower than those for most other developed countries.
- Breast and cervical cancer screening rates have increased, but poor and black women are less likely to be screened and more likely to be diagnosed late (after metastasis).
- Even though hospitalizations can be avoided by regular physician visits, the poor are not reaping such benefits—for example, residents of low-income areas have 4.5 times the rate of hospitalization for asthma as do persons in higher-income communities.
- Primary care physicians and dentists tend to practice in wealthier communities.[37]

The Committee on Monitoring Access to Personal Health Care Services of the Institute of Medicine (1993) concludes that *there is little evidence of progress over the last decade.* While there have been advances—for example, in the rates of breast cancer screening—they have been counterbalanced by the return of diseases that can be avoided, such as tuberculosis and congenital syphilis. Further, with respect to the AIDS epidemic, it appears that access to medical care helps with respect to longevity and quality of life but is not less costly. Particularly disturbing is the growing division between the haves and the have-nots. Even when improvements in access are noted for all, they are generally less for blacks and other minorities. The committee notes growing discrepancies in infant mortality and proportion of low birthweights and suggests that one-third to one-half of the mortality gap between middle-aged blacks and whites might be attributable to access problems.

In summary, trends according to the various measures of access provide a mixed picture. While some trends in realized access (physician and dental visits) suggest continued improvement, other trends in potential access (health insurance coverage) and equity of access according to ethnicity and income show declines. Further, while access to care has apparently been effective in improving some outcomes (deaths from heart attacks, strokes, and low birthweights), we continue to pay increasingly higher prices for medical care—suggesting trends in efficiency leave much to be desired.

# Conclusion: Future Access Indicators and Needed Research

The question underlying the design of a new generation of access indicators is to what extent does medical care contribute to people's health?[38] Issues of effectiveness, efficiency, and equity will all become guiding norms in the development of these indicators.[39]

New measures of realized access should have "a fairly well-recognized service intervention with clear guidelines regarding who should receive the service" and closely linked outcomes.[40] Good examples would be the ratio between the proportion of children vaccinated for a preventable disease such as measles and the incidence of the disease. Further, there should be a source of routine data for the new measures or one should be developed.

The Committee on Monitoring Access to Personal Health Care Services has noted the need to develop access measures concerning HIV/AIDS, substance abuse, migrants, homeless people, people with disabilities, family violence, emergency services, postacute care for the elderly, and prescription drugs.[41] Development of access measures for vulnerable populations is especially important because many of them have interrelated needs.[42] "For instance, the broad group of alcohol and substance abusers can include high risk mothers with fetal alcohol syndrome, intravenous drug users with AIDS, mentally ill substance abusers, drug users who attempt suicide, addictive families suffering domestic abuse, homeless people with substance abuse problems, and substance abusing refugees."[43]

Considerably more research is also needed to further develop the link between realized access measures and outcome measures outlined in Table 1.2. Some of the most important work to improve the effectiveness and efficiency of access will include efforts

- *To promote successful birth outcomes.* We need additional research on the relationships among medical risk factors, the content of prenatal care, and birth outcomes. We also need continued research on the increasing disparity between black and white infant mortality.
- *To reduce the incidence of vaccine-preventable childhood diseases.* We need research on the relationships among race, barriers to vaccination access, and infectious diseases.
- *To promote early detection and diagnosis of treatable diseases.* We need exploration in more depth of why women do not seek breast and cervical cancer screening. We also need research to determine why improvements in the rates of cancer screening among blacks are not reflected in improvements in early diagnosis, mortality rates, and survival compared with rates for whites.

- *To promote functional dentition status.* We need further examination of the continuing differences in use of dental services according to income and ethnicity and the impact of these differences on functional status.
- *To reduce the effects of chronic diseases and prolong life.* We need further attention to the differences in use of high-cost discretionary care according to gender, ethnicity, income, and insurance status and attention to whether these differences represent overuse or underuse of these services.
- *To reduce morbidity and pain through timely and appropriate treatment.* We need to explore methods to better define what constitutes timely and appropriate use of physician services during episodes of acute illness, and research on factors that lead to the hospitalization of people with acute diseases.

## Notes

1. Barbara S. Hulka and John R. Wheat, "Patterns of Utilization: The Patient Perspective," *Medical Care* 23 (1985): 438–460.
2. David M. Bass and Linda S. Noelker, "The Influence of Family Caregivers on Elders' Use of In-Home Services: An Expanded Conceptual Framework," *Journal of Health and Social Behavior* 28 (1987): 184–196; Sylvia Guendelman, "Health Care Users Residing on the Mexican Border: What Factors Determine Choice of the U.S. or Mexican Health System?" *Medical Care* 23 (1985): 438–460; and Alejandro Portes, David Kyle, and William W. Eaton, "Mental Illness and Help-Seeking Behavior Among Mariel Cuban and Haitian Refugees in South Florida," *Journal of Health and Social Behavior* 33 (1993): 283–298.
3. Hulka and Wheat, "Patterns of Utilization."
4. Ronald M. Andersen, Joanna Kravits, and Odin Anderson, *Equity in Health Services: Empirical Analysis in Social Policy* (Boston: Ballinger, 1975).
5. Ronald M. Andersen, *Behavioral Model of Families' Use of Health Services,* Research Series No. 25 (Chicago: Center for Health Administration Studies, University of Chicago, 1968); and Ronald M. Andersen, "Revisiting the Behavioral Model and Access to Medical Care: Does It Matter?" *Journal of Health and Social Behavior* 36 (1995): 1–10.
6. Andersen, *Behavioral Model of Families' Use of Health Services.*
7. Lu Ann Aday, Charles E. Begley, David R. Lairson, and Carl H. Slater, *Evaluating the Medical Care System: Effectiveness, Efficiency, and Equity* (Ann Arbor, Mich.: Health Administration Press, 1993).
8. Aday, Begley, Lairson, and Slater, *Evaluating the Medical Care System;* and R. T. Byrns and G. W. Stone, *Economics* (Glenview, Ill.: Scott, Foresman, 1987); and K. Davis, G. F. Anderson, D. Rowland, and E. P. Steinberg, *Health Care Cost Containment* (Baltimore, Md.: Johns Hopkins University Press, 1990).
9. Lu Ann Aday, "Access to What and Why? Towards a New Generation of Access Indicators," Proceedings of the Public Health Conference on Records and Statistics, DHHS Pub. No. 941214 (Washington, D.C.: U.S. Government Printing Office, 1993), pp. 410–415.
10. S. M. McManus and C. M. Pohl, "Ethics and Financing: Overview of the U.S. Health Care System," *Journal of Health and Human Resources Administration* 16, 3 (1994): 332–349.
11. P. J. Kenkel, "HMO Profit Outlook Begins to Brighten," *Modern Healthcare* 19 (1989): 98; H. Larkin, "Law and Money Spur HMO Profit Status Changes," *Hospitals* 63 (1989): 68–69;

J. S. Coyne and D. M. Meadows, "California HMOs May Provide National Forecast," *Healthcare Financial Management* 45 (1991): 36–39.

12. Aday, Begley, Lairson, and Slater, *Evaluating the Medical Care System.*

13. McManus and Pohl, "Ethics and Financing."

14. Institute of Medicine (U.S.), Committee on Monitoring Access to Personal Health Care Services, *Access to Health Care in America,* ed. Michael Millman (Washington, D.C.: National Academy Press, 1993), p. 4.

15. Joel S. Weissman and Arnold M. Epstein, *Tears in the Safety Net: The Impact of Insurance Status on Access to Care* (New York: Oxford University Press, 1994).

16. Institute of Medicine (U.S.), Committee on Monitoring Access to Personal Health Care Services, *Access to Health Care in America.*

17. Institute of Medicine (U.S.), Committee on Monitoring Access to Personal Health Care Services, *Access to Health Care in America;* and Center for Health Economics Research, *Access to Health Care: Key Indicators for Policy* (Chestnut Hill, Mass.: Center for Health Economics Research, 1993), prepared for the Robert Wood Johnson Foundation, Princeton, N.J.

18. D. M. Eddy, V. Hasselblad, W. McGivney, and W. Hendee, "The Value of Mammography Screening in Women Under 50 Years," *Journal of the American Medical Association* 259 (1988): 1512–1519; L. F. O'Grady, "Breast Cancer," in *Clinical Preventive Medicine,* eds. T. Warner Hudson, Michael A. Reinhart, Steven D. Rose, and Gary K. Stewart (Boston: Little, Brown, 1988): 534–540; and A. I. Mushlin and L. Fintor, "Is Screening For Breast Cancer Cost-Effective?" *Cancer* 69 (1992 Supplement): 1957–1962.

19. M. Marcus, A. L. Koch, M. H. Schoen, and R. Tuominen, "A Proposed New System for Valuing Dental Procedures: The Relative Time-Cost Unit," *Medical Care* 28, 10 (1990): 943–951.

20. K. Davis and D. Rowland, "Uninsured and Underserved: Inequities in Health Care in the United States," *Milbank Quarterly* 61 (1983): 149–176.

21. K. Manton, C. Patrick, and K. Johnson, "Health Differentials Between Blacks and Whites: Recent Trends in Mortality and Morbidity," *Milbank Quarterly* 65, Supplement 1 (1987): 129–199.

22. Davis and Rowland, "Uninsured and Underserved."

23. Valdez R. Burciaga, Aida Giachello, Helen Rodriguez-Trias, Paula Gomez, and Castulo De La Rocha, "Improving Access to Health Care in Latino Communities," *Public Health Reports* 108 (1993): 535–539; and Ronald M. Andersen, Sandra Zelman Lewis, Aida L. Giachello, Lu Ann Aday, and Grace Chiu, "Access to Medical Care Among the Hispanic Population of the Southwestern United States," *Journal of Health and Social Behavior* 22 (March 1981): 78–89.

24. Kim A. Heithoff and Kathleen N. Lohr (eds.), *Effectiveness and Outcomes in Health Care* (Washington, D.C.: National Academy Press, 1993).

25. Aday, Begley, Lairson, and Slater, *Evaluating the Medical Care System.*

26. C. Martini, J. B. Allen, J. Davidson, and E. M. Backett, "Health Indexes Sensitive to Medical Care Variation," *International Journal of Health Services* 7 (1977): 293–309.

27. A. Tarlov, J. Ware, S. Greenfield, E. C. Nelson, E. Perrin, and M. Zubkoff, "The Medical Outcomes Study: An Application of Methods for Monitoring the Results of Medical Care," *Journal of the American Medical Association,* 262 (1989): 925–930; J. E. Ware, "Measuring Patient Function and Well-Being: Some Lessons from the Medical Outcomes Study," in *Effectiveness and Outcomes in Health Care,* proceedings of the invitational conference by the Institute of Medicine, Division of Health Care Services, eds. K. A. Heithoff and K. N.

Lohr (Washington, D.C.: National Academy Press, 1990): 107–119; A. L. Stewart, S. Greenfield, R. D. Hays, et al., "Functional Status and Well-Being of Patients with Chronic Conditions: Results from the Medical Outcomes Study," *JAMA* 262 (1989): 295–930.

28. R. L. Kravitz, S. Greenfield, W. Rogers, W. G. Manning, M. Zubkoff, E. C. Nelson, A. R. Tarlov, and J. E. Ware, "Differences in the Mix of Patients Among Medical Specialties and Systems of Care: Results from the Medical Outcomes Study," *JAMA* 267 (1992): 1617–1623.

29. S. Greenfield, E. C. Nelson, M. Zubkoff, W. G. Manning, W. Rogers, R. L. Kravitz, A. Keller, A. R. Tarlov, and J. E. Ware, "Variations in Resource Utilization Among Medical Specialties and Systems of Care: Results from the Medical Outcomes Study," *JAMA* 267 (1992): 1624–1630.

30. D. G. Safran, A. R. Tarlov, and W. H. Rogers, "Primary Care Performance in Fee-For-Service and Prepaid Health Care Systems: Results from the Medical Outcomes Study," *JAMA* 271 (1994): 1579–1586.

31. Aday, Begley, Lairson, and Slater, *Evaluating the Medical Care System.*

32. Aday, Begley, Lairson, and Slater, *Evaluating the Medical Care System*; and W. G. Manning, A. Liebowitz, and G. A. Goldberg, "A Controlled Trial of the Effect of a Prepaid Group Practice on Use of Services," *New England Journal of Medicine* 310 (1984): 1505–1510.

33. E. Reinhardt, "A Production Function for Physician Services," *Review of Economics and Statistics* 54 (1972): 55–66; K. R. Smith, M. Miller, and F. L. Golladay, "An Analysis of the Optimal Use of Inputs in the Production of Medical Services," *Journal of Human Resources* 7 (1972): 208–255; and D. M. Brown, "Do Physicians Underutilize Aides?" *Journal of Human Resources* 23 (1988): 342–355.

34. M. F. Shapiro, J. E. Ware, and C. D. Sherbourne, "Effects of Cost Sharing on Seeking Care for Serious and Minor Symptoms: Results of a Randomized Controlled Trial," *Annals of Internal Medicine* 104 (1986): 246–251.

35. The Commonwealth Fund, *Managed Care: The Patient's Perspective: A Briefing Note—Karen Davis, President* (New York: Harkness House, 1995), p. 1.

36. Center for Health Economics Research, *Access to Health Care: Key Indicators for Policy,* p. 6, emphasis added.

37. Center for Health Economics Research, *Access to Health Care: Key Indicators For Policy.*

38. Lu Ann Aday, *At Risk in America: The Health and Health Care Needs of Vulnerable Populations in the United States* (San Francisco: Jossey-Bass, 1993).

39. Aday, Begley, Lairson, and Slater, *Evaluating the Medical Care System.*

40. Institute of Medicine (U.S.), Committee on Monitoring Access to Personal Health Care Services, *Access to Health Care in America,* p. 131.

41. Institute of Medicine (U.S.), Committee on Monitoring Access to Personal Health Care Services, *Access to Health Care in America.*

42. Aday, *At Risk in America.*

43. Institute of Medicine (U.S.), Committee on Monitoring Access to Personal Health Care Services, *Access to Health Care in America,* p. 130.

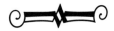

CHAPTER TWO

# PUBLIC POLICIES TO EXTEND HEALTH CARE COVERAGE

E. Richard Brown and Roberta Wyn

The United States remains alone among its leading trading partners in not providing health care coverage to its entire population. With the failure to enact health care reform, health care coverage is continuing to decline and the number of uninsured persons is rising at the rate of more than one million persons each year.

In this chapter, we examine the origins and status of the U.S. system of health care coverage and the options available to extend coverage to the uninsured. First, we describe the current state of health insurance coverage, with an examination of historical trends and the public policies that shaped the current system. Then we examine the major policy options to extend coverage to the remaining uninsured population, focusing in particular on those that received consideration in the recent health care reform debates.

The United States has repeatedly toyed with major reforms to establish a universal social insurance program to provide health care coverage to the entire population. Each time, the nation has failed to come to grips with this issue or has adopted very partial reforms, sometimes enacting programs based on a public assistance, or welfare, approach. After these repeated failures to enact comprehensive reform and despite the partial solutions that have been adopted, the problems of lack of coverage remain a continuing challenge to the U.S. health system and the nation's political institutions.

## The Uninsured

The growing number of people with no health care coverage—no private health insurance, no Medicare or Medicaid coverage, nor coverage through any other source—has become one of the most compelling policy and political issues in the United States. The uninsured have increased from 27 million, 14 percent of the non-elderly population, in 1977 to 41.5 million, 18 percent of the non-elderly population, in 1993. Fourteen states have uninsured rates in excess of 20 percent of their non-elderly populations.[1]

About three in ten of the uninsured are children under age eighteen, and the rest are adults between eighteen and sixty-four years of age. Very few persons above age sixty-five are completely uninsured because of the near-universal coverage provided to the elderly by Medicare. The uninsured are a predominantly lower-income population; 60 percent have incomes below 200 percent of the fed-

**FIGURE 2.1. HEALTH INSURANCE COVERAGE OF THE NON-ELDERLY POPULATION, UNITED STATES, 1993.**

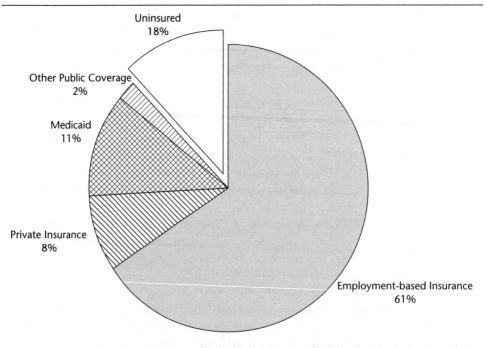

*Source:* Analysis by UCLA Center for Health Policy Research of March 1994 Current Population Survey.

eral poverty level (that is, less than $29,526 for a family of four in 1993). Although 60 percent of the uninsured are non-Latino whites, ethnic minorities—especially Latinos—have disproportionately high uninsured rates.[2]

The overwhelming majority of the uninsured (85 percent) are working adults and their children, including 44 percent of the uninsured who are in families headed by a full-time full-year employee and another 19 percent in families of full-time employees who work less than a full year. The problem is disproportionately centered in small firms; nearly half (48 percent) of uninsured employees work in firms with fewer than 25 workers. But larger firms also contribute to the problem; one in four uninsured employees works in a firm with five hundred or more workers.

The lack of health insurance is a high-profile policy and political issue for several reasons. First, it is widely understood that health insurance coverage is an important determinant of access to health care, for the reasons discussed in the previous chapter. Second, the lack of adequate health insurance coverage puts individuals and families at risk for significant economic losses due to medical expenses. Finally, providers, government, and ultimately employers, employees, and other taxpayers end up paying for uncompensated care provided to uninsured persons. In the absence of comprehensive health care coverage for the working and nonworking population, we have woven a patchwork quilt of community health centers, public indigent-care hospitals and clinics, charity care by private hospitals, and various financing programs for the low-income uninsured.

## Private Health Insurance Coverage

In 1993, in addition to the 18 percent of the non-elderly population who were uninsured, 61 percent were covered by health insurance obtained through employment—their own or a family member's. Another 8 percent were covered by private health insurance purchased without any employer contribution. Approximately 11 percent of the non-elderly population were covered by Medicaid, and another 2 percent by other public programs (see Figure 2.1).[3]

From World War II through the mid 1970s, private health insurance covered a growing proportion of the population. World War II produced several forces that encouraged the expansion of private health insurance, including wage-and-price controls that exempted employee benefits, cost-plus government war contracts, federal tax policies that allowed employers to deduct premiums for health plans from business revenues and allowed employees to deduct employer-paid health insurance premiums from earnings, and labor pressure on employers. In 1945, enrollment in hospital insurance plans had spread to 24 percent of the population, up from 10 percent in 1940. After the war, commercial insurance companies, following the early leadership of Blue Cross, pushed into the employer-sponsored health insurance market, and by 1950, private hospital insurance provided coverage to 51 percent of the population. By 1962, about 70 percent of the entire population had hospital benefits, and 65 percent were covered for physicians' surgical services.[4]

Private health insurance was popular among consumers of health services because it spread the risk of expensive medical conditions across a large population base, reducing the threat of personal bankruptcy in the event of serious health problems and making health services financially more accessible to the covered population. It was also popular among hospitals, physicians, and other health care providers because it created a stable base of revenues that reduced their risks of bankruptcy during recessions and permitted them to expand and introduce new technologies during good years. The growth of private health insurance was the financial foundation for the growth industry that medical care rapidly became.

Employer-funded health insurance, which never achieved universal coverage of the employed population, peaked in the mid 1970s and has declined since that time. The decline in manufacturing and other high-wage and unionized industries has led to a loss of jobs that convey health benefits to workers and their families. The expansion of employment in the retail and service sectors of the economy has not offset this loss because these firms tend to be smaller and, compared with high-coverage industries, to rely more on low-skilled labor employed seasonally or part-time. Full-time full-year employees are about twice as likely to be covered by their own job-based health insurance as are full-time employees who work less than full year. But there is also variation among full-time full-year employees; those who work in firms with five hundred or more employees are twice as likely to have their own employer-funded insurance as those who work in firms with fewer than twenty-five workers.[5]

Private health insurance, even in its period of rapid growth, has not served all sectors of our society. The elderly and the poor were effectively priced out of the market for private coverage. In 1958, while 86 percent of the upper-income third of all U.S. families had some type of private health insurance, only 42 percent of the lower-income third had any coverage at all. Like the lower working class and the poor, the elderly were unable to obtain adequate private hospitalization coverage at a price they could afford. In 1958, only 43 percent of persons aged sixty-five years and over had insurance for hospital care, compared with at least two-thirds of the non-elderly population.[6] Although private health insurance dramatically reduced disparities in the use of health services related to income for the population with coverage, it remained for Medicare and Medicaid to significantly improve access for the elderly and the poor.

# Medicare and Medicaid

By the early 1960s, political pressures to enact public programs to provide for the poor, especially the low-income elderly, had become irresistible.[7] The Kerr-Mills Act, enacted in 1960, provided generous matching federal grants to states to encourage them to develop medical care programs for the elderly poor and the non-elderly disabled and blind. But the program received very uneven implementation by the states, with the bulk of the federal funds going to a handful of states that developed comprehensive programs. Senior-citizen groups, not assuaged by this public assistance program, continued to demand health insurance under Social Security, not a welfare program.[8]

In November 1964, a Democratic landslide electoral victory (the most lop-sided popular vote in this century) gave President Lyndon Johnson both a clear mandate for his Great Society reforms and a Democratic Congress (two-thirds in both houses) to enact them. The next year, Congress established Medicare, a social insurance program for hospital care and voluntary insurance for physician services for the elderly, and Medicaid, a public assistance program for poor people who meet categorical requirements.

Medicare was a landmark in health care reform because, as a contributory program that provided entitlement to health benefits without a means test, it was the first successful enactment of social insurance for health services. Medicaid also was important because of its broad potential scope of benefits and population coverage, despite its public assistance, or welfare, character that rested on means testing.

## Medicare: Improving Access for the Elderly

Medicare has extended coverage to virtually all elderly persons and to many blind and long-term disabled persons for a significant portion of their medical expenses. Medicare, the largest source of public financing for health care services in the United States, was enacted in 1965 to extend acute care health insurance coverage to the elderly population. Legislation enacted during the 1970s extended coverage to blind and long-term disabled persons. Persons aged sixty-five and over with social security benefits are automatically entitled to receive Medicare Part A (coverage for hospital services) and to enroll in Medicare Part B (coverage for physician and other services). In 1993, Medicare covered 36.3 million aged and disabled persons at a cost of $154.2 billion.[9]

Medicare quickly improved access to medical services, especially hospital care, for the elderly. But even under Medicare, an entitlement program with uniform benefits and standards, beneficiary access problems remain. In the program's first few years, more affluent elderly beneficiaries received more physician and hospital services than did the lower-income elderly. Similarly, Anglo beneficiaries received more health services than did African American beneficiaries. Over time, however, both income and racial differentials were reduced. Recent studies show that the vast majority of Medicare beneficiaries report no access problems, but some groups do experience serious access barriers. About one in seven Medicare beneficiaries do not have a usual source of care or have not seen a physician for a medical problem that warranted medical attention. Studies that examine access to specific procedures consistently find differences by race in the rates of selected diagnostic and treatment procedures performed. African American beneficiaries are less likely than Anglo beneficiaries to receive a variety of high-technology procedures.[10]

Lack of coverage for several key benefits limits the effectiveness of Medicare for many types of health services, particularly for lower-income beneficiaries. Medicare does not cover prescription medications and, until recently, did not cover screening mammography or Pap tests. Most notable is the lack of coverage for nonacute long-term care services. Medicare restricts coverage for nursing home stays and home health visits to posthospital use of limited duration, imposing hardships on the elderly who must use extensive personal resources to pay for care or, if eligible, apply to Medicaid.

Medicare cost-sharing provisions also pose financial barriers. Premium costs, deductibles, and coinsurance, as well as physician charges resulting from balance billing, can impose high out-of-pocket costs on beneficiaries. A high proportion of beneficiaries have supplemental coverage to offset these costs, yet poorer beneficiaries and ethnic minorities are less likely to have supplemental coverage. Beneficiaries who had Medicare coverage only—that is, no private Medigap insurance or Medicaid coverage to offset cost-sharing obligations—have lower use of services despite poorer health status.[11] Despite the importance of Medicare coverage, however, out-of-pocket health care expenses as a proportion of mean annual income were similar in 1985 to those in 1965, just before the implementation of Medicare.[12]

## Medicaid: Improving Access for the Poor

Medicaid was enacted in 1965 to provide coverage to poor persons who were eligible for federal-state welfare programs—families with dependent children, the disabled, the blind, and the elderly—and to assist elderly Medicare beneficiaries who could not afford the required cost sharing for Medicare or supplemental insurance. Funding is shared between the federal government and the states, with the federal share ranging from 50 percent up to more than 80 percent. In 1995, Medicaid is expected to cover nearly thirty-seven million persons at a cost of $158 billion.[13] Half of Medicaid beneficiaries are low-income children, about a fifth are low-income women, and the remaining quarter are low-income disabled and elderly persons. Medicaid spending is tilted toward the elderly and disabled, who in 1993 averaged more than $7,000 per recipient annually in Medicaid expenditures, compared with children, who averaged less than $1,000 per recipient.[14]

There is substantial evidence that Medicaid is responsible for significant increases in the use of health services among low-income persons. In 1964, two years before the Medicaid program began operation, poor persons averaged 4.3 doctor visits per year, compared to 4.6 visits for the nonpoor. By the mid 1970s, when nearly all states were operating Medicaid programs, poor adults averaged *more* physician visits than nonpoor adults, and the gap between poor and nonpoor children had been reduced but not eliminated. However, use of greater volumes of services by the poor may not necessarily indicate complete equity in access because of the poorer health status of the low-income population. If we take health status into account when we compare use rates across income groups, the poor continued to have a substantial deficit in physician visits compared to the nonpoor.[15]

Although Medicaid has been shown to provide its beneficiaries with utilization rates that are comparable to those of more affluent groups, its effects are limited by the relatively low proportion of the poor who are eligible for Medicaid. Numerous studies have found that Medicaid beneficiaries, in contrast to uninsured low-income persons, use health services at rates comparable to those of higher-income persons, after adjusting for differences in health status. Among poor and near-poor persons who are sick or in poor health, those who are uninsured during the entire year use far fewer medical services than those who have Medicaid even part of the year.[16]

Prospective studies find that the loss of Medicaid coverage has an adverse impact on the health status of low-income people. The loss of Medicaid has a particularly serious adverse impact on access to health services and on the health status of persons with chronic illnesses, such as diabetes or high blood pressure.[17]

Despite its important contributions, Medicaid's ability to improve access to medical care for the nation's low-income population has been hampered by several factors. State-level discretion in the Medicaid program has resulted in great variation across states in the population covered and the benefits provided. The federal guidelines define mandatory eligible populations and covered benefits but allow states considerable latitude beyond this floor. States vary markedly in the Medicaid income eligibility levels for AFDC recipients and other families. For example, the range in 1992 was, at the upper end, a gross monthly income of $2,057 in Vermont—and, at the lower end, $577 in Missouri. States also differ in the benefits covered in the Medicaid program. Each state defines its own package of benefits beyond the mandatory services defined by federal Medicaid law. For example, coverage for such essential services as physical therapy, occupational therapy, respiratory care services, and corrective eyeglasses are all optional. Reimbursement levels for Medicaid also vary considerably across states, contributing to differences by state in physician participation rates.[18]

Medicaid's limitations in covering the poor were exacerbated by budget cuts during the Reagan administration and ratcheting down by states of income limits for AFDC eligibility. As a result, Medicaid enrollees as a proportion of all poor persons declined from 51 percent in 1981 to 45 percent in 1982. Beginning in the mid 1980s, however, Congress enacted a series of expansions in Medicaid income eligibility in order to extend Medicaid's beneficial effects to more low-income pregnant women and their children. Although only 51 percent of poor children were on Medicaid in 1985, 60 percent were covered by Medicaid in 1994, an important reversal of the trend of a decade earlier.[19]

Most of this increase was aimed at providing financial access for pregnant women to enable them to obtain prenatal care early in their pregnancies so as to improve birth outcomes and the health of their infants. Congress required states to cover pregnant women up to 133 percent of the poverty level, and encouraged states to voluntarily expand coverage up to 185 percent of that level. This extension of Medicaid to a population well above the income eligibility for the AFDC public assistance program partially severed the historical link between Medicaid and welfare. In addition, Congress required states to increase fees for obstetric care to attract an adequate number of providers and appropriated other funds for enhanced perinatal care. By 1994, thirty-four states had expanded coverage of pregnant women beyond federally mandated levels, fifty states had streamlined the eligibility process to at least some extent, and forty-four states offered Medicaid reimbursement for enhanced prenatal services. Nearly one-third of all births in the United States now are paid for by Medicaid, while other programs fund improvements in the supply and accessibility of prenatal care services and nutritional and other supports for mothers and young children.[20]

The Medicaid program's improvements in eligibility for pregnant women to meet specific public health goals provides a valuable example of how public policy may be used directly to improve access. The effects of Medicaid expansion on prenatal care use and birth outcomes are inconsistent. Some studies show improvements in access to care and birth outcomes while others do not. These findings suggest that there are multiple components to providing prenatal care that include, but go beyond, improving financial access. Comprehensive prenatal care should include outreach and educational programs, case management, and supply of providers.[21]

# Public Programs to Extend Coverage

Recent efforts to extend coverage to the uninsured have included both public assistance and social insurance approaches. Proposals for further expansion of Medicaid have involved major changes in this public assistance program, while efforts have continued to enact national or state health insurance based on a social-insurance mode.

## Expanding Medicaid Coverage

In spite of Medicaid expansions during the 1980s, the decline in employer-funded health insurance coverage has continued to add more working people to the rolls of the uninsured. Employer-funded health insurance coverage has fallen steadily for well over a decade. The proportion of the non-elderly population covered by job-based health benefits has recently fallen precipitously—from 66 percent in 1989 to 61 percent in 1993.[22] The private purchase of health insurance, at $4,800 or more per year for a comprehensive family plan, is simply not affordable to most working individuals and families without an employer contribution or government subsidy. The result of this process has been rising numbers of uninsured working families and individuals. When sick or injured, the uninsured not only have difficulty accessing the medical care system; when they finally obtain care, they also become a financial burden to states and local governments as well as to providers whose bills the uninsured cannot pay.

With the failure to enact national health care reform, many states looked to Medicaid, among other methods, to extend coverage to their uninsured residents. Many states have applied for, or are in the process of developing, applications for Medicaid waivers under section 1115 of the Social Security Act. These waivers, which must be approved by the federal Health Care Financing Administration (HCFA), permit states to modify eligibility, payment methods, and other characteristics in their Medicaid programs. More than thirty states have received section 1115 waivers since 1993, and fifteen others had waivers pending as of February 1995.[23] All of the waivers permit states to require Medicaid beneficiaries to enroll in managed care plans, based on the expectation that managed care will enable a state to slow the growth of its Medicaid expenditures. Most of the recent waivers also extend coverage to the working poor and their families who had not previously been eligible for Medicaid, promising to use at least some of the expected savings due to managed care to expand coverage to low-income uninsured persons. Tennessee, for example, has replaced its old fee-for-service Medicaid program with TennCare, a fully capitated managed care program. By May 1995,

TennCare had enrolled 837,000 of the state's 900,000 Medicaid beneficiaries, plus 414,000 previously uninsured residents.[24] Hawaii merged its State Health Insurance Program for the non-Medicaid-eligible uninsured into its Medicaid program, compelling all beneficiaries to enroll in capitated managed care plans. Bruce Vladeck, the HCFA administrator, has estimated that the section 1115 expansions in Oregon, Ohio, Hawaii, Tennessee, Rhode Island, Kentucky, and South Carolina will cover more than a million previously uninsured persons.[25]

These successes notwithstanding, Medicaid managed care programs raise concerns among many different groups. State medical societies, which tend to represent fee-for-service physicians, often object to forcing all Medicaid beneficiaries into managed care plans. These physicians fear a loss of fees that while not necessarily lucrative may be an important source of revenues. Community health centers, a critical part of the health care safety net for the uninsured poor and Medicaid recipients, fear that they will lose current Medicaid fees, which are a major source of their funding. Although many community health centers are developing contracts with managed care plans that enroll Medicaid recipients, they worry that their lost Medicaid fees will not be offset by serving patients enrolled in these plans. Without Medicaid revenues and with expected block grants and cutbacks in other funding programs, there is widespread concern that community health centers and other safety-net providers will not have the financial support they need to continue to serve uninsured patients. Advocates for the uninsured and low-income communities share the concerns of safety-net providers that, without Medicaid revenues, these last-resort providers will lose their financial viability, and the safety net will be shredded.

Advocates for Medicaid beneficiaries worry that managed care will end up reducing access to health services for enrollees because capitation creates incentives for health plans and providers to reduce use of services and because enrollees are locked into their plans for at least several months. They are also concerned that Medicaid HMOs may provide poorer quality care than fee-for-service practices. These concerns have been reinforced by some past experiences. In the 1970s, California's Medicaid beneficiaries suffered from abuses by managed care plans that marketed door-to-door with deceptive sales information, raised serious barriers to obtaining services, and often provided poor quality care. In the 1980s, Medicaid enrollees in Chicago area HMOs experienced similar marketing abuses, failure to provide services, and quality problems.[26]

Despite some very negative experiences, there is a growing body of evidence that overall, managed care plans offer Medicaid beneficiaries access to health services that is at least as good as in the fee-for-service Medicaid program and quality of care that is equal to or better than care in the fee-for-service program.[27] There is little evidence that managed care reduces Medicaid costs—in part because most Medicaid managed care enrollees have not been the higher-cost disabled or elderly for whom substantial savings might be realized and in part because Medicaid expenditures per beneficiary have already been ratcheted down to extremely low levels.

Currently, plans for Medicaid expansion seem to be foundering. The pressure of Medicaid expenditures on state and federal tax resources has generated strong political opposition to further expansion. In 1993, state shares for Medicaid averaged 12.8 percent of state general revenue funds, up from 10.5 percent in 1991; Medicaid was the largest single expenditure item for states after elementary and secondary education spending. Although Medicaid represents only 6 percent of federal expenditures, it is the largest, and fastest growing, of all federal grant-in-aid programs.[28] The political response to these expenditures reflects one of Medicaid's fundamental flaws—it is a program for poor people, who have little or no political voice, rather than a universal program like Medicare, with a broad political base of support. The Republican sweep of state and national offices in the November 1994 election put the brakes on Medicaid expansion and threatens significant cutbacks in this successful program.

## Social Insurance: The Elusive Option

For at least the last half century, Americans have found the concept of government health insurance an appealing way to cover the population.[29] Funded by taxes and administered as a universal national program by the federal government or by a combination of federal and state governments, such a social insurance program would pay physicians, hospitals, and other health care providers, eliminating the need for private health insurance.

Social insurance systems have many advantages. Canada's single-payer system, a social insurance program that has received a great deal of attention in the United States, has been an efficient means to provide universal coverage for comprehensive health benefits. The Canadian system has many advantages that attract people in the United States, including universal coverage, excellent access to primary care, patient freedom to choose personal physicians, a superior record of controlling expenditures for physicians and hospitals, lower administrative costs, lower out-of-pocket costs for patients, less restricted clinical autonomy for physicians, and greater popular satisfaction. Shortages of advanced technologies and long waits for nonurgent surgery in Canada, widely reported in the U.S. press, appear to be relatively minor consequences of the Canadian system to allocate technology. Physicians who have practiced in both Canada and the United States on average prefer the Canadian system. Finally, Canadians are far more satisfied with their health care system than U.S. citizens are with theirs.[30]

Despite these advantages and support, social insurance proposals have not fared well in the United States since the enactment of Medicare. Although the single-payer proposals[31] introduced into the Congress in the recent health care reform effort received substantial support from some unions and consumer-based organizations, they could not overcome the powerful opposition of an array of interest groups representing health care providers, insurers, and business. In November 1994, California voters rejected, by a seventy-three to twenty-seven margin, a Canadian-style single-payer initiative on the election ballot. This initiative had been opposed by a very well funded campaign by insurers, providers, and business. The defeat may have dashed advocates' hopes of demonstrating the political viability of the single-payer approach to health care reform. Given the particular political system and economic structure of the United States, it is uncertain whether national single-payer proposals can be enacted in the near future, despite their popular and policy appeal.[32]

## Reforms to Expand Private Coverage

In addition to expanding the population groups covered through Medicaid, states have also experimented with a wide array of reforms aimed at expanding private coverage to the uninsured population. The recent collapse of national health care reform efforts has increased pressure to implement state rather than national solutions to rising health care costs and access problems. However, states vary in their political and economic capacity to effectively implement reform, and they also lack the legislative authority to enact reforms that would provide universal coverage.

The main approaches that states have pursued to expand private coverage of the uninsured have included the development of risk pools for uninsured subgroups, reform of the insurance laws to increase affordability or access to coverage, the creation of purchase alliances or cooperatives, and in a few states, the passage of legislation mandating coverage. To varying degrees, these approaches build upon the existing employment-based insurance system, strengthening the connection between coverage and work.

### High-Risk Pools

High-risk pools target population groups that are unable to purchase insurance coverage due to preexisting health conditions.[33] Twenty-two states have operational high-risk pools serving at least one hundred persons,[34] with the earliest state-sponsored pools dating back to the mid 1970s. These programs typically require insurers to establish separately administered funds to insure persons who would otherwise be unable to purchase coverage because of their health conditions.

State risk pools have a lot of political appeal because they target people who are in obvious need of coverage, allaying the concerns of those skeptical of the state's role in expanding coverage. But high premium costs, high deductibles, and other cost-sharing provisions of high-risk pools have limited the effectiveness of this approach. Due to the higher costs of covering people with preexisting conditions, premium rates in these pools range from 125 percent to 400 percent of the average in the state.[35] Consequently, only a very small portion of the eligible population has obtained coverage from these pools.[36] Furthermore, risk pools are more expensive to operate than anticipated, further reducing their appeal and effectiveness. Nonetheless, in the absence of more comprehensive reform, these pools expand coverage to a limited population who historically have been denied any coverage or offered coverage at rates that are unaffordable to the target population. For example, in Minnesota, the risk pool serves a disproportionately older and female population,[37] a group that is at risk of coverage loss due to changes in marital and employment status.

## Small-Group and Individual Health Insurance Reform

Almost all states have implemented some type of insurance reform designed to increase the accessibility and affordability of coverage for small groups and individuals.[38] Compared to larger groups, small groups and individuals face higher premiums for health insurance due to higher marketing and administrative costs and more difficulty in managing risk in this market. Consequently, they also face such problems as frequent jumps in premiums, frequent changes in insurance carriers, and medical underwriting (that is, basing premiums on the particular group's expected use of health services).[39] Furthermore, the groups or individuals considered at highest risk may not be able to obtain any coverage.

Small-group and individual insurance market reforms focus on improving the availability and affordability of coverage for groups and individuals considered poor risks. To improve the availability of coverage, these reforms limit or prohibit underwriting to determine eligibility, although underwriting is still used to set rates. Guaranteed renewability of coverage and reinsurance pools are additional elements of reform designed to improve access to coverage. Premium rate restrictions, or more controversial community rating, are used to constrain the cost to enrollees, making coverage more affordable. Community rating averages the cost of coverage across a broader risk pool, lowering the upper bound of premium costs but also raising the lower end of the price range. Premium restrictions narrow the gap between the rates charged for higher- and lower-risk groups, stopping short of full community rating. In 1994, almost all states had enacted legislation that restricted premium rates in the small-group health insurance market, and three had implemented a true community rating system.[40] Although these reforms represent an improvement over the current restrictive practices of the insurance industry, they are not by themselves a sufficient remedy to the health insurance crisis.

## Purchasing Cooperatives

Unlike high-risk pools that target individuals, purchasing cooperatives target small businesses. These cooperatives or alliances of small firms are designed to increase purchasing power and lower administrative costs. Whereas over 85 percent of firms with twenty-five or more employees offer coverage, 73 percent of those with ten to twenty-four employees and only 27 percent of very small firms (those with fewer than ten employees) offer this fringe benefit.[41] The most common reasons given by small firms for not offering health insurance are insufficient profits and the high cost of coverage.[42] The state-sponsored cooperatives enable small businesses to pool the risk of insurance coverage, thus lowering premium costs and improving the businesses' bargaining power in the health insurance market. Although fourteen states have enacted legislation to develop or support the development of these cooperatives, only six have actually implemented such programs as of 1994.[43] Evidence from these programs suggests that they may help small firms continue to provide coverage for employees by offering them somewhat lower premiums than they previously paid, but that they have not been highly successful in attracting firms that do not offer coverage to their employees. In California, for example, only about 14 percent of enrollees in the state's small-group purchasing cooperative had previously been uninsured—less than thirteen thousand persons, or 0.2 percent of California's uninsured population.[44]

## Employer Mandates

The reforms that have been discussed so far create incremental changes in how health services are financed and in the proportion of the uninsured population gaining access to coverage. These reforms make coverage available to employers or individuals whose high risks or small size has made it difficult for them to find coverage at rates available to other employers or individuals. But such reforms do not address the problem of the high cost of health insurance even to those who are best positioned in the market, and this remains the major access barrier for the moderate- and lower-income families and individuals who constitute the majority of the uninsured.

To make health insurance more affordable to this currently uninsured population—as well as to stabilize the employment-based system for financing health insurance—there has been considerable national and state interest in requiring employers to help pay for coverage for their employees. A few states have enacted and one state has implemented such an employer mandate.[45] Employer mandates are appealing to states: they require employers to offer or pay for coverage for their employees, within the mandates of the legislation. Many employees and their families who do not receive employer-funded health insurance now rely on state-funded health insurance coverage or health services programs. For example, in California in 1992, more than six million employees and their dependents not covered by employer-funded health insurance relied on Medi-Cal (California's Medicaid program) coverage or used state- and county-funded indigent medical services at a cost to taxpayers of nearly $4 billion.[46]

Despite the seeming appeal of an employer mandate, only Hawaii has implemented this reform. The ability of states to adopt employer mandates has been thwarted by the federal Employee Retirement Income Security Act (ERISA), which exempts self-insured businesses from state insurance regulations and taxes.[47] Hawaii is the only state that received a Congressional exemption from ERISA for its employer mandate because Hawaii enacted its mandate legislation in 1974, before ERISA itself was enacted. Nationally, more than half of all medium and large firms self-insure (that is, assume all or part of the financial risk of coverage), greatly limiting states' authority over the employer group insurance market.

Both ERISA and the political and economic implications of employer mandates have led the few other states that planned to enact mandate policies to abandon their efforts or place on hold implementation of the mandate.[48] Employer mandates have won the vehement and aggressive opposition of employers, especially interest groups representing small business.

Finally, an employer mandate is not, by itself, a panacea for the lack of universal coverage. Although Hawaii's system of coverage often has been seen as a model for other states,[49] and its uninsured rate is lower than that in most other states, Hawaii has not yet achieved universal coverage. Hawaii's uninsured rate is approximately 13 percent, well below the national average, but Hawaii's mandate excludes part-time and seasonal workers and provides for voluntary rather than mandatory coverage of employees' dependents.[50] Employer mandates will always exclude the nonworking portion of the uninsured population and, depending on the mandate's coverage requirements, a portion of the employed population as well. Thus, this approach is, at best, only a component of any comprehensive reform to achieve universal coverage.

## Facing the New Century: Important Roles for Research and Policy

As we approach the end of the twentieth century, the failures in our system of providing and paying for health care coverage, which contributed to the recent public support for health care reform, show no signs of improvement. If anything, these problems are likely to get worse. Employer-funded health insurance shows no signs of reversing its long-term downward trend. Changes in the labor market—the decline in manufacturing, the increase in service-sector jobs, and the increasing use of temporary and part-time employment arrangements—and the decline in real (inflation-adjusted) income among working families and individuals are eroding the foundation of the nation's private health insurance system. In the long run, these structural changes are likely to undermine our reliance on private employment-based health insurance.

Compounding this declining private insurance coverage, federal cutbacks in Medicaid are likely to limit the program's ability to absorb pregnant women and families who lose job-based coverage and to greatly limit the coverage for the disabled population that currently relies on Medicaid. The growing number and proportions of the population who are completely uninsured place enormous burdens on those individuals and families, who must cope with reduced access and increased personal expense. But this problem also burdens others who help pay for whatever health services remain for the uninsured; this includes employers and employees who pay for private health insurance and state and local taxpayers who bear the financial burden of public hospitals and clinics for the medically indigent.

Health services research will continue to be important to help policy makers and the public understand the impact of these trends. Health services research has played an important role in identifying the gaps in insurance coverage, monitoring the effects of those gaps, and modeling the impact of different reform options on coverage and costs. As the federal government's role in social and public health care programs (such as Medicaid) decreases and as state discretion increases, studies of the effects of these changes, especially the effects on low-income populations, will be particularly important. The private sector also is making major changes in response to rising health care costs—changes that may reduce the affordability of coverage for employees. Many employers are increasing employee contributions for health benefits, especially for family coverage. Low-wage workers may increasingly find their required contributions for health benefits an unaffordable expense, leading to increased uninsured rates. Women may be especially affected by these changes because they are more likely to depend on Medicaid or on coverage through a spouse, two sources of coverage that are particularly vulnerable to cost-saving measures.

Studies of the effects of different types of insurance plans on access and on the process and quality of care will become increasingly more important as managed care and market-based prices dominate the health care field. Managed care cost-saving techniques, such as limitations in hospital stays during normal labor and delivery, are being challenged as too restrictive. As public and private insurers are increasingly turning to managed care, the gaps in knowledge about this approach to financing and delivery become more apparent. Research will be important to assess which aspects of managed care promote effective use of services and which impede appropriate use.

Policy interventions will be needed to shore up growing gaps in coverage. Following the failure of the 103rd Congress to enact comprehensive health care reforms in 1994, access to health care coverage and to health services may decline further with cutbacks and changes that are likely to emanate from the 104th Congress. Although budget cuts in Medicaid and other safety-net programs probably will increase the numbers of uninsured persons, policy solutions are likely to be more difficult to enact and implement because of fiscal restrictions. Yet public policy solutions to these problems of coverage and access cannot be avoided indefinitely as the uninsured population grows. Whether solutions are developed at the state or the federal level, through private-sector insurance and financing or through public programs and taxes, with social insurance programs like Medicare or public assistance programs like Medicaid, the United States cannot escape the need for fundamental reforms that will extend coverage to its entire population.

## Notes

1. Nineteen ninety-three estimates are based on the authors' analysis of March 1994 Current Population Survey; 1977 estimate is from Judith A. Kasper, D. C. Walden, and G. R. Wilensky, "Who Are the Uninsured?" *National Health Care Expenditures Study, Data Preview 1* (Hyattsville, Md.: National Center for Health Services Research, n.d.).
2. Authors' analysis of March 1994 Current Population Survey.
3. Authors' analysis of March 1994 Current Population Survey.
4. M. S. Mueller, "Private Health Insurance in 1973: A Review of Coverage, Enrollment, and Financial Experience," *Social Security Bulletin* 38 (February 1975): 21–40; M. S. Mueller, "Private Health Insurance in 1975: A Review of Coverage, Enrollment, and Financial Experience," *Social Security Bulletin* 40 (June 1977): 3–21; and Cambridge Research Institute, *Trends Affecting the U.S. Health Care System* (Washington, D.C.: Health Resources Administration, 1976), pp. 184–185.
5. Authors' analysis of March 1994 Current Population Survey.
6. Herman W. Somers and Anne R. Somers, *Doctors, Patients and Health Insurance* (Washington, D.C.: Brookings Institution, 1961), pp. 367–368.

7. Theodore R. Marmor, *The Politics of Medicare* (Hawthorne, N.Y.: Aldine de Gruyter, 1970); and Paul Starr, *The Social Transformation of American Medicine* (New York: Basic Books, 1982).

8. Rosemary Stevens and Robert Stevens, *Welfare Medicine in America: A Case Study of Medicaid* (New York: Free Press, 1974).

9. Katherine R. Levit, Cathy A. Cowans, Helen C. Lazenby, Patricia A. McDonnell, Arthur L. Sensenig, Jean M. Stiller, and Darleen K. Won, "National Health Spending Trends, 1960–1993," *Health Affairs* 13 (1994): 14–31.

10. Karen Davis, "Equal Treatment and Unequal Benefits: The Medicare Program," *Milbank Quarterly*, 53 (1975): 449–488; Stephen H. Long and R. F. Settle, "Medicare and the Disadvantaged Elderly: Objectives and Outcomes," *Milbank Quarterly*, 62 (1984): 609–656; C. R. Link, Stephen H. Long, and R. F. Settle, "Equity and the Utilization of Health Services by the Medicare Elderly," *Journal of Human Resources*, 17 (1982): 195–212; Physician Payment Review Commission, *Annual Report to Congress, 1994* (Washington, D.C.: Physician Payment Review Commission, 1994); Mark B. Wenneker and Arnold M. Epstein, "Racial Inequalities in the Use of Procedures for Patients with Ischemic Heart Disease in Massachusetts," *Journal of the American Medical Association* 261 (1989): 253–257; A. Marshall McBean and Marian Gornick, "Differences by Race in the Rates of Procedures Performed in Hospitals for Medicare Beneficiaries," *Health Care Financing Review* 15 (1994): 77–90; and John Z. Ayanian, I. Steven Udvarhelyi, Constantine A. Gatsonis, Chris L. Pashos, and Arnold M. Epstein, "Acute Myocardial Infarction: Process of Care and Clinical Outcomes," *JAMA* 269 (1993): 2642–2646.

11. Marian Gornick, "Physician Payment Reform Under Medicare: Monitoring Utilization and Access," *Health Care Financing Review* 14 (Spring 1993): 77–96.

12. D. Blumenthal, Mark Schlesinger, P. Brown Drumheller, *Renewing the Promise: Medicare and Its Reforms* (New York: Oxford University Press, 1988).

13. Kaiser Commission on the Future of Medicaid, *Medicaid and Federal, State, and Local Budgets* (Washington, D.C.: Kaiser Commission on the Future of Medicaid, March 1995).

14. John K. Iglehart, "Health Policy Report: Medicaid and Managed Care," *New England Journal of Medicine* 332 (1995): 1727–1731.

15. Health Resources Administration, *Health of the Disadvantaged, Chart Book II*, DHHS Pub. No. (HRA) 80–633. (Washington, D.C.: U.S. Government Printing Office, 1980), p. 61; and Lu Ann Aday and Ronald Andersen, "Equity of Access to Medical Care: A Conceptual and Empirical Overview," in *Securing Access to Health Care: The Ethical Implications of Differences in the Availability of Health Services* (Washington, D.C.: President's Commission for the Study of Ethical Problems in Medicine and Biomedical and Behavioral Research, 1983), pp. 19–54.

16. Karen Davis, "Achievements and Problems of Medicaid," *Public Health Reports* 912 (1976): 122–135; Paul Newacheck, "Access to Ambulatory Care for Poor Persons," *Health Services Research* 23 (1988): 401–419; Howard E. Freeman and Christopher R. Corey, "Insurance Status and Access to Health Services Among Poor Persons," *Health Services Research* 28 (1993): 531–541; Gail R. Wilensky and Mark L. Berk, "Health Care, the Poor, and the Role of Medicaid," *Health Affairs* 1 (1982): 93–100; and J. D. Kasper, "Health Status and Utilization: Differences by Medicaid Coverage and Income," *Health Care Financing Review* 7 (Summer 1986): 1–17.

17. Nicole Lurie, N. B. Ward, Martin F. Shapiro, and Robert H. Brook, "Termination from Medi-Cal: Does It Affect Health?" *New England Journal of Medicine* 311 (1984): 480–484; and Nicole Lurie, N. B. Ward, Martin F. Shapiro, C. Gallego, R. Vaghaiwalla, and Robert H.

Brook, "Termination of Medi-Cal Benefits: A Follow-up Study One Year Later," *New England Journal of Medicine* 314 (1986): 1266–1268.

18. See Congressional Research Service, *Medicaid Source Book: Background Data and Analysis,* 1993 update (Washington, D.C.: U.S. Government Printing Office, January 1993), for information regarding variations in eligibility and benefits. See Anne Schwartz, David C. Colby, and Anne L. Reisinger, "Variation in Medicaid Physician Fees," *Health Affairs* 10, 1 (1991): 131–139, for information about variations in provider payment rates.

19. Diane Rowland, B. Lyons, and J. Edwards, "Medicaid: Health Care for the Poor in the Reagan Era," *Annual Review of Public Health* 9 (1988): 427–450; and Sara Rosenbaum and Julie Darnell, *Medicaid Section 1115 Demonstration Waivers: Approved and Proposed Activities as of November 1994* (Washington, D.C.: Kaiser Commission on the Future of Medicaid, 1994).

20. U.S. General Accounting Office, *Medicaid Prenatal Care: States Improve Access and Enhance Services, but Face New Challenges,* GAO/HEHS–94–152BR (Washington, D.C.: U.S. General Accounting Office, May 1994).

21. Linda Loranger and Debra Lipson, *The Medicaid Expansions for Pregnant Women and Children* (Washington, D.C.: Alpha Center, 1995).

22. Authors' analysis of *March 1990 Current Population Survey* and *March 1994 Current Population Survey.*

23. Bruce C. Vladeck, "Medicaid 1115 Demonstrations: Progress Through Partnership," *Health Affairs* 14, 1 (Spring 1995): 217–220.

24. Iglehart, "Health Policy Report: Medicaid and Managed Care."

25. Vladeck, "Medicaid 1115 Demonstrations."

26. U.S. General Accounting Office, *Better Controls Needed for Health Maintenance Organizations Under Medicaid in California,* B–164031 (Washington, D.C.: U.S. General Accounting Office, September 10, 1974); Carol N. D'Onofrio, Patricia D. Mullen, "Consumer Problems with Prepaid Health Plans in California," *Public Health Reports* 92 (1977): 121–134; and U.S. General Accounting Office, *Medicaid: Oversight of Health Maintenance Organizations in the Chicago Area,* GAO/HRD–90–81 (Washington, D.C.: U.S. General Accounting Office, August 27, 1990).

27. Kaiser Commission on the Future of Medicaid, *Medicaid and Managed Care: Lessons from the Literature* (Menlo Park, Calif.: Henry J. Kaiser Family Foundation, 1995); U.S. General Accounting Office, *Medicaid: States Turn to Managed Care to Improve Access and Control Costs,* GAO/HRD–93–46 (Washington, D.C.: U.S. General Accounting Office, March 1993); and Iglehart, "Health Policy Report: Medicaid and Managed Care."

28. Kaiser Commission on the Future of Medicaid, *Medicaid and Federal, State, and Local Budgets.*

29. Starr, *The Social Transformation of American Medicine.*

30. Victor R. Fuchs and J. S. Hahn, "How Does Canada Do It? A Comparison of Expenditures for Physicians' Services in the United States and Canada," *New England Journal of Medicine* 323 (1990): 884–890; Robert G. Evans, J. Lomas, Morris L. Barer, et al., "Controlling Health Expenditures—The Canadian Reality," *New England Journal of Medicine* 320 (1989): 571–577; U.S. Congressional Budget Office, *Single-Payer and All-Payer Health Insurance Systems Using Medicare's Payment Rates,* CBO Staff Memorandum (Washington, D.C.: Congressional Budget Office, April 1993); Steffie Woolhandler and David U. Himmelstein, "The Deteriorating Administrative Efficiency of the U.S. Health Care System," *New England Journal of Medicine* 324 (1991): 1253–1258; Robert J. Blendon and H. Taylor, "Views on Health Care: Public Opinion in Three Nations," *Health Affairs* 8 (Spring 1989): 149–157; U.S. General Accounting Office, *Canadian Health Insurance: Lessons for the United States,*

GAO/HRD–91–90 (Washington, D.C.: U.S. General Accounting Office, June 1991); and G. J. Hayes, S. C. Hayes, and T. Dykstra, "Physicians Who Have Practiced in Both the U.S. and Canada Compare Systems," *American Journal of Public Health* 83 (1993): 1544–1548.

31. Bills introduced into the U.S. Senate by Paul Wellstone and into the House of Representatives by Jim McDermott and John Conyers to create a Canadian-style single-payer system and the bill introduced into the House of Representatives by Pete Stark to make Medicare universally available.

32. Theda Skocpol, "Is the Time Finally Ripe? Health Insurance Reforms in the 1990s," *Journal of Health, Politics, Policy, and Law* 18 (1993): 531–550; Vicente Navarro, "Why Some Countries Have National Health Insurance, Others Have National Health Services, and the U.S. Has Neither," *Social Science and Medicine* 28 (1989): 887–898; and D. J. Rothman, "A Century of Failure: Health Care Reform in America," *Journal of Health, Politics, Policy, and Law* 18 (1993): 271–286.

33. U.S. General Accounting Office, *Health Insurance: Risk Pools for the Medically Uninsurable*, Briefing Report to the Committee on Labor and Human Resources, U.S. Senate, GAO/HRD–88–66–BR (Washington, D.C.: U.S. General Accounting Office, 1988).

34. Deborah J. Chollet, Jo Ann Lamphere, and Debra J. Lipson, *State Health Reform: Recent Public Sector Activity* (Washington, D.C.: National Institute for Health Care Management, 1995).

35. E. Richard Brown and Geraldine Dallek, "State Approaches to Financing Health Care for the Poor," *Annual Review of Public Health* 11 (1993): 377–400.

36. U.S. General Accounting Office, *Health Insurance: Risk Pools for the Medically Uninsurable*, Briefing Report to the Committee on Labor and Human Resources, U.S. Senate, GAO/HRD–88–66–BR (Washington, D.C.: U.S. General Accounting Office, 1988).

37. B. Bruce Zellner, David K. Haugen, and Bryan Dowd, "A Study of Minnesota's High-Risk Health Insurance Pool," *Inquiry* 30 (1993): 170–179.

38. Trish Riley, "State Health Reform and the Role of 1115 Waivers," *Health Care Financing Review* 16 (1995): 139–149.

39. Kenneth Thorpe, "Expanding Employment-Based Health Insurance: Is Small Group Reform the Answer?" *Inquiry* 29 (1992): 128–136.

40. Chollet, Lamphere, and Lipson, *State Health Reform: Recent Public Sector Activity.*

41. Health Insurance Association of America, *Source Book of Health Insurance Data, 1991* (Washington, D.C.: Health Insurance Association of America, 1991), p. 27.

42. G. Kramon, "Small Business Is Overwhelmed by Health Costs," *New York Times* (October 1, 1989): 1, 19; and Small Business Administration, *The State of Small Business: A Report of the President* (Washington, D.C.: U.S. Government Printing Office, 1987).

43. Chollet, Lamphere, and Lipson, *State Health Reform: Recent Public Sector Activity.*

44. Estimate of HIPC enrollees who were previously uninsured from Debra J. Lipson and Jeanne De Sa, *The Health Insurance Plan of California: First Year Results of a Purchasing Cooperative* (Washington, D.C.: Alpha Center, 1995).

45. Milt Freudenheim, "States Shelving Ambitious Plans on Health Care," *New York Times* (July 2, 1995): 1, 14.

46. E. Richard Brown, *Medi-Cal Offsets Declining Private Job-Based Insurance Coverage*, Policy Brief, Los Angeles: UCLA Center for Health Policy Research, 1994.

47. Physician Payment Review Commission, *Annual Report to Congress* (Washington, D.C.: Physician Payment Review Commission), pp. 415–419; and Prospective Payment Assessment Commission, *Medicare and the American Health Care System: Report to the Congress* (Washington, D.C.: Prospective Payment Assessment Commission), pp. 95–119.

48. Freudenheim, "States Shelving Ambitious Plans on Health Care."
49. Deane Neubauer, "Hawaii: A Pioneer in Health System Reform," *Health Affairs* 12 (1993) 31–39.
50. Andrew Dick, "Will Employer Mandates Really Work? Another Look at Hawaii," *Health Affairs* 13 (1994): 343–349; William Glaser, "Employer Mandates: A Failed American Invention," *Health Affairs* 13 (1994): 229–230; and author's analysis of *March 1994 Current Population Survey.*

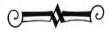

CHAPTER THREE

# MEASURING HEALTH CARE COSTS AND TRENDS

Thomas H. Rice

In 1996, U.S. health care expenditures are expected to eclipse the $1 trillion mark. It is difficult, however, to fathom such a large number. To put it in perspective, suppose that one lined up a trillion dollar bills end to end. They would stretch beyond the sun![1]

This chapter will focus on how these health care expenditures are measured, and then discuss their trends. Although data and measurement may seem a bit pedestrian to the analyst interested in proceeding quickly to policy issues, this is an unfortunate viewpoint. Accurate data on national health care spending are necessary in order to enact appropriate health policy reforms. (A more blunt reason for accurate data that may ring true to the policy analyst comes from computer programming: garbage in, garbage out.) Once these tools are in hand, Chapter Four will provide an analysis of alternative methods of containing health care expenditures.

## Measuring Health Care Expenditures

As just noted, an understanding of measurement issues is essential if one is to fully appreciate many issues that are currently in the forefront of health policy. To give one example, there continues to be a heated debate as to whether or not Canada has been more successful than the United States in controlling the growth of health care expenditures.[2] Resolution of this ostensibly straightforward issue would provide insights about the potential savings, if any, that could accrue from the adoption of a Canadian-style single-payer system in the United States. This section of the chapter discusses a number of key issues concerning the measurement of health care expenditures.

## Expenditures Versus Costs

Most policy discussions employ the term *costs* rather than *expenditures;* indeed, the next chapter will also adopt this convenience. It is important to understand that the two concepts are hardly the same.

Expenditures, of course, mean how much is spent on a particular thing. As discussed in Chapter Four, in a fee-for-service system, expenditures are simply the product of unit prices and the quantity of goods or services purchased. Total expenditures can then be broken down in a number of different ways, such as by type of service (such as hospital expenditures or physician expenditures) or by payer source (such as private insurers, Medicare, or out-of-pocket).

In contrast, costs apply to the production process. More specifically, the term refers to the value of resources used in producing a good or service. There are two distinct definitions of costs: accounting and economic. The *accounting* definition includes only the value of the resources used in production (labor, materials, and capital). The difference between the sales revenue from a good or service and accounting costs is defined as net revenues or profits. This differs from the *economic* definition of costs. To an economist, the term includes not only the value of resources expended in the production process but in addition a so-called normal return on investment.[3] Using their definition, economists predict that in a competitive market, profit levels will be near zero—that is, a typically efficient producer will garner only a normal rate of return on investment.[4] The persistence of economic profit levels far above zero over a long period of time may indicate the existence of market failure, which in turn might call for government policy interventions.

Accounting and economic profits are therefore related to each other. The latter are approximately equal to the former minus a normal rate of return on investment. But both these definitions of costs differ from the definition of expenditures. The distinction is shown in Figure 3.1; for simplicity, we will use the economic definition of costs and compare that to the definition of expenditures. In the figure, the horizontal axis shows the quantity of a particular good or service, and the vertical axis, sales prices and production costs. *MC* refers to marginal costs—the costs of producing the last unit of output; *AC* is average costs of output, and *price* is the selling price. Both of the cost curves include a normal rate of return on investment.

## FIGURE 3.1. DISTINCTION BETWEEN ACCOUNTING AND ECONOMIC PROFITS.

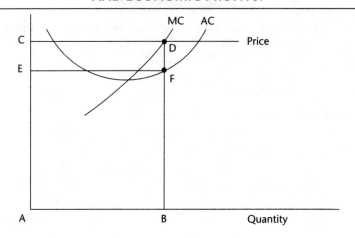

Health care *expenditures* are equal to the rectangle, ABCD, which is simply the selling price multiplied by the quantity sold, AB. In contrast, economic costs are shown by a smaller rectangle, ABEF; this is average costs (AE) multiplied by the quantity sold (AB). In this example, expenditures exceed cost by the rectangle CDEF. This implies that excess profits are being obtained by firms in the industry. Other firms may therefore be stimulated to enter the market in order to reap these profits, which in turn may drive down price and restore profit levels to a normal level. If this does not occur, then some form of government intervention may be necessary to correct market failure.

With these distinctions in mind, we can address the question of whether we should spend most of our efforts analyzing health care costs or expenditures. Although both are useful, analyses of the entire health care system turn out to be considerably easier to conduct using the concept of expenditures. This is because it is extremely difficult to obtain reliable data on costs; private firms are rarely expected to report their internal cost data to any sort of governmental body. One exception is Medicare hospital costs, because such data are collected by the federal government. But for other sectors, such as physician care or pharmaceuticals, and for services that are covered by private insurers rather than Medicare and Medicaid reliable data on costs are exceedingly difficult to obtain. The remainder of this chapter, then, will focus on measurement and trends in health care expenditures rather than costs. First, however, we will discuss measuring changes in unit prices.

## Measuring Health Care Prices

The most common measure of health care prices in the United States is the medical care component of the Consumer Price Index (CPI). The CPI, which is published monthly by the Bureau of Labor Statistics, provides information on the *changes* in the prices charged to urban consumers for a variety of consumer goods and services.[5]

To obtain the index, the CPI begins with a common market basket of goods and services. The monthly price data are obtained from urban localities that represent about 80 percent of the U.S. population.[6] To form the index, each item in the market basket is given a weight representing its relative importance in the spending patterns of urban consumers. An index is then formed that compares the change in prices in a current time period to a base period (usually 1982–1984) whose index value is set to a value of 100. For example, in 1993 the medical care component of the CPI had a value of 201.4, which means that medical care prices were slightly more than double what they were during the base period.

As shown later in the chapter when presenting the trends, the medical care component of the CPI is further subdivided into several categories, making it possible to monitor inflation in various health-related markets. The two main subcategories are medical care services and medical care commodities. Within services, there are separate indexes constructed for physician services, dental services, eye care, other medical professionals, hospital rooms, other inpatient services, and hospital outpatient services. Within commodities, separate indexes exist for prescription drugs, over-the-counter drugs and medical supplies, internal and respiratory over-the-counter drugs, and medical equipment and supplies.

There are a number of limitations to the CPI.[7] First, and perhaps most importantly, the CPI measures changes in prices, not in expenditures. It does not take into account changes in the quantity of services provided, only the price.

Second, the CPI measures changes in prices, not price levels. The index cannot be used to compare differences in health care prices between different parts of the country. Suppose, for example, that in 1993 the medical component of the CPI was 250 in New York City and 200 in Los Angeles. All that one could say is that prices rose faster in New York than Los Angeles since the base year in which the index was set to 100. It cannot be concluded that health care prices are lower in Los Angeles than New York (that may or may not be true).

Third, the CPI measures prices charged, not the prices received by producers. This is a critical distinction because of the prevalence of discounts offered by providers to managed care plans such as preferred provider organizations (PPOs). In some of the more competitive parts of the country, such as California, providers' list charges or billed charges are illusory; almost no one pays them. However, these prices are exactly what is measured by the CPI.[8] What this means is that the CPI might overstate the amount of medical care inflation in certain parts of the country because, over time, the true price of care has deviated further and further below the billed charge.

Fourth, the CPI measures changes in price for a *fixed market basket of consumer goods.* In fact, the entire notion of the CPI is based on the existence of such an apples-to-apples comparison. By using a standard market basket of goods, it is possible to determine how price alone has changed. But this also leads to two problems: people *do* change their consumption habits over time, so the market basket being measured by the CPI may become increasingly irrelevant, and the CPI does not take into account changes in the quality of goods and services produced. In that regard, increases in per diem hospital charges over the last twenty years are likely to be exaggerated by the CPI because much of the increase is due to enhancements in the types of services and facilities available to hospital patients.

Fifth, the CPI measures only changes in consumers' expenditures (premiums plus out-of-pocket payments). If, as in the case of hospital care, most expenditures are not paid out-of-pocket, then the index will not capture the majority of underlying inflation. This could bias the index figures because there has been a gradual movement away from out-of-pocket expenditures toward more employer and government payments, which are not included in the CPI.

The above caveats are not meant as criticisms; a differently configured index would raise a host of other problems. Rather, the limitations of the CPI must simply be understood when using the index.

## Measuring Expenditures

This section is divided into two parts: U.S. expenditures and international comparisons.

***U.S. Expenditures.*** There are many sources of data on U.S. health expenditures; space does not permit a separate discussion of each. Rather, we will focus on the primary source—the national health accounts produced by the Office of the Actuary of the Health Care Financing Administration (HCFA), which is housed in the U.S. Department of Health and Human Services. Trends in these data will be presented later in the chapter.

Data on U.S. national health expenditures are published regularly—usually on an annual basis—in the *Health Care Financing Review.*[9] The data for one year can be viewed best as a matrix. Each row of the matrix represents the group spending the money, whereas each column indicates the providers of services receiving the funds.[10] (An example will be presented later in Table 3.5.) A particular cell in the matrix therefore represents how much a particular type of payer (for example, private insurers) spends on a particular service (for example, hospital care).

Because these same data are compiled annually, by comparing the matrices of several years one can calculate the rate of change in expenditures in various components of the health care area.

When viewing the matrix, it might appear that the data come from a single, consistent source. They do not. Rather, literally dozens of sources are used to piece the matrices together. Some of the data are collected in a relatively systematic fashion, but others are not. For example, data from the Medicare program (one of the matrix rows) is systematically collected by HCFA through the Medicare Statistical System (MSS). One file in the MSS, the Hospital Insurance Claims File, contains information on each beneficiary's spending for Part A (hospital) services, while the Supplementary Medicare Insurance File includes similar data for Part B (primarily physician) services. Although somewhat more unwieldy, Medicaid data are also collected in a consistent format by HCFA from the states.

But because there are no national data collection requirements for private insurers, other aspects of the matrices have to be pieced together from multiple data sources. Some are more systematic than others, however. Hospital expenditures, for example, largely come from a single source: the American Hospital Association's annual survey of hospitals. But out-of-pocket expenditures come from any number of sources: a consumer expenditures survey conducted by the Bureau of Labor Statistics, periodic surveys of nursing homes conducted by the National Center for Health Statistics, surveys about home health care conducted by the Visiting Nurse Association, physician and dentist surveys conducted by the American Medical Association and the American Dental Association, data about outpatient clinic services collected by the Bureau of the Census, and information about community health centers collected by the Health Resources and Services Administration.[11] As discussed at the end of the chapter, the lack of a consistent data source may make it difficult to successfully administer certain types of health care reforms, such as national expenditure targets.

Over the years, there have been various revisions made to the national health accounts. The most noteworthy ones, which applied to the estimates beginning in 1988, employed new data sources and provided a greater level of data. An account of the changes made as well as a detailed discussion of the data sources that are currently being used can be found in the summer 1990 issue of the *Health Care Financing Review.*[12]

There are, nevertheless, a number of problems that still exist, most of which are caused by a lack of source data. Some of these are that:

• The accounts are unable to distinguish among some inpatient and outpatient expenditures (for example, care given by salaried physicians is counted as hospital rather than physician expenditures).

- Premium expenditures by consumers (such as Medicare Part B payments or private insurance premiums) are included as payments made by insurers rather than as out-of-pocket expenditures by consumers.
- Some capital expenditures are double-counted.

These and other issues, as well as recommendations for improving the accounts, are discussed in a report published by a HCFA technical advisory panel.[13]

***International Comparisons.*** The primary source of data on international health care spending for two dozen developed countries is collected by the Organization for Economic Cooperation and Development (OECD), which is based in Paris. These data are published in periodic articles published by *Health Affairs,* the *Health Care Financing Review,* and occasionally by other outlets.[14] Data from the OECD database will be presented later in the chapter.

The previous discussion about U.S. health expenditures focused on the lack of a consistent data source. As can be imagined, the lack of consistent data is an even greater problem when one is comparing data from two dozen countries. Those who compile the OECD data have attempted to make the data reliable by disseminating definitions of key terms as well as common accounting principles to all member countries. Nevertheless, one must use a great deal of caution in using the data because of differences in definitions, sources of data, and accuracy among the different countries.

Some of the areas of particular concern include the following:

- How different countries distinguish between health and social services.[15] Some countries, for example, may classify certain domiciliary care to the elderly as health while others might not.
- How countries distinguish between hospital and long-term care. In some countries, the distinction between the two is much finer than in the United States, with more long-term care being provided in hospitals.
- Accurately converting different currencies to a common unit. This is typically done through purchasing power parities, which are "indices that relate the prices of a market basket of goods in one country to the prices in a comparative group of countries."[16] For this reason, it is probably safer to rely on figures pertaining to the *proportion* of a country's national income devoted to health than to an absolute monetary amount.
- Underreporting of certain categories of expenditures by some countries, due in part to data limitations.

Schieber and Poullier, who have published the OECD data for many years, have responded to various criticisms of the data by noting, "These data have the advantage of being based on an internationally accepted functional classification; receiving direct comment and input from the statistical offices of the countries; and having methodology, sources, and underlying assumptions widely disseminated."[17]

# Trends in Health Care Expenditures

This section is divided into three parts: trends in prices, U.S. expenditures, and international expenditures.

## Prices

Table 3.1 presents the values for the major components of the CPI from 1975 to 1993, while Table 3.2 provides the corresponding annual rates of change.[18] Tables 3.3 and 3.4 present similar data for the items that make up the medical care component of the CPI.

Tables 3.1 and 3.2 show that since 1975, medical care prices have grown far faster than others in the U.S. economy. Between 1975 and 1993, they rose more than fourfold, whereas the index as a whole—and the other components listed—all increased by less than threefold. The pattern is even sharper in the eight-year period since 1985: medical prices rose by 77 percent, more than twice as fast as any other component.

Tables 3.3 and 3.4 show the patterns within the medical care sector. In general, the prices of medical care services grew more quickly than the prices of medical care commodities. The largest growth rate was for hospital rooms, which increased almost sixfold during the 1975–1993 period. As mentioned earlier, however, one should be skeptical about this number because the CPI does not do a good job of accounting for the changing nature of the hospital product.

## U.S. Expenditures

Table 3.5 provides 1993 data on U.S. health expenditures from the U.S. national health accounts. The rows provide information on the source of funds, while the columns indicate the provider of services that received the funds. Some noteworthy aspects of the data include the following:

- Government expenditures account for 43 percent of total health expenditures, three-fourths of which are federal.
- Although out-of-pocket costs constitute an average of 20 percent of total expenditures, this figure varies tremendously by type of service. The figure ranges

## TABLE 3.1. CONSUMER PRICE INDEX FOR ALL ITEMS: UNITED STATES, 1975–1993.

| | | | Consumer Price Index | | | |
|---|---|---|---|---|---|---|
| Year | All Items | Medical Care | Food | Apparel and Upkeep | Housing | Energy | Personal Care |
| 1975 | 53.8 | 47.5 | 59.8 | 72.5 | 50.7 | 42.1 | 57.9 |
| 1976 | 56.9 | 52.0 | 61.6 | 75.2 | 53.8 | 45.1 | 61.7 |
| 1977 | 60.2 | 57.0 | 65.6 | 78.6 | 57.4 | 49.4 | 65.7 |
| 1978 | 65.2 | 61.8 | 72.0 | 81.4 | 62.4 | 52.5 | 69.9 |
| 1979 | 72.6 | 67.5 | 79.9 | 84.9 | 70.1 | 65.7 | 75.2 |
| 1980 | 82.4 | 74.9 | 86.8 | 90.9 | 81.1 | 86.0 | 81.9 |
| 1981 | 90.9 | 82.9 | 93.6 | 95.3 | 90.4 | 97.7 | 89.1 |
| 1982 | 96.5 | 92.5 | 97.4 | 97.8 | 96.9 | 99.2 | 95.4 |
| 1983 | 99.6 | 100.6 | 99.4 | 100.2 | 99.5 | 99.9 | 100.3 |
| 1984 | 103.9 | 106.8 | 103.2 | 102.1 | 103.6 | 100.9 | 104.3 |
| 1985 | 107.6 | 113.5 | 105.6 | 105.0 | 107.7 | 101.6 | 108.3 |
| 1986 | 109.6 | 122.0 | 109.0 | 105.9 | 110.9 | 88.2 | 111.9 |
| 1987 | 113.6 | 130.1 | 113.5 | 110.6 | 114.2 | 88.6 | 115.1 |
| 1988 | 118.3 | 138.6 | 118.2 | 115.4 | 118.5 | 89.3 | 119.4 |
| 1989 | 124.0 | 149.3 | 125.1 | 118.6 | 123.0 | 94.3 | 125.0 |
| 1990 | 130.7 | 162.8 | 132.4 | 124.1 | 128.5 | 102.1 | 130.4 |
| 1991 | 136.2 | 177.0 | 136.3 | 128.7 | 133.6 | 102.5 | 134.9 |
| 1992 | 140.3 | 190.1 | 137.9 | 131.9 | 137.5 | 103.0 | 138.3 |
| 1993 | 144.5 | 201.4 | 140.9 | 133.7 | 141.2 | 104.2 | 141.5 |

*Source:* U.S. Department of Health and Human Services, Public Health Service, *Health United States, 1993,* DHHS Pub. No. (PHS) 94–1232 (Hyattsville, Md.: Public Health Service, May 1994), p. 221 (modified by author).

from only three percent for hospital care to over 60 percent for drugs and other nondurables.

• Private insurance pays a substantial proportion (over 35 percent) of expenditures for hospital, physician, dental, and other professional services but relatively little (less than 15 percent) for nursing homes, home health, and vision care.

More can be learned by examining trends in U.S. expenditures over time, which are shown in Table 3.6. Since 1975, annual rates of change in health ex-

## TABLE 3.2. ANNUAL CHANGE IN CONSUMER PRICE INDEX FOR ALL ITEMS: UNITED STATES, 1975–1993.

*Average Annual Percentage Change*

| Year | All Items | Medical Care | Food | Apparel and Upkeep | Housing | Energy | Personal Care |
|------|-----------|--------------|------|--------------------|---------|--------|----------------|
| 1975–1980 | 8.9 | 9.5 | 7.7 | 4.6 | 9.9 | 15.4 | 7.2 |
| 1975–1976 | 5.8 | 9.5 | 3.0 | 3.7 | 6.1 | 7.1 | 6.6 |
| 1976–1977 | 6.5 | 9.6 | 6.3 | 4.5 | 6.7 | 9.5 | 6.5 |
| 1977–1978 | 7.6 | 8.4 | 9.9 | 3.6 | 8.7 | 6.3 | 6.4 |
| 1978–1979 | 11.3 | 9.2 | 11.0 | 4.3 | 12.3 | 25.1 | 7.6 |
| 1979–1980 | 13.5 | 11.0 | 8.6 | 7.1 | 15.7 | 30.9 | 8.9 |
| 1980–1985 | 5.5 | 8.7 | 4.0 | 2.9 | 5.8 | 3.4 | 5.7 |
| 1980–1981 | 10.3 | 10.7 | 7.8 | 4.8 | 11.5 | 13.6 | 8.8 |
| 1981–1982 | 6.2 | 11.6 | 4.1 | 2.6 | 7.2 | 1.5 | 7.1 |
| 1982–1983 | 3.2 | 8.8 | 2.1 | 2.5 | 2.7 | 0.7 | 5.1 |
| 1983–1984 | 4.3 | 6.2 | 3.8 | 1.9 | 4.1 | 1.0 | 4.0 |
| 1984–1985 | 3.6 | 6.3 | 2.3 | 2.8 | 4.0 | 0.7 | 3.8 |
| 1985–1990 | 4.0 | 7.5 | 4.6 | 3.4 | 3.6 | 0.1 | 3.8 |
| 1985–1986 | 1.9 | 7.5 | 3.2 | 0.9 | 3.0 | −13.2 | 3.3 |
| 1986–1987 | 3.6 | 6.6 | 4.1 | 4.4 | 3.0 | 0.5 | 2.9 |
| 1987–1988 | 4.1 | 6.5 | 4.1 | 4.3 | 3.8 | 0.8 | 3.7 |
| 1988–1989 | 4.8 | 7.7 | 5.8 | 2.8 | 3.8 | 5.6 | 4.7 |
| 1989–1990 | 5.4 | 9.0 | 5.8 | 4.6 | 4.5 | 8.3 | 4.3 |
| 1990–1991 | 4.2 | 8.7 | 2.9 | 3.7 | 4.0 | 0.4 | 3.5 |
| 1991–1992 | 3.0 | 7.4 | 1.2 | 2.5 | 2.9 | 0.5 | 2.5 |
| 1992–1993 | 3.0 | 5.9 | 2.2 | 1.4 | 2.7 | 1.2 | 2.3 |

*Source:* U.S. Department of Health and Human Services, Public Health Service, *Health United States, 1993,* DHHS Pub. No. (PHS) 94–1232 (Hyattsville, Md.: Public Health Service, May 1994), p. 221 (modified by author).

penditures have typically just exceeded double-digit rates. The largest growth rates (not shown in table) were experienced by home health care, followed by other professional services; the smallest rates of growth were for research and construction.

Analysts have not stopped at analyzing past trends in expenditures; they have also used simulation models to project what expenditures will be in future years.[19] One set of projections was computed by the Congressional Budget Office (CBO). It concluded that, even adjusting for inflation, per capita health care expenditures

## TABLE 3.3. CONSUMER PRICE INDEX FOR ALL ITEMS AND FOR MEDICAL CARE COMPONENTS: UNITED STATES, SELECTED YEARS, 1975–1993.

| Item and Medical Care Component | Consumer Price Index | | | | | | |
|---|---|---|---|---|---|---|---|
| | 1975 | 1980 | 1985 | 1990 | 1991 | 1992 | 1993 |
| CPI, all items | 53.8 | 82.4 | 107.6 | 130.7 | 135.2 | 140.3 | 144.5 |
| Less medical care | 54.3 | 82.8 | 107.2 | 158.8 | 133.8 | 137.5 | 141.2 |
| CPI, all services | 48.0 | 77.9 | 109.9 | 139.2 | 146.3 | 152.0 | 157.9 |
| All medical care | 47.5 | 74.9 | 113.5 | 162.8 | 177.0 | 190.1 | 201.4 |
| Medical care services | 46.6 | 74.8 | 113.2 | 162.7 | 177.1 | 190.5 | 202.9 |
| Professional medical services | 50.8 | 77.9 | 113.5 | 156.1 | 165.7 | 175.8 | 184.7 |
| Physician services | 448.1 | 76.5 | 113.3 | 160.8 | 170.5 | 181.2 | 191.3 |
| Dental services | 53.2 | 78.9 | 114.2 | 155.8 | 167.4 | 178.7 | 188.1 |
| Eye care | — | — | — | 117.3 | 121.9 | 127.0 | 130.4 |
| Services by other medical professionals | — | — | — | 120.2 | 126.6 | 131.7 | 135.9 |
| Hospital and related services | — | 69.2 | 116.1 | 178.0 | 196.1 | 214.0 | 231.9 |
| Hospital rooms | 38.3 | 68.0 | 115.4 | 175.4 | 191.9 | 208.7 | 226.4 |
| Other inpatient services | — | — | — | 142.7 | 158.0 | 172.3 | 185.7 |
| Outpatient services | — | — | — | 138.7 | 153.4 | 1668.7 | 184.3 |
| Medical care commodities | 53.3 | 75.4 | 115.2 | 163.4 | 176.8 | 188.1 | 195.0 |
| Prescription drugs | 51.2 | 42.5 | 120.1 | 181.7 | 199.7 | 214.7 | 223.0 |
| Nonprescription drugs and medical supplies | — | — | — | 120.6 | 126.3 | 131.2 | 135.5 |
| Internal and respiratory over-the-counter drugs | 51.8 | 74.9 | 112.2 | 146.9 | 152.4 | 158.2 | 163.5 |
| Nonprescription medical equipment and supplies | — | 79.2 | 109.6 | 138.0 | 145.0 | 150.9 | 155.9 |

*Source:* U.S. Department of Health and Human Services, Public Health Service, *Health United States, 1993,* DHHS Pub. No. (PHS) 94–1232 (Hyattsville, Md.: Public Health Service, May 1994), p. 222 (modified by author).

## TABLE 3.4. AVERAGE ANNUAL CHANGE IN CONSUMER PRICE INDEX FOR ALL ITEMS AND FOR MEDICAL CARE COMPONENTS: UNITED STATES, SELECTED YEARS, 1975–1993.

| Item and Medical Care Component | *Average Annual Percentage Change* | | | | | |
|---|---|---|---|---|---|---|
| | *1975–80* | *1980–85* | *1985–90* | *1990–91* | *1991–92* | *1992–93* |
| CPI, all items | 8.9 | 5.5 | 4.0 | 4.2 | 3.0 | 3.0 |
| Less medical care | 8.8 | 5.3 | 3.7 | 3.9 | 2.8 | 2.7 |
| CPI, all services | 10.2 | 7.1 | 4.8 | 5.1 | 3.9 | 3.9 |
| All medical care | 9.5 | 8.7 | 7.5 | 8.7 | 7.4 | 5.9 |
| Medical care services | 9.9 | 8.6 | 7.5 | 8.9 | 7.6 | 6.5 |
| Professional medical services | 8.9 | 7.8 | 6.6 | 6.1 | 6.1 | 5.1 |
| Physician services | 9.7 | 8.2 | 7.3 | 6.0 | 6.3 | 5.6 |
| Dental services | 8.2 | 7.7 | 6.4 | 7.4 | 6.8 | 5.3 |
| Eye care | — | — | — | 3.9 | 4.2 | 2.7 |
| Services by other medical professionals | — | — | — | 5.3 | 4.0 | 3.2 |
| Hospital and related services | — | 10.9 | 8.9 | 10.2 | 9.1 | 8.4 |
| Hospital rooms | 12.2 | 1.2 | 8.7 | 9.4 | 8.8 | 8.5 |
| Other inpatient services | — | — | — | 10.7 | 9.1 | 7.8 |
| Outpatient services | — | — | — | 10.6 | 10.0 | 9.2 |
| Medical care commodities | 7.2 | 8.8 | 7.2 | 8.2 | 6.4 | 3.7 |
| Prescription drugs | 7.2 | 10.6 | 8.6 | 9.9 | 7.5 | 3.9 |
| Nonprescription drugs and medical supplies | — | — | — | 4.7 | 3.9 | 3.3 |
| Internal and respiratory over-the-counter drugs | 7.7 | 8.4 | 5.4 | 4.5 | 3.8 | 3.4 |
| Nonprescription medical equipment and supplies | — | 6.7 | 4.7 | 5.1 | 4.1 | 3.3 |

*Source:* Adapted from U.S. Department of Health and Human Services, Public Health Service, *Health United States, 1993,* DHHS Pub. No. (PHS) 94–1232 (Hyattsville, Md.: Public Health Service, May 1994), p. 222.

# TABLE 3.5. PERSONAL HEALTH CARE EXPENDITURES, BY TYPE OF EXPENDITURE AND SELECTED SOURCES OF PAYMENT, 1993.

| Source of Payment | Total | Hospital Care | Physician Service | Dental Service | Other Professional Services | Home Health Care | Drugs and Other Medical Nondurables | Vision Products and Other Medical Durables | Nursing Home Care | Other Personal Care |
|---|---|---|---|---|---|---|---|---|---|---|
| Personal health care expenditures | 782.5 | 326.6 | 171.2 | 37.4 | 51.2 | 20.8 | 75.0 | 12.6 | 69.6 | 18.2 |
| Out-of-pocket payments | 157.5 | 9.1 | 26.2 | 18.7 | 21.2 | 4.3 | 47.4 | 7.6 | 23.0 | 0.0 |
| Private health insurance | 258.0 | 117.8 | 84.1 | 16.8 | 15.8 | 2.5 | 18.4 | 0.9 | 1.7 | 0.0 |
| Other private | 30.0 | 16.8 | 2.7 | 0.2 | 3.6 | 2.5 | 0.0 | 0.0 | 1.3 | 2.8 |
| Government | 337.0 | 182.9 | 58.1 | 1.7 | 10.6 | 11.4 | 9.2 | 4.2 | 43.6 | 15.3 |
| Federal | 259.0 | 149.2 | 45.0 | 1.0 | 7.3 | 9.8 | 4.7 | 4.0 | 28.3 | 9.5 |
| State and local | 78.1 | 33.7 | 13.1 | 0.8 | 3.3 | 1.5 | 4.4 | 0.2 | 15.3 | 5.8 |

Note: Amounts in billions of dollars.

Note: 0.0 denotes amounts less than $50 million.

Source: Katherine R. Levit, Cathy A. Cowans, Helen G. Lazenby, et al., "National Health Spending Trends, 1960–1993," Health Affairs 13 (Winter 1994), p. 22. Reprinted by permission.

will rise by almost 70 percent between 1990 and the year 2000, at which point health expenditures will constitute 18 percent of gross domestic product (GDP). Although one might be skeptical of these predictions, anyone familiar with the health care reform debate of 1992–1994 will recall the power wielded by the CBO's estimates of the costs of alternative health care reform proposals.

One problem with projecting health expenditures into the future is that, over time, the estimates become increasingly farfetched. A recent analysis of these issues was recently conducted by Warshawsky. He concluded, "Even the most conservative projects, which assume either robust economic growth, improved demographic trends, or some moderation in health care price inflation, foresee the health care sector consuming more than a quarter of national output by [the year] 2065. If, on the other hand, current relative price trends continue, economic growth remains anemic, demographic trends continue or worsen, or the health care sector becomes a major user of capital, [simulation models] predict that health care expenditures will comprise *between a third to a half of national output.*"[20]

Aside from a number of technical assumptions, the problem with believing these projections is that they assume, on some level at least, a continuation of current expenditure trends. This is unlikely to be the case as health care continues to crowd out other expenditures. Nevertheless, the increasing ability of new medical technologies to improve people's health,[21] coupled with the inability of the

## TABLE 3.6. ANNUAL PERCENTAGE CHANGE IN NATIONAL HEALTH EXPENDITURES, BY SOURCE OF FUNDS: UNITED STATES, SELECTED YEARS, 1975–1993.

| Year | All Health Expenditures | Private Funds | Public Funds |
|------|------|------|------|
| 1975–1993 | 11.4 | 10.8 | 12.2 |
| 1975–1980 | 12.9 | 12.1 | 14.3 |
| 1980–1985 | 11.6 | 12.2 | 10.7 |
| 1985–1993 | 9.3 | 8.5 | 10.4 |
| 1985–1987 | 7.9 | 7.3 | 8.9 |
| 1987–1989 | 11.0 | 11.4 | 10.4 |
| 1989–1990 | 11.6 | 10.6 | 13.2 |
| 1990–1991 | 8.5 | 5.6 | 12.6 |
| 1991–1992 | 8.6 | 6.9 | 10.8 |
| 1992–1993 | 7.8 | 7.2 | 8.5 |

*Source:* Adapted from U.S. Department of Health and Human Services, Public Health Service, *Health United States, 1993,* DHHS Pub. No. (PHS) 94–1232 (Hyattsville, Md.: Public Health Service, May 1994), p. 223.

## TABLE 3.7. TOTAL HEALTH EXPENDITURES AS A PERCENTAGE OF GROSS DOMESTIC PRODUCT: OECD COUNTRIES, SELECTED YEARS, 1980–1992.

| Country | 1980 | 1985 | 1986 | 1987 | 1988 |
|---|---|---|---|---|---|
| Australia | 7.3 | 7.7 | 8.0 | 7.8 | 7.7 |
| Austria | 7.9 | 8.1 | 8.3 | 8.4 | 8.4 |
| Belgium | 6.6 | 7.4 | 7.7 | 7.7 | 7.7 |
| Canada | 7.4 | 8.5 | 8.8 | 8.9 | 8.8 |
| Denmark | 6.8 | 6.3 | 6.0 | 6.5 | 6.5 |
| Finland | 6.5 | 7.3 | 7.4 | 7.5 | 7.3 |
| France | 7.6 | 8.5 | 8.5 | 8.5 | 8.6 |
| Germany | 8.4 | 8.7 | 8.6 | 8.7 | 8.8 |
| Greece | 4.3 | 4.9 | 5.4 | 5.2 | 5.0 |
| Iceland | 6.4 | 7.0 | 7.8 | 7.9 | 8.5 |
| Ireland | 9.2 | 8.2 | 8.1 | 7.7 | 7.3 |
| Italy | 6.9 | 7.0 | 6.9 | 7.4 | 7.6 |
| Japan | 6.6 | 6.5 | 6.6 | 7.0 | 6.8 |
| Luxembourg | 6.8 | 6.8 | 6.7 | 7.3 | 7.2 |
| Netherlands | 8.0 | 8.0 | 8.1 | 8.3 | 8.2 |
| New Zealand | 7.0 | 6.5 | 6.7 | 7.0 | 7.1 |
| Norway | 6.6 | 6.4 | 7.1 | 7.4 | 7.7 |
| Portugal | 5.9 | 7.0 | 5.9 | 5.6 | 6.3 |
| Spain | 5.6 | 5.7 | 5.6 | 5.7 | 6.0 |
| Sweden | 9.4 | 8.9 | 8.6 | 8.6 | 8.6 |
| Switzerland | 7.3 | 8.1 | 8.1 | 8.3 | 8.4 |
| Turkey | 4.0 | 2.8 | 3.5 | 3.6 | 3.8 |
| United Kingdom | 5.8 | 6.0 | 6.1 | 3.4 | 6.1 |
| United States | 9.3 | 10.8 | 10.9 | 11.1 | 11.5 |
| OECD Average | 7.0% | 7.2% | 7.3% | 7.4% | 7.5% |

*Source:* George J. Schieber, Jean-Pierre Poullier, and Leslie M. Greenwald, "Health System Performance in OECD Countries, 1980–1992," *Health Affairs* 13 (Fall 1994), p. 101. Reprinted by permission.

| 1989 | 1990 | 1991 | 1992 | Growth Rate 1980–1992 | Growth Rate 1991–1992 |
|---|---|---|---|---|---|
| 7.8 | 8.2 | 8.5 | 8.8 | 1.6 | 3.5 |
| 8.5 | 8.4 | 8.6 | 8.8 | 0.9 | 2.3 |
| 7.6 | 7.6 | 87.1 | 8.2 | 1.8 | 1.2 |
| 9.0 | 9.4 | 10.0 | 10.3 | 2.8 | 3.0 |
| 6.5 | 6.3 | 6.6 | 6.5 | −0.4 | −1.5 |
| 7.4 | 8.0 | 9.1 | 9.4 | 3.1 | 3.3 |
| 8.7 | 8.9 | 9.1 | 9.4 | 1.8 | 3.3 |
| 8.3 | 8.3 | 8.4 | 8.7 | 0.3 | 3.6 |
| 5.1 | 5.3 | 5.3 | 5.4 | 1.9 | 1.9 |
| 8.5 | 8.2 | 8.4 | 8.5 | 2.4 | 1.2 |
| 6.9 | 7.0 | 7.4 | 7.1 | −2.1 | −4.1 |
| 7.6 | 8.1 | 8.4 | 8.5 | 1.8 | 1.2 |
| 6.7 | 6.6 | 6.7 | 6.9 | 0.4 | 3.0 |
| 6.9 | 7.2 | 7.3 | 7.4 | 0.7 | 1.4 |
| 8.1 | 8.2 | 8.4 | 8.6 | 0.6 | 2.4 |
| 7.2 | 7.3 | 7.7 | 7.7 | 0.6 | 0.0 |
| 7.4 | 7.5 | 8.0 | 8.3 | 1.9 | 3.8 |
| 5.4 | 5.4 | 5.9 | 6.0 | 0.1 | 1.7 |
| 6.3 | 6.6 | 6.5 | 7.0 | 1.9 | 7.7 |
| 8.6 | 8.6 | 8.5 | 7.9 | −1.4 | −7.1 |
| 8.4 | 8.4 | 9.0 | 9.3 | 22.0 | 3.3 |
| 3.9 | 4.0 | 4.7 | 4.1 | 0.2 | −12.8 |
| 6.0 | 6.2 | 6.6 | 7.1 | 1.7 | 7.6 |
| 11.9 | 12.6 | 13.2 | 13.6 | 3.2 | 3.0 |
| 7.4% | 7.6% | 7.9% | 8.1% | 1.2% | 1.4% |

U.S. Congress to approve health care reform containing strong cost control measures, provides credence to the belief that health expenditures will continue to grow rapidly in the years to come.

## International Expenditures

Table 3.7 shows total health expenditures as a percentage of GDP in OECD countries over the period 1980–1992. The 1992 figure for the United States, 13.6 percent, is considerably higher than the figure for any other country; only Canada also exceeded the 10 percent mark. The table also shows how these figures have grown; U.S. growth exceeded that of all other countries; the 3.2 percent annual rate was almost three times that of the typical country. Not shown in the table are per capita expenditures expressed in dollars. In 1992, the U.S. figure was about $3,100, a full 50 percent higher than the next highest figure (for Switzerland).[22]

# Future Issues

The major issue regarding measuring health care expenditures and their trends is the availability of accurate data. The United States does not have a system in place that allows it to compute expenditures for the entire health care sector in a consistent and timely fashion. Such a data set would be extremely beneficial and perhaps even essential for enacting certain types of health care reform.

The problem, in a nutshell, is this: the U.S. government does not require private insurers to collect and release data on expenditures. The availability of such data, if provided in a consistent format, would increase the country's flexibility to adopt various types of reform.

The next chapter discusses two kinds of reforms that are designed to control health expenditures: expenditure targets, which apply to a fee-for-service system, and premium caps, which pertain to capitated systems. Both systems would require timely data on health expenditures on a subnational (for example, statewide) basis for all payers. (The current dearth of statewide data is one important impediment to enacting major health care reforms.) Current data systems, however, would support the implementation of neither. In this regard, the Physician Payment Review Commission, in its 1994 Annual Report to Congress, recommended that premium caps should serve as only a "backup or standby approach to cost containment" until the necessary databases can be produced to support the implementation of such an approach to health care reform.[23]

# Notes

1. Dollar bills are six inches, or half a foot, long. Lining up one trillion of them would therefore stretch 500 billion feet, or over 94 million miles. The sun, by contrast, is *only* 93 million miles from earth.
2. See, for example, Robert G. Evans et al., "Controlling Health Expenditures—The Canadian Reality," *New England Journal of Medicine* 320 (March 2, 1989): 571–576; versus Judith Feder et al., "Canada's Health Care System," *New England Journal of Medicine* 317 (July 30, 1987): 320–325. Also see the debate between Morris Barer and his colleagues on the one hand and Edward Neuschler on the other in *Health Affairs* 20, 3 (Fall 1991).
3. Roger L. Miller and Roger E. Meiners, *Intermediate Microeconomics* (New York: McGraw-Hill, 1986), pp. 319–320.
4. There are other distinctions in the definitions of costs used by economists and accountants. Specifically, economic profits equal an organization's cash flow minus a normal rate of return on investment. For a discussion of these issues, see Paul J. Feldstein, *Health Care Economics* (New York: Wiley, 1988), pp. 451–455; and Richard A. Brealey and Stewart C. Myers, *Principles of Corporate Finance* (New York: McGraw-Hill, 1988), p. 264.
5. For more information on the index, including some important revisions made in 1977, see U.S. Department of Labor, Bureau of Labor Statistics, *Handbook of Methods*, BLS Bulletin No. 2285 (Washington, D.C.: U.S. Department of Labor, April 1988).
6. U.S. Department of Health and Human Services, *Health United States, 1993*, DHHS Pub. No. (PHS) 94–1232 (Hyattsville, Md.: U.S. Department of Health and Human Services, Public Health Service, May 1994), p. 273.
7. See Feldstein, *Health Care Economics,* pp. 55–64, for a thorough discussion of the issue.
8. Feldstein, *Health Care Economics,* pp. 59–60.
9. Suzanne W. Letsch, Helen C. Lazenby, Katharine R. Levit, and Cathy A. Cowans, "National Health Expenditures, 1991," *Health Care Financing Review* 14 (Winter 1992): 1–30.
10. Office of National Cost Estimates, "Revisions of the National Health Accounts and Methodology," *Health Care Financing Review* 11 (Summer 1990): 42–54.
11. Office of National Cost Estimates, "Revisions of the National Health Accounts and Methodology."
12. Office of National Cost Estimates, "Revisions of the National Health Accounts and Methodology."
13. Susan G. Haber and Joseph P. Newhouse, "Recent Revisions to and Recommendations for National Health Expenditures Accounting," *Health Care Financing Review* 13 (Fall 1991): 111–116.
14. George J. Schieber, Jean-Pierre Poullier, and Leslie M. Greenwald, "Health System Performance in OECD Countries, 1980–1992," *Health Affairs* 13 (Fall 1994): 100–112; George J. Schieber, Jean-Pierre Poullier, and Leslie M. Greenwald, "U.S. Health Expenditure Performance: An International Comparison and Data Update," *Health Care Financing Review* 13 (Summer 1992): 1–87.
15. George J. Schieber and Jean-Pierre Poullier, "International Health Spending: Issues and Trends," *Health Affairs* 10 (Spring 1991): 106–116.
16. Schieber and Poullier, "International Health Spending: Issues and Trends," p. 108.
17. Schieber and Poullier, "International Health Spending: Issues and Trends," p. 107.
18. The starting date of 1975 was chosen because it is well after the enactment of Medicare and Medicaid in 1965. Although price and expenditure data are available before these dates, trends would be colored by inclusion of these programs.

19. Two recent examples: Congressional Budget Office, "Projections of National Health Expenditures" (Washington, D.C.: Congressional Budget Office, October 1992); and Sally T. Sonnefeld, Daniel R. Waldo, Jeffrey A. Lemieux, and David R. McKusick, "Projections of National Health Expenditures Through the Year 2000," *Health Care Financing Review* 13 (Fall 1991): 1–27.

20. Mark J. Warshawsky, "Projections of Health Care Expenditures as a Share of the Gross Domestic Product: Actuarial and Macroeconomic Approaches," *Health Services Research* 29 (August 1994): 293–313, p. 311, emphasis added.

21. For a list and discussion of some of these recent technologies, see William B. Schwartz, "In the Pipeline: A Wave of Valuable Medical Technology," *Health Affairs* 13 (Summer 1994): 70–79.

22. Schieber, Poullier, and Greenwald, "Health System Performance in OECD Countries, 1980–1992."

23. Physician Payment Review Commission, *Annual Report to Congress* (Washington, D.C.: Physician Payment Review Commission, 1994), p. xliii.

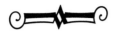

CHAPTER FOUR

# CONTAINING HEALTH CARE COSTS

Thomas H. Rice

The failure of the Clinton administration's health care reform plan and all competing proposals during the 103rd Congress suggests that the debate on how to best control growing health care costs in the United States will broaden. Once the Clinton plan was introduced, most discussion focused on whether premium caps were necessary to control costs or whether, alternatively, relying on managed competition would be sufficient. A host of other options, such as supply and technology controls, utilization review, the use of fee schedules, expenditure targets, and single- and all-payer systems, were put on the back burner.

Now that the reform debate—at least at the federal level—will be starting again almost from scratch, it is an opportune time to reconsider the many available options that attempt to control costs. This chapter is aimed at contributing to the continuing debate. It has three purposes: to provide a framework for assessing alternative cost containment strategies, to review previous research on the success and failure of these strategies, and to present directions for future research that may help clarify the most effective future cost containment options for the United States to pursue.

# Framework

Before embarking on an analysis of alternative cost containment strategies, it is useful to provide a framework that groups together similar strategies.[1] The framework developed here relies on two equations. Equation 1 applies to the fee-for-service system:

$$E = \sum_{j=1}^{J} (P_j \, Q_j)$$

Equation 2 applies to capitated systems:

$$E = \sum_{j=1}^{J} (C_j \, N_j)$$

In both equations:

$E =$ total health expenditures

$P =$ unit prices for services

$Q =$ quantity of services

$C =$ cost of services per person

$N =$ number of persons

$j \ =$ index representing each payer

Equation 1 states that total expenditures are equal to the product of the price of services and the quantity of services, summed over all payers. In other words, it is the sum of $P$ times $Q$ for Medicare, Medicaid, Blue Cross and Blue Shield, each private insurer, and so on. In contrast, Equation 2 is oriented toward the person, not the service. In this equation, total expenditures are simply the product of costs per person and the number of persons, again summed over all payers. Here, total expenditures would equal the number of Medicare beneficiaries times cost per beneficiary, plus the number of Blue Cross enrollees times the cost per enrollee, and so on.

The equations employ summation signs in order to illustrate the potential for cost shifting. To illustrate, suppose that one payer, Medicare, successfully controls both $P$ and $Q$. That clearly would result in lower Medicare costs but would not necessarily contain systemwide health care costs. This is because hospitals and physicians might respond to Medicare's controls by trying to increase their $P$s or $Q$s to the patients of other payers. The same thing could happen in relation to

Equation 2. A strong health alliance might cut a particularly good deal with a health maintenance organization (HMO), with the HMO responding by charging more to groups outside of the alliance.[2]

The framework provided simply defines the determinants of health expenditures; what may be hidden is how much the success of alternative cost containment strategies hinges on how they affect consumer and provider behavior. In Equation 1, for example, it might appear that a reasonable strategy for controlling expenditures would be to lower the prices of services paid to physicians. But this would not be successful if physicians responded to these price controls by inducing their patients to obtain more services (in which case, $P$ would go down, but $Q$ would go up).

The same is true of the capitation strategies related to Equation 2. The most obvious approach for controlling expenditures would appear to be to control costs per person. However, if this is accomplished by paying HMOs less, they may in turn respond by seeking to enroll only the healthiest people or by lowering the quality of care that they provide.

In analyzing cost containment strategies, then, we must be aware of the ability of providers (and others) to game the system to meet their own goals. Strategies that are difficult to game will tend to be the most successful ones. As an example, one could argue that some hospital rate-setting programs were moderately successful in containing costs because it was difficult for hospitals to game the system by increasing admission rates and length-of-stay; rather, the decisions were made by physicians rather than hospitals, and physician payment rates were not affected by the rate-setting programs. In contrast, certificate-of-need programs were less successful in controlling costs because hospitals were able to respond to restrictions on growth in the number of beds by increasing the purchase of equipment and engaging in other activities that were not regulated (or that were tolerated by the regulators). Thus, in the analysis of the cost-containment strategies, we will focus on how they influence provider and consumer behavior, which in turn will strongly influence their ultimate success or failure.

Before proceeding any further, one other caveat is necessary. This chapter focuses on ways of containing costs, but it must be remembered that cost containment is not society's only goal with regard to health services: access and quality of care also matter. Consequently, if analysts find that a particular strategy is effective in controlling costs, they must also consider any spillover effects—such as decreased quality—that may also result. Only by considering both benefits and costs can we make the best policy decisions for reforming our health care system.

## Analysis of Cost Containment Strategies

This section uses the framework presented above to review evidence regarding the cost containment potential of various fee-for-service and capitated cost containment strategies. Although it addresses over a dozen such strategies, there are still others that cannot be included due to space limitations.

### Fee-for-Service Options

Fee-for-service options[3] can be divided into three types, each corresponding to a term in Equation 1: $P$, $Q$, or $E$. The following discussion will be divided accordingly.

***Price Options.*** One type of cost containment strategy that has been attempted at various times in the United States is controlling the unit prices paid to providers. On the hospital side, examples include state hospital rate-setting programs and the use of diagnosis-related groups (DRGs). On the physician side, both the Medicare and Medicaid programs have, at various times, attempted to control their costs by freezing (or even lowering) physician payment rates. There is also some experience in this regard from Canada.

Before reviewing the available evidence, it is useful to outline the overall advantages and disadvantages of the price control options. There appear to be two possible advantages. First, controlling price typically involves less administrative effort (and expense) than controlling the quantity of services. Rather than examining the appropriateness of every provider and every service, it is only necessary to ensure that payment rates conform to regulated amounts. Second—and related to this—price regulation tends to be less intrusive; it does not entail the type of micromanagement often entailed in the quantity-related options discussed next.

There are some disadvantages, however. First, controlling price addresses only one component of total expenditures. As we shall see, price-based strategies can be circumvented if providers are able to increase the quantity of services they provide. Second, these strategies can diminish the efficiency of the market. If the wrong price is chosen, the wrong quantity or mix of services may be provided.

Several states adopted hospital rate-setting programs in the 1970s and 1980s. These programs varied on a number of dimensions, the most important of which were whether they were voluntary or mandatory and whether they applied to some or all payers. Most (but not all) were aimed at giving hospitals incentives to spend less by controlling hospital charges per day.

Of the twenty-five state-level programs that were in effect by the end of the 1970s, only eight were mandatory as opposed to voluntary, and only four—in Maryland, Massachusetts, New Jersey, and New York—applied to all payers.[4] Most research on the subject has found that it was these four programs that were most effective, with savings on the order of 10 to 15 percent.

It might seem surprising that a gross strategy like limiting hospital payments per day would work, but apparently it did. This is likely to have been the case because of the difficulty a hospital would have in gaming the system. If a hospital wanted to raise more revenue under an all-payer mandatory rate-setting program that set daily payment rates, it would have two choices: increase the number of admissions or increase length of stay. But neither of these options is typically available to hospitals because these decisions are made by physicians, whose fees were not subject to these controls. Consequently, as much as a hospital might have wished to raise more revenue, it might not have had the ability to do so.

The implementation of the Medicare DRG system made such gaming even more difficult (although it led to its own gaming, of course). Under the DRG system, hospitals are paid a fixed amount of money for a particular diagnosis, irrespective of how much is spent on treating a particular patient.[5] Hospitals therefore cannot benefit by trying to keep patients longer. One other avenue for garnering more revenue is to increase the number of admissions, but this has not happened for two reasons: the physician rather than the hospital makes the admission decision, and hospitals have found it profitable to treat patients on an outpatient basis, which is paid for separately, outside the DRG system.

There remain two other avenues for increasing revenues under DRGs: earning more from treating Medicare patients on an outpatient basis and shifting costs to other payers. Although Medicare outpatient costs have risen rapidly, this increase has not been sufficient to cut into Medicare savings very deeply.[6]

The same cannot be said about the shift to other payers. According to the Prospective Payment Assessment Commission (ProPAC), the congressional commission that studies hospital payment under Medicare, there has been a large increase in cost shifting to private payers since the enactment of DRGs.[7] The magnitude of cost shifting practice is shown in Table 4.1. In 1990, Medicare paid hospitals less than 90 percent of the costs associated with treating program patients, and Medicaid only 80 percent. In contrast, private insurers paid hospitals about 28 percent more for their patients' care than it actually cost to provide.

Because of cost shifting, a researcher from the Health Care Financing Administration has concluded that DRGs have done little if anything to control national health care spending.[8] This is not necessarily an indictment of DRGs, however. If other payers were to adopt DRGs, it is possible that systemwide hospital spending would be better controlled.

### TABLE 4.1. HOSPITAL PAYMENTS-TO-COST RATIOS, 1990.

|  | Payment-to-Cost Ratio (percent) | Payment Under or over Cost ($ billions) |
|---|---|---|
| **Below-cost payments** | | |
| Medicare | 89.6 | −8.2 |
| Medicaid | 80.1 | −4.6 |
| Uncompensated care | 21.0 | −9.6 |
| Total | | −22.4 |
| **Above-cost payments** | | |
| Private insurers | 127.6 | 22.5 |
| Other government payers | 106.4 | 0.2 |
| Total | | 22.7 |

*Source:* Prospective Payment Assessment Commission, *Optional Hospital Payment Rates, Congressional Report C-92–03* (Washington, D.C.: Prospective Payment Assessment Commission, 1992).

The above conclusions about the successes and failures of hospital price controls are further supported by the experience with physician controls. Most studies indicate limited cost savings when physician payments are frozen or reduced, because physicians respond by providing a greater quantity of services.[9] In making its projections about physician payment costs under the new Medicare Fee Schedule that was implemented starting in 1992, the Congressional Budget Office concluded that for every 1 percent reduction in physician fees, the volume of services would rise by 0.56 percent.[10]

Why might these physician controls be less effective than hospital controls? Because physicians have greater ability to game the payment system. If their payment rates drop, physicians can attempt to increase the volume of services they provide and may very well succeed. Hospitals do not tend to have this ability. Nevertheless, physicians' ability to generate additional billings is probably limited. This is illustrated by the experience of the Canadian provinces, which have tightly controlled physician fees since the early 1970s. Although the quantity of services provided has risen faster in Canada than in the United States over this time period, it was not nearly enough to compensate for the lower fees.[11] And in a country like the United States, where there are multiple payers, an effective way for a payer to control physician spending is to pay so little to doctors that they do not want to treat such patients. This, of course, is what has happened in many state Medicaid programs. Canadian provinces have not suffered from this problem because there is only one payer; the provinces are the only game in town.

***Quantity Options.*** The next group of fee-for-service cost containment strategies covers those aimed at service quantity or utilization. Examples include certificate-of-need programs, technology controls, utilization reviews, and practice guidelines (to name just a few). Their primary advantage over the price options is that they can focus on reducing the waste in the system. For example, if a particular procedure is inappropriate for a patient with a given diagnosis, quantity options can focus on that particular problem.

There are two disadvantages. Like the price options, quantity options target only one component of expenditures. If providers can game utilization controls by increasing prices, then the savings from these programs will be diminished. In addition, these strategies often are cumbersome from an administrative standpoint, involving much bureaucracy, paperwork, and undue oversight over the practice of medicine.

The earliest examples of quantity controls were certificate-of-need (CON) programs. These programs, which became commonplace in the early 1970s, were aimed at controlling expenditures by reducing the amount of hospital resources available—both beds and equipment. Typically, hospitals needed permission for proposed investments in excess of $100,000. Local boards, called health systems agencies, ruled on hospital requests for additional resources.

Many studies have been conducted on CON, and almost all reach the same conclusion: it did not succeed in saving money.[12] Although there was some effect on the number of hospital beds, capital equipment per bed rose even more quickly than before.[13] There are a number of reasons for this failure, but the fundamental one is this: the entities making the decisions on hospitals' applications—local health systems agencies and, ultimately, states—were not financially accountable for the increased costs associated with approving hospitals' requests. In other words, why turn a hospital request down when the costs would be borne by such payers as Medicare, Blue Cross, or commercial insurers? On the contrary, board members would have every incentive to approve requests by their local hospitals, since that would be viewed as helpful to their communities and constituencies.

This is not to say that technology controls cannot work—they probably can. But they need to be implemented on a broader geographical level by an entity that is at risk for additional health care spending. The Canadian provinces provide such an example.

Despite claims to the contrary, there is no single Canadian health care system. Rather, each province has its own, but each must conform to various federal requirements if it is to receive federal contributions. One of the key points, often overlooked in the literature, is that provinces are 100 percent at risk for additional health care spending because annual federal contributions are fixed. Unlike the U.S. Medicaid program, where the federal government at least matches additional state spending, provinces do not receive a penny more if they spend more on health care than anticipated.

Since provinces are also responsible for financing a host of other nonhealth programs, they must be judicious in allotting their tax revenues to health care. One way they have done this is by controlling the diffusion of medical technologies. If a hospital wants to expand or purchase equipment, it needs the province's permission, and provinces have not been eager to grant requests. As shown in Table 4.2, the United States has far more of most technologies than Canada, when measured on a per capita basis. Canadians often claim that they have achieved this by regionalizing their technologies, thereby making their system more efficient. Others contend, however, that the result is rationing. Indeed, evidence from a General Accounting Office study of Ontario shows that Canadians are subject to waiting lists for most kinds of elective surgery.[14]

Up to this point, the discussion of quantity has focused not on services but on hospital beds and technologies. Most recent efforts in the United States, however, have been aimed at particular services. Most commonly this is done through utilization review (UR). UR programs are usually implemented by third-party payers as a way to reduce the provision of unnecessary or inappropriate services. Examples include preadmission certification of hospital stays, concurrent and retrospective review of stays, management of high-cost patients, requiring second opinions before embarking on surgery, and profiling of physicians' practices.

Evidence so far indicates that some mild savings may be derived from these programs, particularly preadmission certification of hospital stays.[15] The evidence on other programs, particularly second opinions for surgery, is less optimistic.[16] One issue for those who are concerned about controlling future health care costs

### TABLE 4.2. AVAILABILITY OF SELECTED MEDICAL TECHNOLOGIES (UNITS PER MILLION PERSONS).

|                                         | Canada (1989) | United States (1987) |
| --------------------------------------- | ------------- | -------------------- |
| Open-heart surgery                      | 1.3           | 3.7                  |
| Cardiac catheterization                 | 2.8           | 6.4                  |
| Organ transplantation                   | 1.2           | 2.4                  |
| Radiation therapy                       | 4.8           | 10.3                 |
| Extracorporeal shock wave lithotripsy   | 0.5           | 1.9                  |
| Magnetic resonance imaging              | 1.1           | 11.2                 |

*Source:* Dale A. Rublee, "Medical Technology in Canada, Germany, and the United States: An Update," *Health Affairs* 13 (Fall 1994), p. 115.

is that UR programs are almost universal now, meaning that we may have already garnered about as much saving as can be extracted.

The wave of the future is now on developing UR for the outpatient setting, particularly through physician profiling. But the savings potential of these programs is still untested. There is strong reason to believe that UR for the outpatient setting will be much more difficult to implement, given the huge numbers of physicians and the difficulty in knowing whether a physician who is a high spender is less efficient or more profligate or, alternatively, has a more severely ill group of patients than his or her peers.

The most recent UR efforts have focused on developing practice guidelines. These are written protocols designed to instruct physicians on what procedures are appropriate for patients with particular diagnoses. The guidelines are largely being developed by researchers under the auspices of a federal agency, the Agency for Health Care Policy and Research, although some medical specialty groups are doing so as well. One intent of the guidelines is to increase quality by reducing the amount of regional variation in health care use. It has been widely documented that different parts of the country have very different surgery rates for certain procedures and that these differences cannot be readily explained by differences in patient health status.[17]

Development of practice guidelines is still in its infancy, so we cannot know the extent to which they can control costs. There is reason to be skeptical, however. Just as practice guidelines could reduce resource use by physicians who provide too many services, they could just as well *increase* spending by physicians who currently provide fewer services than are recommended by the guidelines. The issue, then, is whether the guidelines are likely to prescribe a quantity of services that is greater or less than what is currently being provided. A General Accounting Office study on treatment of cancer patients provides evidence that there are more physicians who are providing less treatment than is suggested by the guidelines. It concluded that "20 percent of those with Hodgkin's disease, 25 percent of those with one type of lung cancer, 60 percent of those with rectum cancer, 94 percent of colon cancer patients—did *not* receive what [the National Cancer Institute] considers state-of-the-art treatments. This is especially troubling in that all these treatments have been proven to extend patients' survival in controlled experiments, many of which were concluded 10 or more years ago."[18]

***Expenditure Options.*** The final group of fee-for-service options are those that directly target expenditures. Some examples include Medicare Volume Performance Standards, hospital global budgets, and national and subnational health budgeting. The overriding advantage of expenditure controls is somewhat tautological— they directly aim at controlling health care expenditures. (The extent to which they can succeed, however, depends in large measure on whether all health care spending is targeted, or just a component of total spending, such as hospital or physician expenditures.) The primary disadvantage is that the implementation of such controls may result in a less efficient health care system. A related disadvantage is that these controls could reduce the quality of services provided.

The primary example of expenditure controls in the United States is Medicare Volume Performance Standards (VPS). This system was part of the 1989 physician payment reforms adopted by Congress, reforms that also resulted in the new Medicare fee schedule based on resource-based relative values. Congress recognized that simply redistributing physician fees to provide higher payments to primary care physicians and lower payments to specialists, while more equitable, would not by itself control burgeoning program expenditures. That was left to the VPS system.

Under the system, each year Congress sets a target rate of increase in Medicare Part B physician expenditures. If actual spending increases exceed the target, the next year's physician fee update is normally reduced by that amount (although Congress can, of course, do whatever it wants when the time comes). Conversely, if the growth in spending is less than the target, physicians would get more. Suppose, for example, that the target for 1995 were a 10 percent increase in spending. If actual spending increased by 12 percent, the target would have been exceeded. Most likely, this would be extracted the next time Congress updated Medicare physician fees. If physicians were due a 5 percent cost-of-living increase, they would likely be granted only 3 percent.

The VPS system has been criticized as being too blunt an instrument to affect individual physicians' behavior. Because it applies nationally (with separate targets and fee updates only for surgery versus all other services), individual physicians who increased the volume of services they provided would not pay the price by experiencing a decline in their fees. This would only happen if all physicians behaved this way. But if some physicians do not increase their volume while other physicians do, then the first group would suffer—their volume $(Q)$ did not climb, but their fees $(P)$ will have fallen due to the behavior of other physicians. The VPS system may therefore contain a perverse incentive to increase the volume of services—which is exactly what it was supposed to prevent. (One way to improve the incentives would be to target smaller groups of physicians by having separate targets for each specialty, state, or state-specialty combination.[19])

Fortunately, this type of behavior does not appear to have become prevalent—the volume of services, by and large, has been approximately equal to the target, and surgeons have kept well below the target, which in turn has resulted in large fee increases for surgical procedures.[20] One possible explanation—which has not been confirmed by researchers—is that physicians could be moving more of their practices toward privately insured patients, because private insurer fees are far higher than Medicare's. In any case, since the VPS system is not broken, it is unlikely to be the subject of any fixes in the near term.

To find an example of expenditure controls applied to the hospital level, we must again look to Canada. In each of the provinces, hospitals are paid an annual global budget, which is negotiated by the provinces with each individual hospital. If a hospital exceeds its budget, there is no guarantee that it will be compensated.

Hospital global budgets seem to have worked in the sense that hospital spending in Canada has risen much less quickly than in the United States.[21] The primary way in which this has been achieved is that Canadian hospitals now have only about half as many nonphysician personnel as do their U.S. counterparts.[22] (Capital expenditures have also been controlled, but for different reasons—they are not included in the global budgets.) One perverse effect is that Canadian hospitals seem to prefer long-staying patients who might belong in nursing homes because these patients occupy a bed but use few other resources. Another fear is that the lack of resources is diminishing the quality of care in Canadian hospitals. What little available evidence there is, however, indicates that inpatient outcomes appear to be similar in the two countries.[23]

The two strategies just discussed, Medicare VPS and hospital global budgets, do not constitute comprehensive cost control policies because they are aimed at only one component of health care expenditures. A broader strategy might be to target all (or most) health expenditures at the same time, through a system of national or subnational (regional) budgeting. This section of the chapter focuses on fee-for-service strategies, whereas the next part examines premium controls, which would more logically be applied to capitated systems.

The typical way of controlling total expenditures in a fee-for-service system is through expenditure targets. Generally under such a system, unit prices are adjusted to ensure that expenditures meet targets. This differs from the VPS system in two primary ways: it applies to all payers, not just to Medicare, and it applies to most of the health care system, not just physician payment. Although we have the most experience—both domestic and international—with using expenditure targets for paying physicians, it could nevertheless be applied to other services, such as hospitalization. In such a case, DRG payments per admission could be tied to meeting a particular growth in inpatient expenditures.

The advantage of such a system, of course, is that it would control expenditures directly. There are several possible disadvantages, however: it might result in an inefficient use of resources, it could potentially harm quality, and it requires massive amounts of data in a timely fashion that currently are not being produced.

With regard to efficiency, in the long run, prices are based on the cost of producing a good or service in a competitive market. If prices are too high, then the incentive would be to overproduce the good; if they are too low, the incentive would be to underproduce. Under an expenditure target system, prices would change not due to demand and supply considerations but rather to how closely total expenditures conformed to a target. The good news is that prices would tend to fall when quantity got too high, so it might be argued that the system is self-correcting. The bad news is that there is no assurance that health care inputs would be used efficiently by producers when the market mechanism is circumvented. Even more troubling is the possibility that the mix of services produced would not be based on what consumers would like to buy.

This touches on the second potential problem—quality. Suppose that Congress set an austere budget level, necessitating a subsequent decline in unit prices. This might dissuade providers from delivering necessary services for fear that they would exceed the expenditure target, which in turn could result in diminished quality. Because adequate data systems do not yet exist for monitoring quality, there is a strong possibility that it would be sacrificed in favor of controlling expenditures.

Finally, there is the data problem. To make expenditure targets work, it is necessary to have up-to-date information about the quantity of services provided to all patients. It is through this information that total expenditures are tallied and updates are made to provider prices. In the United States, however, we have no formal mechanism for obtaining utilization and expenditure data on a timely basis for privately insured patients. It would take several years to develop such a system, and the process has not yet even started. Thus, the fee-for-service method that would have the greatest likelihood of controlling costs also perhaps suffers from the most shortcomings. This illustrates that there are indeed no easy answers for controlling costs under a fee-for-service system.

## Capitation Options

Equation 2 showed that three things are necessary for controlling expenditures under a capitated system: controlling costs per person $(C)$, the number of persons $(N)$, and the shifting of costs between payers. This section will focus on the first component; cost shifting has already been addressed, and controlling the number of persons (say, by denying eligibility for coverage), although clearly a cost containment strategy, is inconsistent with the notion of health care reform.

This section will address three overlapping strategies for controlling costs under a capitated system: HMOs, managed competition, and premium controls.

*HMOs.* Unlike many so-called competitive strategies, HMOs offer the United States an extensive experience base. They have been a part of the U.S. health care system for decades and have been growing so rapidly that about one-fifth of the insured non-elderly population are HMO members.[24] HMOs are given an incentive to control costs by the fact that they are paid on a capitation basis. That is, they receive a fixed payment (called prepayment) to provide an enrollee's care for a specific length of time, and this payment is unrelated to how much the HMO actually spends. Thus, if they spend less by being more efficient (for example, avoiding unnecessary hospitalization), then they get to keep more money. But how much they charge in premiums is kept in check by competitive pressures; if an HMO charges too much in premiums, fewer people are likely to enroll.

Much of the early evidence through the 1970s focused on group and staff model HMOs; it indicated that they could provide substantial savings—as much as 30 percent or 40 percent over fee-for-service.[25] Less evidence was available on independent practice associations, or IPAs, in which physicians continue to practice privately and see both HMO and non-HMO patients. More recent evidence, however, has seriously questioned whether HMOs (as presently structured) can achieve such a high level of savings.[26] There are two primary reasons to be skeptical of the applicability of early savings estimates to the present. First, most new HMO enrollment is in IPAs,[27] which have not yet demonstrated their cost containment potential (at least to most researchers). In IPAs, physicians are not subject to the corporate culture of large group-practice HMOs, and they are often paid on a modified fee-for-service basis. In group and staff model HMOs, there is often a strong corporate culture to conserve resources, and physicians are typically paid on a modified salary basis. Second, most current research studies have shown that HMO savings are partly attributable to favorable selection.[28] That is, healthier people are more likely to join HMOs, a circumstance partly responsible for HMO savings. In considering all of the literature, the Congressional Budget Office has concluded, "Compared with traditional (unmanaged) indemnity plans, CBO's most recent findings indicate that group/staff HMOs reduce use of services by 21.9 percent for privately insured patients, and IPAs reduce use by an average of 3.6 percent."[29]

Although such savings are significant, HMOs by themselves may not be sufficient to solve the health care cost problem. One reason is that they are subject to the same forces that raise the costs of fee-for-service medicine—overall growth in input costs, and the development and diffusion of expensive medical technologies. Even less evidence is available on how HMOs affect the quality of care provided. Although most early studies of HMO quality found it to be equal to or superior to that provided in the fee-for-service sector, some recent studies on the topic provide at least some cause for concern.[30] One significant finding from the RAND Health Insurance Study was that the people who did best in HMOs were those who were best off from a socioeconomic standpoint—perhaps because they were most able to effectively voice their concerns.[31]

*Managed Competition.*  Analysts have recognized for years that pure competition is unlikely to work very well in the health care sector. There are many reasons for this; two will be listed here. First, the market is a very complicated one, with people having relatively poor information about their alternative choices and about the implications (on their health and pocketbooks) of making these choices. A second is biased selection; insurers may compete on the basis of choosing the healthiest people, leaving sicker people with no source of insurance.

Advocates of managed competition believe that the marketplace can be trusted in the health care market so long as the players conform to certain rules.[32] To facilitate consumer understanding, health plans would be required to provide specific minimum benefits, or in some proposals, conform to standardized benefits. The latter would aid consumers in comparison shopping between alternative plans. Furthermore, certain practices on the part of insurers—"cherry picking" the healthiest people, charging unaffordably high premiums to unhealthy individuals and groups, and denying coverage for preexisting conditions—would be prohibited. And to make consumers think twice before purchasing extravagant insurance policies, employers could not pay more of the premiums for any such policies. Some proposals would also tax health plans that were more expensive than the cheapest approved plan in an area. All of this would be carried out through consortiums called health insurance purchasing cooperatives, or health alliances.

There is no way to know whether managed competition can succeed in controlling health care costs; it has never been tried on a widespread basis. The degree to which it works will depend on the answers to two broad questions: Are consumer insurance purchasing decisions sensitive to differences in premiums? and, Will health plans successfully exert pressure on providers to keep costs down?

In a previous article, I have argued that by itself, managed competition is unlikely to successfully control costs.[33] Three reasons were given. First, consumers may continue to join health plans with rich benefit packages. Estimates of the so-called elasticity of demand for insurance purchase are relatively low. Furthermore, the people most likely to respond are those who are relatively healthy. Those who are unhealthy are more attached to their providers and may not be very responsive to the price mechanism with regard to health plan choice.

Second, managed competition relies on HMOs to control costs, but it is not clear that large systemwide savings will occur even if more of the population joins up. The reasons for this were discussed above in the section on HMOs. And third, providers may continue to have strong bargaining power in their negotiations with health plans. This will be particularly true if health alliances do not include all or even most of the population in their geographic areas. (Under most health care reform proposals, only individuals and small businesses would be included in the alliances.) The reason that providers are likely to continue to have negotiating power is that they are swiftly merging with each other, in order to obtain countervailing market power. Simply put, the best way for providers to deal with a monopolist purchaser—the health alliances—is to become monopolistic themselves.

It is important to point out that other researchers would disagree with this analysis. Many point to the experience of the CalPERS program, a purchasing consortium of California public employers, which has been able to successfully control the premiums charged to members by competing health plans.[34] The competitive marketplace in California also provides evidence that competition may be successful in holding down cost increases. Zwanziger, Melnick, and Bamezai have shown that, as a percentage of per capita income, per capita hospital costs in California fell between 1982 and 1990, whereas they rose for the nation as a whole. This is attributed to increased competition brought about by selective contracting carried out by HMOs and PPOs.[35]

Thus, there is little agreement about whether relying on competitive health care reform solutions will succeed in controlling costs. Because of this doubt, many analysts, including those who framed the Clinton administration proposal, believe that to ensure cost control, it is necessary to couple managed competition with limits on insurance premiums;[36] this cost containment strategy is examined next.

***Premium Controls.*** After the employer mandate, perhaps the most contentious element of the health care reform debate in 1994 centered around the premium controls that were included in the Clinton administration proposal. Advocates contended that these controls were necessary because there was no assurance that the other elements of the proposal—which was loosely based on managed competition—would control health care costs. Detractors stated that enacting such controls would not only be unwieldy and unfair but would also stifle the exact type of product and managerial innovation that competition is supposed to foster.

The extent to which premium controls would succeed in containing overall health care costs depends, for the most part, on how broadly they are applied. Most proposals, including the Clinton administration's, controlled the total amount of premiums for benefits that were included in the standardized benefit package. Although this would include most health care costs, it would leave out two key components: spending on supplemental insurance plans that provide coverage for patient deductibles and coinsurance, and out-of-pocket costs for uncovered services.

A host of issues arise from the implementation of premium controls. One of the central ones concerns what is being targeted: premium levels, premium increases, or both. (The Clinton administration targeted both premium levels and increases). A troubling aspect of controlling the rate of increase in premiums is that it would penalize plans that come in with low bids initially and later need to raise them for whatever reason.[37] An even greater problem concerns how to allocate budgets across geographical areas. Ideally, one would prefer to have differences across geographic areas to reward areas that have been more successful in controlling costs, but it may be impossible to know whether a high-spending area is less efficient or just happens to have a sicker population. This, in turn, raises a fundamental implementation issue: Do we have sufficiently accurate data to allocate budgets across state or substate areas? In its 1994 report to Congress, the Physician Payment Review Commission said that we did not and that the implementation of premium controls should therefore wait until the necessary data systems are in place.[38]

## Future Research Issues in Cost Containment

Before addressing future research issues, it is necessary to ask a more basic question: Are health care costs in the United States too high? Unfortunately, it is impossible to know the answer to this question. To answer it, we would have to know the benefits (both tangible and intangible) that we derive from medical care services and compare them to the benefits and costs of alternative uses of our resources. The necessary information is not available to make such macro-level comparisons, and probably never will be.

There are, nevertheless, good reasons to continue the study of how to contain U.S. health care costs. First, the fact that other countries spend so much less raises the possibility that there may be effective cost control options available. Second, it is a truism that every dollar spent on health means that there is a dollar less to spend on other goods and services that the country and its citizens may want. The concern that health spending may be crowding out the purchase of other desirable things becomes even more acute as the proportion of national income devoted to health continues to move toward the 20 percent mark. Third, and related to this, there are strong reasons to believe that the availability of new and effective medical technologies (such as gene therapy) will result in even greater jumps in spending levels.[39] It would seem prudent that we understand what options are available to control these and other costs before health care spending absorbs too much more of national income.

If it is accepted that continued research on cost containment methods is appropriate, the next question is what areas of inquiry would be most fruitful. On the domestic front, there should be continued study of the effects of competition on health care costs. Different parts of the country are experimenting with different competitively driven cost containment strategies; research should continue on which of these approaches are most effective in controlling costs. In this regard, federally sanctioned state demonstration projects are extremely desirable because they allow researchers to assess whether particular methods work on a large-scale basis. In addition, research on particular components of competitive approaches (for example, risk-adjustment formulas and health alliances) should continue so that the tools are available to implement selective competitive reforms if there is a political will to do so.

Obviously, regulatory approaches should be studied as well. In this regard, premium caps and expenditure targets have received the most attention recently; again, state or other large-scale demonstration projects would provide much needed evidence of how well such approaches work in the United States. Nevertheless, some types of approaches (such as single-payer) would be difficult to test in the United States, even on a small scale. For that reason, more research on how other countries have implemented cost containment—and the effects of these approaches—is warranted. Of special note in this regard is how these countries are grappling with the rising costs associated with many new medical technologies.

With the creation of the Agency for Health Care Policy and Research in the Department of Health and Human Services in the late 1980s, there has been a movement toward more funded research in the areas of medical effectiveness and clinical outcomes. The infusion of more federal monies into this branch of health services research has, in most analysts' minds, been a good thing because of the dearth of available information on what medical interventions work the best. It is hoped, however, that this will not diminish the importance of general health services research, which seeks to address some of the larger concerns that have been addressed in this chapter.

## Notes

1. The framework presented in this chapter is new but draws on somewhat different ones that I have published previously. See Thomas Rice, "An Evaluation of Alternative Policies for Controlling Health Care Costs," in *Building Blocks for Change: How Health Care Reform Affects Our Future*, eds. Jack A. Meyer and Sharon Silow-Carroll (Washington, D.C.: Economic and Social Research Institute, 1993), pp. 19–41; and Thomas Rice, "Containing Health Care Costs in the United States," *Medical Care Review* 49 (Spring 1992): 19–65.

2. There is some evidence to indicate that this has happened in the California public employees' health benefits plan, CalPERS. See Service Employees International Union, *The CalPERS Experience and Managed Competition* (Washington, D.C.: Service Employees International Union, March 1993).

3. This discussion draws upon my previous work (see note 1).

4. John L. Ashby, Jr., "The Impact of Hospital Regulatory Programs on Per Capita Costs, Utilization, and Capital Investment," *Inquiry* 21 (Spring 1984): 45–59.

5. So-called outlier payments are made for patients who become much more expensive than the typical patient with that diagnosis. Even with the formula, hospitals still usually lose money on long-staying patients. Thus, there is little or no incentive on the part of the hospital to keep patients for a very long time just so that it can reap outlier payments.

6. George S. Chulis, "Assessing Medicare's Prospective Payment System for Hospitals," *Medical Care Review* 48 (Summer 1991): 167–206.

7. Prospective Payment Assessment Commission, *Optional Hospital Payment Rates, Congressional Report C–92–03* (Washington, D.C.: Prospective Payment Assessment Commission, 1992).

8. George S. Chulis, "Assessing Medicare's Prospective Payment System for Hospitals."

9. For a review of early evidence from several natural experiments, see Jon Gabel and Thomas Rice, "Reducing Public Expenditures for Physician Services: The Price of Paying Less," *Journal of Health, Politics, Policy, and Law* 9 (1985): 595–609.

10. Sandra Christensen, "Volume Responses to Exogenous Changes in Medicare's Payment Policies," *Health Services Research* 27 (April 1992): 65–79.

11. Morris L. Barer, Robert G. Evans, and Roberta J. Labelle, "Fee Controls as Cost Controls: Tales from the Frozen North," *Milbank Quarterly* 66 (1988): 1–64.

12. Bruce Steinwald and Frank A. Sloan, "Regulatory Approaches to Hospital Cost Containment: A Synthesis of the Empirical Evidence," in *A New Approach to the Economics of Health Care*, ed. Mancur Olson (Washington, D.C.: American Enterprise Institute for Public Policy Research, 1981), pp. 273–308.

13. Another effect was that hospitals increased the purchase of equipment that cost less than the CON threshold ($100,000), and sometimes split the costs of more expensive equipment in order to circumvent the regulations.

14. U.S. General Accounting Office, *Canadian Health Insurance: Lessons for the United States*, Pub. No. HRD–91–90 (Washington, D.C.: U.S. General Accounting Office, June 1991).

15. There is a perception among employees (or employee benefit managers) that management of high-cost patients can result in very large savings because only the most costly patients are targeted. See Jon Gabel, S. Fink, C. Lippert, et al., *Trends in Managed Care* (Washington, D.C.: Health Insurance Association of America, 1989). However, this has never been verified with claims data.

16. Phoebe A. Lindsey and Joseph P. Newhouse, "The Cost and Value of Second Surgical Opinion Programs: A Critical Review of the Literature," *Journal of Health, Politics, Policy, and Law* 15 (Fall 1990): 543–570.

17. This research was originally conducted by Dr. John Wennberg and his colleagues. For a review of the literature, see Pamela Paul-Shaheen, Jane Deane Clark, and Daniel Williams, "Small Area Analysis: A Review and Analysis of the North American Literature," *Journal of Health, Politics, Policy, and Law* 12 (Winter 1987): 741–809.

18. U.S. General Accounting Office, *Cancer Treatment, 1975–1985: The Use of Breakthrough Treatments for Seven Types of Cancer*, Pub. No. PEMD–88–12BR (Washington, D.C.: U.S. General Accounting Office, 1988), p. 4.

19. Thomas Rice and Jill Bernstein, "Volume Performance Standards: Can They Control Growth in Medicare Services?" *Milbank Quarterly* 68 (1990): 295–319; and M. Susan Marquis and Gerald F. Kominski, "Alternative Volume Performance Standards for Medicare Physicians' Services," *Milbank Quarterly* 72 (1994): 329–357.

20. Physician Payment Review Commission, *Annual Report to Congress* (Washington, D.C.: Physician Payment Review Commission, 1993), pp. 229–230.

21. Organization for Economic Cooperation and Development Secretariat, "Health Care Expenditure and Other Data," *Health Care Financing Review* 11 (1989 Annual Supplement): 111–194.

22. Joseph P. Newhouse, Gerard Anderson, and Leslie L. Roos, "Hospital Spending in the United States and Canada: A Comparison," *Health Affairs* 7 (Winter 1988): 6–24; and Allan A. Detsky, Sidney R. Stacey, and Claire Bombardier, "The Effectiveness of a Regulatory Strategy in Containing Hospital Costs: The Ontario Experience, 1967–1981," *New England Journal of Medicine* 309 (July 21, 1983): 151–159.

23. Leslie L. Roos, Elliott S. Fisher, Ruth Brazauskas, et al., "Health and Surgical Outcomes in Canada and the United States," *Health Affairs* 11 (Summer 1992): 56–72.

24. U.S. Department of Health and Human Services, *Health United States, 1993,* DHHS Pub. No. (PHS) 94–1232 (Hyattsville, Md.: U.S. Department of Health and Human Services, Public Health Service, May 1994).

25. Harold S. Luft, *Health Maintenance Organizations: Dimensions of Performance* (New York: Wiley, 1981); and Willard G. Manning, Arleen Leibowitz, George A. Goldberg, et al., "A Controlled Trial of the Effect of a Prepaid Group Practice on Use of Services," *New England Journal of Medicine* 310 (June 7, 1984): 1505–1410.

26. For a recent literature review and synthesis, see Robert H. Miller and Harold S. Luft, "Managed Care Plan Performance Since 1980," *Journal of the American Medical Association* 271 (May 18, 1994): 1512–1519.

27. Congressional Budget Office, *The Effects of Managed Care on Use and Cost of Health Services* (Washington, D.C.: Congressional Budget Office, 1992).

28. Miller and Luft, "Managed Care Plan Performance Since 1980."

29. Congressional Budget Office, *The Effects of Managed Care and Managed Competition* (Washington, D.C.: Congressional Budget Office, February 1995), p. 8.

30. See, for example, Haya R. Rubin, Barbara Gandek, William H. Rosers, et al., "Patients' Ratings of Outpatient Visits in Different Practice Settings," *JAMA* 270 (August 18, 1993): 835–840; Dolores G. Clement, Sheldon M. Retchin, Randall S. Brown, and MeriBeth H. Stegall, "Access and Outcomes of Elderly Patients Enrolled in Managed Care," *JAMA* 271 (May 18, 1994): 1487–1492; and Dana G. Safran, Alvin R. Tarlov, and William H. Rogers, "Primary Care Performance in Fee-for-Service and Prepaid Health Systems," *JAMA* 271 (May 25, 1994): 1579–1586.

31. John E. Ware, Jr., et al., "Comparison of Health Outcomes at a Health Maintenance Organization with Those of Fee-for-Service," *Lancet* (May 3, 1986): 1017–1022.

32. This is the theme of the writings of Professor Alain Enthoven. See, for example, Alain C. Enthoven, "The History and Principles of Managed Competition," *Health Affairs* 12 (1993 Supplement): 24–48.

33. Thomas Rice, E. Richard Brown, and Roberta Wyn, "Holes in the Jackson Hole Approach to Health Care Reform," *JAMA* 270 (September 15, 1993): 1357–1362.

34. U.S. General Accounting Office, *California Public Employees' Alliance Has Reduced Recent Premium Growth* (Washington, D.C.: U.S. General Accounting Office, November 1993).

35. Jack Zwanziger, Glenn A. Melnick, and Anil Bamezai, "Costs and Price Competition in California Hospitals," *Health Affairs* 13 (Fall 1994): 118–126.

36. See, for example, Paul Starr and Walter A. Zelman, "Bridge to Compromise: Competition Under a Budget," *Health Affairs* 12 (1993 Supplement): 7–23.

37. This would be especially problematic for plans that were burdened with an unfavorable (that is, sick) group of enrollees, particularly if there is not a sufficiently sensitive risk-

adjustment formula to account for differences in the health status of enrollees among alternative plans.

38. Physician Payment Review Commission, *Annual Report to Congress* (Washington, D.C.: Physician Payment Review Commission, 1994).

39. William B. Schwartz, "In the Pipeline: A Wave of Valuable Medical Technology," *Health Affairs* 13 (Summer 1994): 70–79.

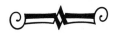

CHAPTER FIVE

# THE COST OF PHARMACEUTICALS

Stuart O. Schweitzer and William S. Comanor

The cost of pharmaceuticals has been a continuing issue in U.S. society and the subject of intense policy debates for over thirty years. In the late 1950s, the Kefauver committee of the U.S. Senate held a series of hearings that focused on the prices charged and the profits earned by leading pharmaceutical companies. At the heart of these debates was the question of whether drug prices were too high. To answer this question, the committee suggested that prices should be "appraised in the light of certain yardsticks or standards, principal among which are (i) unit production costs, (ii) prices in different markets (as in different countries), and (iii) profits."[1] The committee went further and proposed that "the most obvious, and in many ways the most satisfactory, standard in appraising the price of a given product is the relationship to price of unit direct costs, sometimes referred to as "production" or "manufacturing" costs."[2]

On these grounds, the committee concluded that the prices of many pharmaceuticals were excessive.

Many of these same concerns are raised today. For example, at 1993 hearings before the Senate Special Committee on Aging, Chairman David Pryor stated: "Millions of older Americans go to bed at night wondering if they will be able to afford their medications. . . . New drugs are selling in the United States at prices which are simply staggering. Unless I have read from the wrong economics textbook, this appears to be market failure at its worst. . . . Where the market has not, will not, or cannot work, we must take prudent actions to assure that drugs are priced reasonably."[3]

Despite major changes in the U.S. health care system since the 1950s, public discourse concerning the pharmaceutical industry has changed very little. The issue of pharmaceutical costs is of long standing. Our purpose here is to discuss this question and consider some possible answers.

Although aggregate expenditures on pharmaceuticals depend on both prices and quantities, there has been little discussion of the latter. Presumably, most critics consider quantities of prescribed pharmaceuticals to be medically determined, and direct their attention to the prices charged for these products. In our discussion of pharmaceutical policy, however, we consider quantities as well as prices.

First, we review trends in drug prices and expenditures in the United States and also compare U.S. drug prices to those in other countries. Next, we examine the intertemporal relationship between price increases and quality changes to determine whether pharmaceutical prices have increased after correcting for therapeutic improvements. Then we describe the factors affecting drug prices in the United States. Of particular importance here are the roles of therapeutic advance and competition. Finally, we discuss a series of policy options for containing pharmaceutical expenditures. Some of these are directed at consumers, some at physicians, and still others at manufacturers. Current efforts to control pharmaceutical costs are a blend of all three approaches.

## The Problem of Drug Expenditures

The expenditure shares of pharmaceuticals and other components of the U.S. health care system from 1960 through 1990 are shown in Figure 5.1. During this thirty-year period, the proportion of total health expenditures devoted to pharmaceuticals has actually declined. In 1990, pharmaceuticals' share was 8.2 percent—down nearly 50 percent from their 1960 share of over 15 percent.[4] Clearly, this decline in market share was not due to lower drug expenditures but rather to a far larger rise in expenditures on other health services.

The rates of price increase for the hospital, physician, dentist, and drug segments, as reported by the U.S. Bureau of Labor Statistics (BLS), are shown in Figure 5.2. While here we review the published figures, later we discuss questions concerning BLS measurement methods. The data in Figure 5.2 show that the reported rate of increase in pharmaceutical prices from 1960 to 1980 was substantially below that of the other components of the health care system and, indeed, was negative at the start of this period. Therefore, pharmaceutical price increases actually *moderated* the overall rate of increase of health care costs between

## FIGURE 5.1. PERSONAL HEALTH EXPENDITURES, 1960–1990.

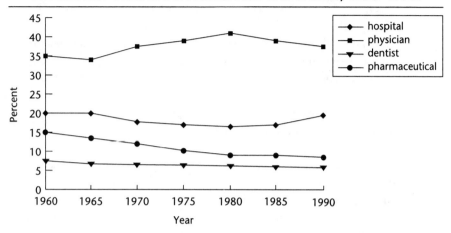

1960 and 1980. However, by 1980, the rate of price increase for pharmaceuticals accelerated and was as rapid as that for hospital services and higher than that of either physician or dental services. Still, the rate of pharmaceutical price increase never exceeded the rates of increase of the other components.[5]

If pharmaceuticals constitute only a small portion of overall health care expenditures, and if price increases have been relatively moderate for many years and no higher than those found in other sectors, what is the reason behind the

## FIGURE 5.2. ANNUAL RATE OF PRICE INCREASE BY SECTOR, 1960–1990.

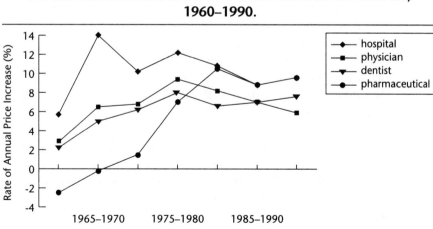

continued public and congressional concern with drug prices? One answer to this query is that the prices charged for pharmaceuticals are still much higher than production costs, so that it would be possible to reduce prices substantially and still cover these costs. To be sure, high pharmaceutical margins cover high research and marketing costs that accompany the continued introduction of new drugs. At the same time, these are costs that generally have already been paid, and consumers may not see a link between the purchased product and what they are asked to pay. Further obscuring this linkage is the apparent willingness of most pharmaceutical companies to sell the same or similar drugs at much lower prices.

Another reason for public concern with pharmaceutical prices lies in the fact that many insurance plans cover less than 100 percent of the charges for drugs. Although over four-fifths of health care costs in the United States are paid by government or private insurers, third-party coverage for pharmaceuticals has historically been lower than that of hospital and physician services. At the time of the Kefauver hearings, there was virtually no insurance coverage for drugs, and even as recently as 1986, patients paid directly for over 75 percent of their drug costs.[6]

Although insurance coverage for health care services has broadened in recent years, pharmaceutical coverage still lags behind the other segments of the medical care sector. In 1992, patients paid directly for 28 percent of their pharmaceutical expenses, but at the same time, the out-of-pocket shares of hospital and physician charges were only 5 and 18 percent, respectively.[7] The higher share of pharmaceutical expenditures paid directly implies that consumers are less sheltered from the burden of paying for drugs than from paying for other services, making pharmaceutical prices more visible to consumers.

International comparisons of drug prices have also contributed to public concern that drugs are overpriced in the United States. For example, the U.S. General Accounting Office (GAO) recently published studies comparing U.S. drug prices with those in the United Kingdom and Canada.[8] These reports indicate that prices for the same branded products are generally higher in the United States than elsewhere. Despite the criticism implicit in these results, the GAO studies are subject to conceptual and methodological problems that limit any conclusions to be drawn.

In the first place, these studies fail to account for generic substitution in any comprehensive way. Thus, while their comparison of relative prices for a particular branded drug may be correct, observed differences in the prices facing consumers are overstated to the extent that consumers substitute lower-priced generics for branded products more frequently in one country than in another. In fact, the use of generics is more widespread in the United States than elsewhere so that merely comparing the prices of specific branded products gives a misleading picture of the relative consumer costs of filling prescriptions.

For example, suppose that half of U.S. prescriptions for cimetidine are filled by the generic version, the price of which is $104 per hundred, while the price of the branded product, Tagamet, is $167. The average price is then $135.50. Suppose further that the price of Tagamet in Canada is $150, and the generic price is $100. But if the generic's market share is only 20 percent in Canada, the average price will be $140, which is higher than the average United States price, even though prices of the same products are lower in Canada.

A second problem with the GAO approach is that it relies on wholesale prices, which do not account for the many discounts and rebates present in the United States. Even if these prices accurately describe charges to individual pharmacies, they may not reflect transaction prices to other classes of buyers, who in fact constitute a substantial segment of demand. This factor is important to the extent that discounting is more widespread in the United States than in Britain or Canada. In that case, the observed relative cost of pharmaceuticals in the United States is biased upward. One implication of this is that manufacturer list prices are poor proxies for retail prices, so analyses of the cost of pharmaceuticals to consumers should focus on retail prices directly and not on published manufacturer prices.

Finally, the most serious problem with the GAO studies is their failure to deal with different drug consumption patterns in the three countries studied. Not only are drugs used differently in each country, but even the same drugs are taken in different forms and dosages.[9] The GAO approach sidestepped the entire question and considered a narrower question: Are wholesale prices higher in the United States than in Britain or Canada for the specific items that are major-selling U.S. drugs? Note that this approach may compare prices of highly popular U.S. products with those of less commonly used products in other countries.

In response to the GAO reports, Danzon carried out a more complete analysis of international drug price comparisons.[10] She includes all drugs sold in each of nine countries, incorporating over-the-counter drugs that substitute for prescribed drugs, and uses data on average transaction prices at the manufacturer level. She finds that price differences between countries depend greatly on the way in which the comparison is framed, particularly on which country's quantity weights are used to construct the price index. Comparisons also differ depending on whether one compares prices per gram of active ingredient or prices per *standard unit* (that is, per capsule or milliliter of liquid). Still, by most measures, average U.S. drug prices exceed those in most other countries; although for some products, U.S. prices are actually lower. However, there is no consistency in these results.

Before concluding this discussion of pharmaceutical prices, the important distinction between the prices set by pharmaceutical manufacturers and prices ultimately paid by consumers must be noted. The difference between these two prices is the distribution margin, which includes the costs and profits of both the dispensing pharmacy and the wholesaler, if one is involved in distributing the product. In many discussions of the cost of pharmaceuticals, there is the implicit assumption that distribution margins are constant across products so that whatever price is charged by the manufacturer is passed on to consumers, with merely a fixed amount added to cover distribution costs.

However, that picture is not generally accurate in the United States. Steiner, particularly, has pointed to "the inverse association between the margins of manufacturers and [those of] retailers."[11] His study provides empirical evidence on this relationship as well as the reasons for its presence. Salehi and Schweitzer[12] have found that the same relationship applies to pharmaceuticals. On the one hand, branded pharmaceuticals, which typically embody a high manufacturing margin, have lower distribution margins. On the other hand, generic products, with relatively low margins at the manufacturing stage, have much higher distribution margins. As a result, price differences between branded and generic products are greater at the manufacturing stage of production than at retail.

## Pharmaceutical Prices over Time

The problem of high pharmaceutical prices arises not only from high prices relative to production costs and the perception of high U.S. prices relative to those found elsewhere but also from recent rapid rates of price increase. In this section, we review the available evidence on the latter issue.

Measuring pharmaceutical price increases is a more complicated matter than appears on the surface. The BLS computes the overall Consumer Price Index (CPI) and its constituent parts as a Laspeyre index, which compares the cost of a given bundle of goods (often referred to as the market basket) purchased at current prices to the cost of that same quantity purchased at base-year prices.[13] Even then, however, the index must be adjusted when the composition of the market basket changes to reflect current expenditure patterns. With regard to health care, newer treatments for old problems, such as coronary artery disease or renal failure, have totally replaced techniques in use only a few years ago. And in many cases, there are new therapies available for problems that were previously untreatable. If new and improved drugs replace older ones but at a higher price, the appropriate price index should account for quality improvement as well as price increases. When the BLS fails to account adequately for quality improvement, measures of price changes are biased upward.

The method used by the BLS for measuring price changes is designed to track prices for a fixed market basket, or one that changes slowly. When items in the market basket change through shifts in consumer demand, the BLS uses a linking technique through which the price index of a new market basket replaces the index for an older one. For example, when a new product such as a more powerful antihypertensive drug replaces an established but less expensive one, price indexes with the old and the new product are each calculated, and the new index (with the higher-priced product) is scaled downward to equal the older one. The index including the new item then replaces the prior index in future calculations. No attempt is made to assess whether an improved drug is more or less expensive than would be justified by the quality change represented by its introduction. The price index merely tracks the prices of all items making up the market basket and then recalculates the price index when a new product is included.

Failure to capture the effect of quality change is especially serious for pharmaceuticals, where the turnover of products is rapid and new products frequently are improved versions of older ones but with greater efficacy, fewer side effects, or a more convenient regimen. The question of whether increases in drug prices exceed, fall behind, or accurately reflect quality changes is left unanswered.

A related problem arises because the BLS does not acknowledge that generic drugs represent products that are equivalent to established ones (as certified by the Food and Drug Administration) although offered at a much lower price. Because the BLS treats a generic drug as an entirely *different* product, requiring its own New Drug Application, its introduction is merely linked into the price index, thereby ignoring any price decline that follows from its introduction. Grilliches and Cockburn estimate that failure by the BLS to properly account for the introduction of generics led in one case to a reported price *increase* of 14 percent over a forty-five-month period, while the correct figure was a *decrease* of 48 percent.[14]

A third difficulty with the BLS index occurs because of the lag in including new drugs in the index, which is frequently four months or longer.[15] In introducing more imitative new drugs, firms often use a penetration strategy. A new drug is initially priced below existing products to penetrate the market and gain an increased market share, and only later is the price increased. If a new product is introduced into the price index only after a lag, the effect of the initially low price is missed and only the subsequent price *rise* is captured. Thus, the inability of the BLS index to account for the quality improvement of new drugs, its failure to acknowledge the price reductions associated with equivalent generic products, and the lag in incorporating new products all tend to overstate reported rates of change of drug prices.

## Determination of Drug Prices

While previous sections considered actual trends of pharmaceutical prices, we now turn to the causative factors that determine these prices. The research and development costs required to introduce a new drug are substantial—frequently in the hundreds of millions of dollars per drug. These costs include not only the direct costs of research and testing but also the time costs incurred while waiting for the FDA to approve a new product. But these outlays are typically made before a single prescription is filled. Therefore, they represent a classic example of sunk costs that do not vary with output. R&D costs, like those on fixed plant and equipment, have already been spent before the product is sold, so they cannot influence actual market prices. Whether these costs are high or low, the optimal prices charged by the manufacturing company in the short run are the same.

Similarly, most marketing costs are made in the early years of a product's life cycle and designed to introduce it to the medical community. Like research costs, they do not generally vary with output and therefore also represent fixed costs. As a result, the only variable costs in this industry lie at the manufacturing stage. For large, research-intensive companies, however, production costs may be only about 30 percent of the value of the product.[16] Marginal costs for most drugs are quite low and actually explain little about the prices charged.

Research and development, marketing, and manufacturing costs are all factors that reflect conditions on the supply side of the market. But as they are fixed and insensitive to the level of output, none of them has a major impact on pharmaceutical prices. Instead, prices depend predominantly on demand-side considerations. The prices charged for pharmaceuticals are determined largely by how valuable they are to consumers and what consumers are willing to pay for them. The critical factor is willingness to pay, which in turn depends on various considerations. In this section, we consider the relevant factors and review some available evidence on their importance.

### Therapeutic Advance

The demand-side factor most important in determining pharmaceutical prices is a product's therapeutic advance as compared with products already on the market. Doctors and patients are willing to pay larger amounts for medically improved products as compared to those without a substantial therapeutic advance. And with an increased willingness to pay, sellers can set higher prices without driving their customers away.

To explore the importance of this factor, one of the authors examined the price premium for new products as compared to their existing rivals.[17] The results

## TABLE 5.1. PRICES FOR NEW PHARMACEUTICALS RELATIVE TO EXISTING DRUGS.

| FDA Designation of Therapeutic Advance | Ratio of Median Prices of New Drug to Existing Drugs | |
|---|---|---|
| | Acute | Chronic |
| Important therapeutic advance | 2.97 | 2.29 |
| Modest therapeutic advance | 1.72 | 1.19 |
| Little or no therapeutic advance | 1.22 | 0.94 |

*Source:* John Z. Lu and William S. Comanor, "Strategic Pricing of New Pharmaceuticals," UCLA Research Program in Pharmaceutical Economics and Policy, Working Paper 95–1, February 15, 1995.

are given in Table 5.1 for new products used for both acute and chronic conditions.

These data show that the launch prices of drugs that embody an important therapeutic gain are priced about two and one-half times above those of existing substitutes. Drugs with moderate gains are priced about one and one-half times above, and products with little or no therapeutic advance are generally priced at or about the same level as existing products.

Not only do therapeutic improvements affect relative launch prices but they also influence the rate of price advance following introduction. One observes two distinct patterns of drug prices for new products. For some new products, prices at introduction are set above those of rival products, but these prices are held relatively constant over time. This is called a skimming strategy and is typically used for more innovative products. For other products, the initial price is set below those of competing products to gain market share, and then the price is raised over time. For the most part, sellers of largely imitative products follow a penetration strategy. Price levels for highly innovative products are generally fairly stable after introduction, although not so for more imitative products.

## Competitive Forces

When a new product is introduced, whether it embodies a small or large therapeutic advance, there are typically existing products used for the same or similar indications. These alternate products are those that physicians would prescribe in the absence of the new product and are thereby the rival products with which a new one must compete. Note that this concept of relevant market, resting on specific therapeutic indications, is far narrower than the conventional classification of a therapeutic category. Those classifications, such as antibiotics or hypertensives, are so broad that they include pharmaceuticals with very different indications, which do not actually compete with one another.

When there are alternative products available for the same or similar indications, prescribing physicians must select among rival drugs. Any price differences that may exist among these rivals have a material influence on doctors' and patients' willingness to pay for specific drugs. In this case, sellers can seek to increase sales by cutting prices, and the more rival products there are competing in a market, the more price cutting actually occurs. Lu and Comanor found that launch prices are substantially lower when there are more branded rivals in direct competition, and subsequent price changes are lower as well. Despite the common disdain of imitative products,[18] they play the essential role of promoting more competitive behavior and leading to lower final prices. New imitative products are an important competitive factor in the pharmaceutical marketplace.

Generic pharmaceuticals also have an important impact on price levels. Generic producers typically start production after the relevant patent has expired. They do so by gaining FDA approval of an Abbreviated New Drug Application that merely requires the demonstration of bioequivalence to the original product. Production costs of generic producers are frequently higher than those of the original producers, yet these manufacturers set prices generally much below those of the original seller, confirming our thesis that prices are set more by demand than cost considerations. The prices set by generic producers are also affected by the number of sellers. As their numbers increase, price competition becomes more vigorous, and prices decline below levels found when there is only a single entrant. A recent study of anti-infectives found that the largest price effects occurred when the fourth and fifth firms entered.[19] Average prices per prescription declined from nearly $30 with two or three sellers to roughly $17 with the presence of a fourth rival, and then to $9.25 when a fifth firm entered.

These reported declines in average prices took place despite the fact that prices charged for the original branded products typically *increase* when entry occurs.[20] The original manufacturers do not generally compete on the basis of price with generic entrants; they find it more profitable to concentrate on that segment of the market that includes brand-loyal customers. Such buyers are physicians and patients who know a particular brand and prefer it, so they continue to use it despite the presence of a lower-priced substitute. When generic manufacturers enter production, the price differential expands as the prices charged for the original branded products increase.

The entry of generic producers affects not only the prices charged by the original manufacturer for the same product but also the prices set for new products with the same or similar indications. Indeed, the introductory launch price of a new product is generally affected by the presence or absence of generic competition for substitute products. Again, rather than compete directly over price with generic producers, manufacturers typically cede that segment of the market to them and set higher prices to customers in the remaining segments. In effect, generic rivalry over substitute products leads to higher rather than lower launch prices and also to faster rather than slower rates of subsequent price increase. Generic competition is thus a two-edged sword, resulting in lower prices in some market segments but higher prices in others.

## Buyer Characteristics

Another major factor affecting consumers' willingness to pay for particular drugs is the mechanism by which payments are made. For uninsured patients who purchase pharmaceuticals much as they do other consumer goods, demand may be fairly price elastic. While the patient is limited to the prescribed product, he or she can sometimes influence prescribing decisions by calling attention to the prices of alternate products. Where generic versions of the drug are available, patients may also ask the pharmacist to substitute it for the branded product. And the patient always has the option of not filling the prescription, which occurs in a large number of cases.[21] For all of these reasons, producers may encounter substantial price resistance if they set prices much above anticipated values.

However, this resistance is attenuated when buyers have substantial insurance coverage. In that case, the out-of-pocket costs of prescribed pharmaceuticals may be minimal or quite low, and any economic reason to limit consumption removed. Demand conditions then depend on the conduct of managed care organizations and other third-party payers, and also on the nature of the contractual agreements that govern their payments.

Where payers simply agree to cover the pharmaceutical costs of insured patients, perhaps with a deductible and coinsurance provision, demand may become rather price inelastic. Judgments as to what products are prescribed are made exclusively by physicians whose decisions may depend on marketing and other idiosyncratic factors and who are not likely to be constrained by their patients' economic circumstances. And the more inelastic is consumer demand, the higher product prices will be. Increased insurance coverage of pharmaceuticals would then lead directly to higher prices.

However, there are other circumstances where expanded insurance coverage may lead to more elastic demand conditions; these circumstances involve a shift from patient-driven to payer-driven competition.[22] The central factor here is the conduct of third-party payers. When insurance companies and HMOs institute formularies, which are restrictive lists of approved products, and indicate to both doctors and patients that they will pay only for those drugs, they gain a direct influence on prescribing decisions. Furthermore, the drug's price can be a major determinant of whether or not it is included in the formulary. In these circumstances, pharmaceutical coverage will lead to more rather than less elastic demands. Of critical importance is whether third-party payers can affect prescribing decisions.

Where generic products are available in the market, the conduct of third-party payers can affect prices even without influencing prescribing decisions. That is because pharmacists can substitute generics for prescribed branded drugs, and patients can be encouraged through various incentives to buy generics. In these circumstances, the price elasticity of demand for branded drugs will increase (in absolute value) and the affected producers will respond by setting lower prices. While there are few empirical studies that explore these factors, we know that the structure of demand conditions for pharmaceuticals is not a simple matter and depends on the complex relationships among patients, physicians, and third-party payers. Depending on the behavior of all of these parties, demand elasticities are determined, and so are prices set in the marketplace.

Before concluding this section, we note that insurance coverage for prescription drugs has been steadily increasing, so there is an increasing distinction between patient costs and prices. Furthermore, there has been a general shift from overall deductibles to fixed co-payments, which implies improved insurance coverage. These factors suggest that demand conditions in pharmaceutical markets will increasingly depend on the conduct of managed care providers and other third-party payers. And the prices that are set will depend largely on what commitments are made by these payers to offer drugs to their subscribers.

## Differential Pricing

Where prices depend on demand conditions, and also where there are clear distinctions among types of buyers, we expect to find different prices charged to different buyers. The economist's model of price discrimination provides a clear description of this process and indicates that prices will depend primarily on the relevant price elasticities of demand. Where these elasticities differ among classes of consumers, final prices will differ as well. There is considerable evidence that this pattern is pervasive throughout the pharmaceutical industry.

While pharmaceutical companies establish a list price for each drug, many sales are made by discounting that price, and these discounts can be substantial. A survey of drug prices in one area found that the average price charged for a selection of well-known products sold to hospitals was only 19 percent of that charged to a local pharmacy.[23] Since hospital demands for specific products are likely to be more elastic than those of individual pharmacies, who must stock a large number of products to fill individual prescriptions, hospital prices will be much lower than those charged to pharmacies. Where prices are demand driven, differences in demand elasticities are reflected in differences in actual prices.

These discounts may also differ between individual and chain store pharmacies and between hospitals and HMOs. A critical fact about the pharmaceutical industry is that there is no single price for an individual product even at a specific point in time; prices depend on the demand conditions presented by particular buyers.

When generic products enter the marketplace, they typically appeal more to some buyers than to others. In particular, HMOs and hospital pharmacies are more likely to use generic products, as they have the knowledge and expertise required to evaluate them, in contrast to individual physicians. One expects therefore that generic rivals will make greater sales to some buyers than to others. That being so, original producers will respond to generic competition more strongly in some market segments than in others. By setting much lower prices where generic competition exists, but keeping prices at their original levels or even higher where generic competition is less important, the original sellers of many products have been able to maintain a large proportion of their original sales without substantially depressing revenues.

The evidence that major pharmaceutical firms have pursued this type of strategy is that they have generally maintained market shares following patent expiration and generic entry. By the sixth year after patent expiration, average market shares for thirty-five products between 1984 and 1987 were fully 62 percent in physical units and 85 percent in dollar sales as compared to their previous levels.[24] The strategy of charging lower prices where they face strenuous competition but setting higher prices where they do not has been used by many companies to maintain sales and market shares. Once again, buyers' willingness to pay is the critical factor that determines pharmaceutical prices.

## Approaches for Containing Pharmaceutical Costs

While pharmaceutical companies have sought to maintain or expand revenues, health care providers have looked for methods to limit drug expenditures and control costs. Some approaches have attempted to reduce the quantity of drugs provided but most have looked for means to lower the prices paid for specific products or to redirect patients toward lower-priced alternatives. These methods can be divided into those focused on consumer behavior, physician prescribing patterns, and manufacturer actions. At this point, we review some measures that have been used.

Consumer behavior can be altered through economic incentives or education. Economic incentives typically involve cost sharing, through which patients bear more of the financial consequences of their actions by paying a larger share of drug costs. As the cost of drugs to consumers increases, it is presumed that the quantity purchased will decline, with patients either going without the prescribed drugs or shifting to less expensive alternatives such as generic products or over-the-counter options.

Cost sharing is sometimes criticized as being an overly blunt instrument, that is, as discouraging the use of necessary as well as unnecessary therapies. The RAND Health Insurance Study examined the effect of cost sharing on the consumption of prescribed drugs. Leibowitz and her colleagues reported that pharmaceutical expenditures by individuals without cost sharing were as much as 60 percent higher than for those with cost sharing.[25] The findings were similar for patients at a large HMO, although at a smaller magnitude.[26] A cost-sharing requirement of $1.50 per prescription reduced the number of prescriptions filled by 10.7 percent, and doubling the co-payment led to an additional 10.6 percent reduction in the number of filled prescriptions. Furthermore, the authors found that consumers were more likely to reduce consumption of discretionary rather than essential drugs in response to increased cost sharing. These findings are tempered, however, by their observation that the cost per prescription rose in response to higher cost sharing. This change may have occurred because consumers purchased a greater quantity of drug per prescription, as their cost is related to the prescription rather than the quantity of product actually purchased.

An alternative to economic incentives in dealing with consumer behavior is patient education. An example of this type of program is informing patients that generic drugs are equivalent to branded products, thereby lowering costs. Another is explaining to patients that the extensive use of certain drugs, such as antibiotics, is unnecessary and may even be harmful, thereby lowering the quantity purchased. While such programs can reduce consumer demand for specific products, they are unlikely to limit the aggregate demand for pharmaceuticals to a substantial extent. Many patients still expect a prescription at the conclusion of a physician visit, and physicians respond accordingly.

Despite the presence of consumer-oriented programs, most efforts at cost containment for pharmaceuticals are directed at those who make decisions on drug therapies: physicians, hospitals, and managed care providers. Because physicians, particularly those in private practice, have few incentives to limit pharmaceutical costs, apart from satisfying their patients, physician-directed policies are not very different from those aimed at consumers. When financial constraints are removed from patients, they are also removed from their physicians.

However, physicians are also the subject of education programs that seek to improve the quality of prescribing and reduce overall drug expenditures. These programs are present especially in HMOs or other managed care programs and have great potential because the pace of new drug introductions is rapid and physicians have difficulty keeping abreast of new therapeutic options. Without such programs, the primary means that physicians have to learn about new products is from pharmaceutical company marketing efforts, which are designed to increase rather than reduce spending on pharmaceuticals.

Even if physicians have few incentives to restrain costs, that is not so for organizations that actually pay for pharmaceuticals. Hospitals, HMOs, and government reimbursement plans have long adopted formularies designed explicitly to restrict the drug choices available to physicians. By specifying reimbursable drugs within a particular class, payers seek to reduce costs. These lists of approved drugs depend in principle on the relative cost and effectiveness of alternative products. Generic versions of drugs are generally favored, and newer, more expensive drugs are often excluded.[27] While nearly all formulary programs permit exceptions, the burden of obtaining an exemption is often great enough to discourage a physician from doing so unless he or she feels that a nonlisted drug is absolutely necessary.

Formularies, however, have the potential for increasing rather than decreasing health care costs if they are so restrictive that patients are prescribed less effective drugs. Even expensive drugs are generally less costly than physician visits or hospital episodes, so using suboptimal drugs may be penny-wise but pound-foolish. The question of whether or not a formulary lowers or raises drug or overall health care costs depends on the relative prices of the drugs included and excluded from the formulary, the number of patients who use the more expensive product when it is not necessary, and the treatment ramifications for patients who are switched to a less expensive drug when they need the more expensive one. Sloan, Gordon, and Cocks found that limiting the number of drugs through a formulary appeared to have been a very good idea for gastrointestinal disease patients and for those with asthma, but a bad one for coronary disease patients.[28] In the latter case, total medical costs actually increased with the adoption of the formulary. Other studies have also shown that Medicaid formularies are not effective in either lowering drug expenditures or reducing overall health care costs.[29] Apparently, formularies have not been able to discourage consumption of expensive drugs whose use is unnecessary while allowing such use when appropriate.

A more direct approach toward cost containment is the exercise of payer's monopsony power to limit the prices charged by pharmaceutical manufacturers for their specific health programs. Such actions are frequently adopted by governments that provide coverage for pharmaceuticals in their national programs. Increasingly, foreign governments or insurance funds have sought to reduce drug prices as a means of cost control. In most countries, the question is not whether to fix prices, but how to do so, and in particular, how to set prices without removing the incentive to develop new and improved pharmaceuticals. A typical response is to permit a product's use and reimburse its costs in accord with its relative therapeutic benefits. Note that this objective leads ideally to the same prices as those set in a competitive market. Regulatory objectives are thereby similar to those enforced by competitive markets.

Australia has progressed further than other countries in attempting to calculate the cost effectiveness of new drugs and set reimbursement prices accordingly.[30] Canada uses this model at the national level as well. Britain, however, incorporates the profitability of the pharmaceutical company into its calculation of the National Health Service price for new products.

Similarly, managed care programs in the United States affect the prices they pay for pharmaceuticals purchased on behalf of their patients. For this reason, pharmaceutical manufacturers now provide managed care plans with studies of the cost-effectiveness of new products while at the same time demonstrating clinical effectiveness and safety for the FDA. As a result of their actions, managed care programs typically pay less for pharmaceuticals than do individual patients.

The most serious question raised in any discussion of drug cost containment is whether success can be achieved without sacrificing the vitality and viability of the industry, whose hallmark is a large investment in R&D for new products. If cost containment is pursued too severely, will that effort diminish the returns from innovation such that lower spending levels on research and development will ensue? Or are returns already sufficiently high that little will be lost? While we acknowledge that some trade-off exists between cost containment and research spending, we know little about the terms of this trade-off and therefore little about how much reduced spending on pharmaceuticals might occur. More research is needed before we can reach a firm conclusion on this matter.

## Conclusions and Directions for Future Research

Our picture of drug price control is a mixed one. The share of health expenditures devoted to pharmaceuticals is relatively low, and there is a history of moderate price increases—though with some acceleration in recent years. Furthermore, there have been rapid changes recently in the market for drugs, with increasing importance for provider-driven rather than patient-driven competition. These changes will have a growing impact on both average rates of price increase and patterns of price dispersion for pharmaceuticals. The increasing Balkanization of pharmaceutical markets also means that average price levels will convey less and less information about what is actually taking place. Not only are traditional measures of price changes inadequate, tending to inflate reported rates of increase, but also international comparisons yield inconclusive results.

A critical policy issue for the cost of pharmaceuticals is whether uniform pharmaceutical prices should be mandated for different classes of customers. If this type of proposal were enacted, either through legislation or judicial decisions, pricing practices would change sharply. Berndt has pointed out that under these conditions the vigor of competition in many pharmaceutical markets would diminish sharply, and we could expect higher overall prices.[31] That type of policy change would increase the cost of pharmaceuticals.

This overview of the major factors determining the cost of pharmaceuticals illustrates three important areas where additional information would assist policy analysts. The first is the need to improve understanding of the relationship between drug prices and quality levels. Preliminary data show that prices are positively affected by a drug's therapeutic advance—but the extent of this relationship is not well studied. This question is especially important because of our present inability to account for quality improvement in measures of pharmaceutical price increases.

Second, we know little about how quality levels of drugs are determined. Until recently, the FDA assigned a three-level quality improvement score to each drug for which marketing approval was sought. That designation was crude at best and sometimes contradicted by the marketplace. However, the FDA currently does not provide even these designations, and there is no agreed-upon measure of the extent of therapeutic improvement in new drugs.

And third, we need a better understanding of the degree of competition in pharmaceutical markets. That factor is especially critical for we are now observing another wave of consolidation in this industry. A better understanding of the appropriate breadth of pharmaceutical markets is needed. How much rivalry is there within therapeutic categories? Across therapeutic categories? An understanding of how pharmaceutical markets are structured and interact is essential to creating appropriate public policy for this industry.

## Notes

1. United States Senate, *Administered Prices Drugs: Report of the Committee on the Judiciary, United States Senate, Made by Its Subcommittee on Antitrust and Monopoly* (Washington, D.C.: U.S. Government Printing Office, 1961), p. 6.

2. United States Senate, *Administered Prices Drugs,* p. 6.

3. United States Senate, *Hearings Before the Special Committee on Aging,* November 16, 1993 (Washington, D.C.: U.S. Government Printing Office, 1994), pp. 3–4.

4. U.S. Department of Health and Human Services, *Health United States, 1992* (Washington, D.C.: U.S. Government Printing Office, 1993).

5. U.S. Department of Health and Human Services, *Health United States, 1992.*

6. Health Insurance Institute of America, *Source Book of Health Insurance Data, 1989* (Washington, D.C.: Health Insurance Institute of America, 1989).

7. Health Insurance Institute of America, *Source Book of Health Insurance Data, 1993* (Washington, D.C.: Health Insurance Institute of America, 1993).

8. U.S. General Accounting Office, *Prescription Drugs: Companies Typically Charge More in the United States Than in Canada,* GAO/HRD–92–110 (Washington, D.C.: U.S. General Accounting Office, September 30, 1992); and U.S. General Accounting Office, *Prescription Drugs: Companies Typically Charge More in the United States Than in the United Kingdom,* GAO/HEHS–94–29 (Washington, D.C.: U.S. General Accounting Office, January 12, 1994).

9. Lynn Payer, *Medicine and Culture: Varieties of Treatment in the United States, England, West Germany, and France* (New York: Viking Penguin, 1988).

10. Patricia Danzon, "International Drug Price Comparisons: Uses and Abuses," University of Pennsylvania, unpublished manuscript presented to the American Enterprise Institute Conference on Competitive Strategies in the Pharmaceutical Industry, October 27–28, 1993.

11. Robert L. Steiner, "The Inverse Association Between the Margins of Manufacturers and Retailers," *Review of Industrial Organization* 8 (December 1993): 717–740, see p. 717.

12. H. Salehi and S. Schweitzer, "Economic Aspects of Drug Substitution," *Health Care Financing Review* 6, 5 (Spring, 1985): 59–68.

13. Paul J. Feldstein, *Health Care Economics,* 4th ed. (Albany, N.Y.: Delmar, 1993).

14. Zvi Grilliches and Iain Cockburn, "Generics and New Goods in Pharmaceutical Price Indexes," *American Economic Review* 84, 5 (December 1994): 1213–1232.

15. Grilliches and Cockburn, "Generics and New Goods."

16. William S. Comanor and Stuart O. Schweitzer, "Pharmaceuticals," in *Structure of American Industry,* 9th ed., eds. Walter Adams and James W. Brock (Englewood Cliffs, N.J.: Prentice Hall, 1994), p. 179.

17. John Z. Lu and William S. Comanor, "Strategic Pricing of New Pharmaceuticals," UCLA Research Program in Pharmaceutical Economics and Policy, working paper 95–1, February 15, 1995.

18. David A. Kessler, Janet L. Rose, Robert J. Temple, et al., "Therapeutic Class Wars— Drug Promotion in a Competitive Marketplace," *New England Journal of Medicine* 331 (November 17, 1994): 1350–1353.

19. Steven N. Wiggins and Robert Maness, "Price Competition in Pharmaceutical Markets," unpublished paper, October 1993, p. 5.

20. Richard Frank and David Salkever, "Pricing Patent Loss and the Market for Pharmaceuticals," *Southern Economic Journal* 50 (October 1992): 165–179.

21. J. K. Cooper, D. W. Love, and P. R. Raffoul, "Intentional Prescription Nonadherence (Noncompliance) by the Elderly," *American Geriatrics Society* 30 (1982): 329; and L. T. Clark, "Improving Compliance and Increasing Control of Hypertension: Needs of Special Hypertensive Populations," *American Heart Journal* 121 (1991): 664.

22. David Dranove, Mark Shanley, and William D. White, "Price and Concentration in Hospital Markets: The Switch from Patient-Driven to Payer-Driven Competition," *Journal of Law and Economics* 36 (April 1993): 179–204.

23. *Los Angeles Times* (January 30, 1994).

24. Office of Technology Assessment, *Pharmaceutical R&D: Costs, Risks and Rewards*, OTA–H–522 (Washington, D.C.: U.S. Government Printing Office, February 1993).

25. A. Leibowitz, W. G. Manning, and J. P. Newhouse, "The Demand for Prescription Drugs as a Function of Cost-Sharing," *Social Science and Medicine* 21 (1985): 1063.

26. B. L. Harris, A. Stergachis, and L. D. Ried, "The Effect of Drug Co-Payments on Utilization and Cost of Pharmaceuticals in a Health Maintenance Organization," *Medical Care* 28, 10 (1990): 907–917.

27. H. G. Grabowski, S. O. Schweitzer, and S. R. Shiota, "The Medicaid Drug Lag: Adoption of New Drugs by State Medicaid Formularies," *Pharmacoeconomics* 1, Supplement (1992): 32–40.

28. F. A. Sloan, G. S. Gordon, and D. L. Cocks, "Do Hospital Drug Formularies Reduce Spending on Hospital Services?" *Medical Care* 31, 10 (October 1993): 851–867.

29. See S. O. Schweitzer and S. R. Shiota, "Access and Cost Implications of State Limitations on Medicaid Reimbursement for Pharmaceuticals," *Annual Review of Public Health* 13 (1992): 399–410; and William J. Moore and Robert J. Newman, "Drug Formulary Restrictions as a Cost-Containment Policy in Medicaid Programs," *Journal of Law and Economics* 36 (April 1993): 71–97.

30. Office of Technology Assessment, *Pharmaceutical R&D*.

31. Ernst R. Berndt, *Uniform Pharmaceutical Pricing: An Economic Analysis* (Washington, D.C.: American Enterprise Institute, 1994).

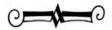

# CHAPTER SIX

# MEASURING OUTCOMES AND HEALTH-RELATED QUALITY OF LIFE

Patricia A. Ganz and Mark S. Litwin

In his 1988 Shattuck lecture, Paul Ellwood set the stage for the inclusion of patient-perceived outcomes in the evaluation of health care delivery. In discussion of the destabilizing effects of the restructuring of the health care system in the 1970s, he notes, "The health care system has become an organism guided by misguided choices; it is unstable, confused, and desperately in need of a central nervous system that can help it cope with the complexities of modern medicine. The problem is our inability to measure and understand the effect of the choices of patients, payors, managers, and physicians on the patient's aspirations for a better quality of life."[1] Further, he advocates use of a technology of patient experience, drawing on a common patient-understood language of health outcomes. He proposes, "Outcomes management would draw on four already rapidly maturing techniques. First, it would place greater reliance on standards and guidelines that physicians can use in selecting appropriate interventions. Second, it would routinely and systematically measure the functioning and well-being of patients, along with disease-specific clinical outcomes, at appropriate time intervals. Third, it would pool clinical and outcome data on a massive scale. Fourth, it would analyze and disseminate results from the segment of the data base most appropriate to the concerns of each decision maker."[2]

Later, Ellwood goes on to say, "The centerpiece and unifying ingredient of outcomes management is the tracking and measurement of function and well-being or quality of life. Although this sounds like a hopelessly optimistic undertaking, I believe that we already have the ability to obtain crucial, reliable data on quality of life at minimal cost and inconvenience."[3]

Ellwood's support for the active inclusion of quality-of-life data as a key component of outcomes management provides important support for the advancement of this field; however, more than six years later, this form of outcome assessment is still in its infancy. Despite its appeal, quality-of-life data must be collected prospectively and cannot be retrieved from administrative databases that are commonly used by health services researchers. During the past decade, patient-rated assessments of health-related quality of life have been included more frequently in research and clinical settings, and we are now on the verge of seeing some results.

## Defining and Measuring Quality of Life

Great energy has traditionally been spent by clinicians and other health care professionals attempting to lengthen the duration of survival in patients with various chronic diseases.[4] During the last few decades, dramatic advances in diagnosis, management, and the overall understanding of the mechanisms of human disease have refined the treatment approaches to many medical conditions so that patients are now living longer with their diseases. This is particularly true in oncology, where certain patients live for years after their initial diagnosis.[5]

Historically, evaluation of the success of medical therapies has focused on specific clinical parameters and survival. However the recent surge of interest in more patient-centered endpoints has generated great support for the medical outcomes movement. Not only clinicians but also payers and managers have become interested in assessing outcomes in order to begin to measure quality of care. Indeed, some would argue that the thrust of the outcomes movement comes largely from outside the biomedical establishment as clinicians are held more and more accountable to external authorities. To understand better how medical outcomes fit into the framework of health services research, it is necessary to focus on the assessment of quality of care.

In the well-known Donabedian model,[6] health care quality is examined in three parts: structure, process, and outcomes of care. *Structure of care* refers to how medical and other services are organized in a particular institution or delivery system. It may include such variables as specialty mix in a multiphysician medical group, access to timely radiological files in a hospital, availability of pharmacy services in a hospice program, or convenience of parking at an outpatient surgery center. It may also involve factors such as nonmedical support services like coordination of care, social work, home care, daily assistance for the disabled, or clothing and housing for the socially disadvantaged. *Process of care* refers to the content of the medical and psychological interactions between patient and provider. It may include variables such as whether or not a blood culture is ordered for a baby with a fever, the nature of the treatment prescribed for a patient with abdominal pain, how much compassion a doctor demonstrates when presenting a negative diagnosis to a patient, how many times a psychologist interrupts a client during a session, or whether a nurse regularly turns a bedridden patient to prevent bedsores. *Outcomes of care* refer to specific indicators of what happens to the patient once care has been rendered. These may include clinical variables, such as blood sugar levels in a diabetic, blood pressure measurements in a hypertensive, abnormal chest x-rays during treatment for pneumonia, kidney function after transplantation, or pain after treatment for cancer. They may also include complications of treatment, such as bleeding after colonoscopic biopsies, allergic reactions to antibiotics or iodinated contrast material injections, graft occlusion after cardiac bypass surgery, infant mortality following emergency cesarean delivery, or hospital death rates.

Besides the Donabedian variables, medical outcomes researchers often study health-related quality of life (HRQL). The general concept of quality of life encompasses a wide range of human experience, including access to the daily necessities of life such as food and shelter, intrapersonal and interpersonal responses to life events, and activities associated with professional fulfillment and personal happiness.[7] A subcomponent of overall quality of life relates to health, and HRQL focuses on the patient's own perception of health and the ability to function as a result of health status or disease experience. The World Health Organization defines health as a state of complete physical, mental, and social well-being and not merely the absence of disease.[8] Because disease may affect both quantity and quality of life, the various components of well-being must be addressed when treating patients. Figure 6.1 presents a framework described by Patrick and Bergner for the theoretical relationships among HRQL concepts, disease, the environment and prognosis.

While quantity of life is relatively easy to assess as survival or disease-free interval (measured in days, months, or years), the measurement of quality of life presents more challenges, primarily because it is less familiar to most clinicians and researchers. Proper measurement of such variables is often quite costly. To quantify what is essentially a subjective or qualitative phenomenon, the principles of psychometric test theory are applied.[9] This discipline provides the theoretical underpinnings for the science of survey research. Typically HRQL data are collected with self-administered questionnaires, called instruments. These instruments contain questions, or items, that are organized into scales. Each scale measures a

## FIGURE 6.1. CONCEPTUALIZATION OF HRQL.

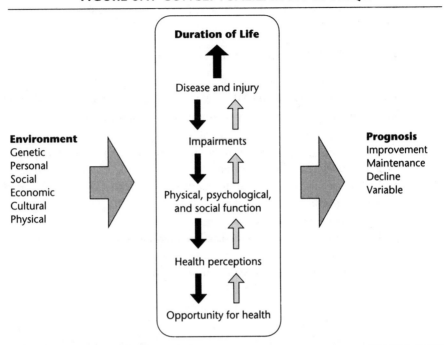

*Source:* Adapted from D. Patrick and M. Bergner, "Measurement of Health Status in the 1990s," *Annual Review of Public Health* 11 (1990), p. 174.

different aspect, or domain, of HRQL. Some scales comprise dozens of items, while others may include only one or two items.

HRQL instruments may be general or disease specific. General HRQL domains address the essential or common components of overall well-being, while disease-specific domains focus on the impact of particular organic dysfunctions that affect HRQL.[10] Generic HRQL instruments typically address general health perceptions, sense of overall well-being, and function in the physical, emotional, and social domains. Disease-specific HRQL instruments focus on special or more directly relevant domains, such as anxiety about cancer recurrence, dizziness from antihypertensive medications, or suicidal thoughts during depression therapy.

There are many available HRQL instruments. Many psychologists, sociologists, and statisticians devote their entire professional careers to the activity of developing and validating these instruments. At least one medical journal, *Quality of Life Research,* is dedicated exclusively to presenting this research. Hence, an abundance of literature exists on general HRQL, and a significant body of work has been published on HRQL in patients with various conditions.[11]

## Approaches to the Measurement of HRQL

The Southwest Oncology Group (SWOG) has described six principles for HRQL research in cancer clinical trials, and these principles can be applied to other clinical or research settings. They recommend the following:[12]

- Always measure physical functioning, emotional functioning, symptoms, and global quality of life separately.
- Include measures of social functioning and additional protocol-specific measures if resources permit.
- Use patient-based questionnaires.
- Use categorical rather than visual analog scales.
- Select brief questionnaires, not interviews.
- Select HRQL measures with published psychometric properties.

Using the SWOG guidelines, one can confidently select a set of instruments to assess HRQL in longitudinal or cross-sectional studies of patients with malignant or benign conditions. While there are some single instruments that are multidimensional, the SWOG investigators have proposed a battery approach, in which the various components of HRQL are measured with different scales to assure that each domain receives adequate attention. Ideally, the instruments should be self-administered by the patient independent of interviewers; however, at times a patient may need assistance in completing a questionnaire. Self-assessment of HRQL frees patient responses from interviewer bias. Although many instruments utilize visual analog scales, many quality-of-life researchers believe that items with specific response sets from which to choose, such as Likert scales, provide more accurate information that is easier to interpret.[13] Longer instruments can provide greater precision, but they also increase the chance that patients will tire of the exercise and not provide reliable or valid answers. This is particularly true in the multicenter clinical trial setting. Hence, shorter instruments are generally preferable when obtaining HRQL measurements under such circumstances. In general, it is easier and more efficient to use established instruments that have already undergone psychometric validation. HRQL data collected using published instruments allow the researcher to compare the study results to data from other samples or diverse populations with various chronic diseases. Nevertheless, sometimes it is necessary to develop new questionnaire items to ensure that a particular concept is adequately evaluated. Under such circumstances new scales can be tested for reliability and validity during the course of data collection.

***Psychometric Validation of HRQL Instruments.*** The development and validation of new instruments and scales is a long and arduous process. It is not undertaken lightly. Simply drawing up a list of questions that seem appropriate is fraught with potential traps and pitfalls. Two important characteristics to assess in new instruments are reliability and validity. Reliability is the term used to indicate that a test instrument measures the same thing on repeated testing. Validation is more complex and can be represented by criterion validity, in which the test instrument is compared to a gold standard measure, or by construct validity, through which components of the test instrument are highly correlated with other instruments that measure similar content areas. Reliability and validity should be established before using an instrument, and therefore, it is preferable to utilize established HRQL instruments if they are available and conceptually appropriate.

When scales and instruments are developed, they are first pilot tested to ensure that the target population can understand and complete them with ease. Pilot testing reveals problems that might otherwise go unrecognized by researchers. For example, many terms that are commonly used by medical professionals are poorly understood by patients. This may result in missing data if patients leave questions blank. Furthermore, since older patients may have poor eyesight, pilot testing in this group often identifies easily corrected visual barriers such as type size and page layout. In addition, self-administered instruments with complicated skip patterns (for example, "If you answered yes to item 16b, continue with item 16c; if you answered no to item 16b, skip to item 19a") may be too confusing for even the most competent patients to follow. This, too, can result in missing data and introduce difficulties in the analysis. Pilot testing is a necessary and valuable part of instrument development. It serves as a reality check for scale developers.

***Caveats on the Collection of HRQL Data.*** Once an instrument is thoroughly pilot tested and found to be reliable and valid, it must be administered in a manner that minimizes bias. Quality-of-life data cannot and should not be collected from patients directly by the treating health care provider. Patients often provide socially desirable responses under such circumstances.[14] This introduces measurement error. No matter how objective the treating clinician may claim to be, it is impossible for him or her to collect objective and unbiased outcomes data through direct questioning. Variations in phrasing, inflection, eye contact, rapport, mood, and other factors are difficult or impossible to eliminate. Data must be gathered by disinterested third parties using established psychometric scales and instruments.

## Future Directions in the Application of HRQL Assessment

There is a need for basic descriptive information on the HRQL of different patient groups, simply from an epidemiological perspective. Characterization of the fundamental elements of HRQL for these individuals requires study of their health perceptions and how their daily activities are affected by both their general health and their specific illness. Physical and emotional well-being form the cornerstone of this approach, but research must also extend to issues such as eating and sleeping habits, anxiety and fatigue, depression, rapport with the clinician, presence of a spouse or partner, and social interactions. Characterization of all domains must address not only the actual functions but also the relative importance of these issues to patients.

Beyond the descriptive analysis, HRQL outcomes must be compared in patients undergoing different types of therapy for the same condition. From the perspective of health policy, both general and disease-specific HRQL should be measured to facilitate comparison among different common diseases or conditions. HRQL outcomes may also be correlated with medical variables such as comorbidity or sociodemographic variables such as age, race, gender, education, income, insurance status, geographic region, and access to health care. In this context, HRQL may be linked with many factors other than the traditional medical ones.

Research initiatives must rely on the use of established HRQL instruments with accepted psychometric characteristics, using independent data collection procedures. The basic science of measurement of HRQL is now well established[15] and is being widely adopted. However, the integration of HRQL among other health services outcomes is still in its infancy. Indeed, the potential value of these methods in health management organizations has yet to be fully realized. This affords a unique opportunity for simultaneous, coordinated introduction of such measurement techniques in both the clinical and administrative spheres.

## Quality-Adjusted Life Years

One popular technique used to evaluate new or established therapies is cost-effectiveness analysis. It is performed by developing a probability model of the possible medical outcomes of different interventions for a given condition. For each outcome in the model, expenses are identified, and the results are compared, typically as cost per year of life saved.[16] Years of life saved, or life years (LYs), are calculated for a population, not for individuals.[17]

For example, if one treatment produces on average six years of survival with HRQL at a low level, and an alternative treatment produces on average three years of survival with HRQL at a relatively higher level, then the duration of survival must be adjusted for these differences before the two treatments can be compared. Hence, before the final analysis, LYs are adjusted for HRQL to account for different health states that may result from various treatments. These are called quality-adjusted life years (QALYs). By using QALYs, researchers recognize that a year of time spent in one health state is not necessarily equivalent to the same year spent in a different health state. Because medical treatments for the same illness may produce various health states, it is important to adjust for these differences.

The primary appeal of these approaches to summarizing the quality of various health states is their simplicity. By using QALYs, clinicians, managers, payers, and investigators can compare outcomes and health services utilization among different individuals or populations with a uniform unit of measurement that is easily quantified. However, these approaches raise important ethical concerns for the physician providing care to an individual patient.[18] While a wide range of variables contribute to the physician's recommendations for treatment (or no treatment), there is nothing more relevant to decision making than the patient's own assessment of quality of life. Even when a treatment may be life-saving, ethical principles suggest that the patient's preference regarding treatment must be respected. If the patient feels that his or her quality of life is so poor that no treatment would make it better, then we must respect the patient's wishes.

To provide better information to patients facing such decisions, it will be important to have HRQL outcome data on individual treatments to facilitate clinical decision making. Specific examples of currently available information include the finding that HRQL is better when chemotherapy is given continuously rather than intermittently in women with advanced breast cancer,[19] or that the HRQL of women receiving breast conservation treatment is no different than for women undergoing mastectomy.[20] In addition, new information has recently become available to understand HRQL in men treated for localized prostate cancer.[21] However, there are limited data of this type. We need to expand our database on HRQL outcomes to enable the provision of information to managers, payers, health care executives, and policy makers involved in the process of distributing limited health care resources, as well as to physicians and patients involved in clinical decision making.

# Contributions from the Literature

In this section, we review seminal research in health services where HRQL methods were developed or incorporated as important outcomes. Although not exhaustive, it provides a historical framework for research in this area.

## Alameda County Human Population Laboratory Studies

Three decades ago, Lester Breslow and his colleagues recruited a probability sample of adults from Alameda County, California, to examine the health status and well-being of a community. This research program conceptualized health in broader terms than the traditional categories of disability and disease. Their work drew heavily on the World Health Organization (WHO) definition of health to guide their assessment of the population, focusing on the physical, emotional, and social dimensions of well-being.[22] Although they examined some social indicators (for example, employment, income, marital status) in their study sample, the focus of their work was on the self-reported evaluation of the three dimensions of well-being identified in the WHO definition of health. The measurement methods available at the time were less developed psychometrically than now; however, these investigators consistently demonstrated the reliability and validity of their self-report surveys and were able to evaluate these three dimensions of health. They established the feasibility of asking people about their HRQL, and demonstrated equal response rates to personal interview, telephone, and mailed questionnaires as strategies for data collection. Further, they showed that data from the three administration strategies were nearly interchangeable.

In addition to the conceptual and methodological pioneering work of this group, this research program made several critical observations: those who were employed were healthier than those who were out of work or retired; separated persons were less healthy than those in other marital status groups;[23] there was a positive association between physical health status and mental health status, independent of sex, age, or income adequacy; there was a positive association between socioeconomic status and mental health;[24] certain common health habits (hours of sleep, exercise, abstention from alcohol and tobacco, and so on) were positively related to physical health status;[25] and these personal health habits were related to subsequent mortality[26] and disability.[27]

## RAND Health Insurance Study

The RAND Health Insurance Study (HIS) was one of the first large health services research intervention trials. This study was conceived in the early 1970s, at a time when there was considerable discussion about national health insurance reform and new approaches to limiting the rapidly expanding health care budget.[28] The HIS randomly assigned 2,005 families (3,958 individuals who were between fourteen and sixty-one years of age) to health insurance plans that provided free care, varying degrees of co-payments, or care through a health maintenance organization.[29] In addition to examining the cost of care and utilization of services, this comprehensively designed study examined a number of important health outcomes. The outcomes included physiologic measures (such as blood pressure or far vision), parameters that reflect health habits (such as smoking, weight, and cholesterol level), and self-reported measures of health status (such as physical functioning, role functioning, mental health, social contacts, and health perceptions). The requirement for reliable and valid measures of health status in the RAND HIS led to one of the most extensive explorations of the conceptualization of health and the methodologies required for the measurement of HRQL.

Although it is not possible in this chapter to examine all of the advances in measurement of HRQL that were developed as part of the RAND HIS, a few key concepts and measures will be described. The methodological aspects of this work were spearheaded by John E. Ware, Jr., and are best captured in a paper published in 1984.[30] Ware noted that the "attention of society, government and health care providers has broadened beyond survival and biomedical status into the areas of behavioral and psychosocial outcomes. There also seems to be a shift in the objectives of health care toward more socially relevant health and quality of life outcomes and increased awareness of the interest in the psychological and economic costs of disease and disability."[31] He also noted the methodological advances that made it possible to have patients evaluate these matters through self-report measures. Ware carefully clarifies that "quality of life encompasses personal health status and other factors such as family life, finances, housing and jobs," such aspects being the content of much of the social indicators research movement; however, not all of these factors are expected to be influenced by the health care system.[32] Therefore, he suggests that it is more important to consider the concept of health status as separate from the larger arena of quality of life, with health representing proper functioning and well-being, harking back to the WHO definition of health.[33] In this explication of a framework for measurement of health-related quality of life, Ware identifies the following dimensions (see Figure 6.2): disease, personal functioning, psychological distress and well-being, general health perceptions, and social/role functioning.

Using this framework, the RAND investigators developed a number of large questionnaire batteries to examine each dimension of HRQL. These questionnaires were developed specifically for the HIS, were tested and validated as part of the HIS, and were then used as critical outcome measures. Detailed descriptions of these measures are available as separate reports prepared through the RAND Corporation and also through many publications. One of the most widely used measures is the Mental Health Inventory (MHI) described by Veit and Ware in 1983.[34] In contrast to existing psychological measures designed to diagnose mental illness, the MHI was developed to look at psychological distress and well-being in general populations. Ware and associates drew heavily on existing measures

## FIGURE 6.2. FRAMEWORK FOR MEASURING HEALTH STATUS.

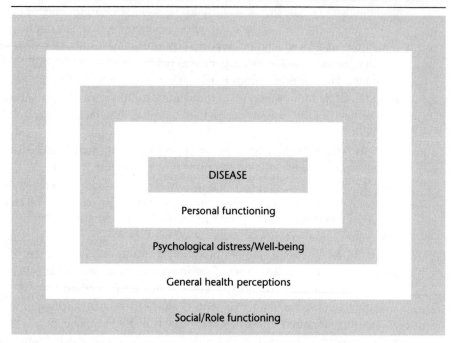

Source: Adapted from J. E. Ware, Jr., "Conceptualizing Disease Impact and Treatment Outcomes," *Cancer* 53 Supplement (1984), p. 2317.

of well-being in the development of the MHI. However, they performed much additional work to conceptualize the issues of importance to this domain of HRQL and were careful in separating mental health from physical health. What resulted was a thirty-eight–item index of mental health that could be separated into two main constructs: *psychological distress* (anxiety, depression, loss of behavioral or emotional control) and *psychological well-being* (general positive affect and emotional ties). Elegant psychometric evaluation of this measure was completed as part of the HIS.[35]

There are many important legacies from the RAND Health Insurance Study. From the point of view of quality-of-life research, the conceptualization of HRQL as a key outcome of health care is critical. In addition, the HIS developed many reliable and valid tools for measurement of the dimensions of health-related quality of life. However, in addition to the tools themselves, data from this study also provide important reference points for the relative value of specific changes in scores. That is to say, what does a change in quality-of-life score mean? Data on life events captured in the RAND HIS in relation to change scores for the measures of health-related quality of life provide intervention-based validity for the quality-of-life scores. The reader is referred to a review by Testa and Nackley[36] for an excellent discussion of this issue.

## Medical Outcomes Study

The Medical Outcomes Study (MOS), summarized in Table 6.1, is another example of a major health services research study that in its design and conceptualization included health-related quality of life as a key outcome of care.[37] Many of the key investigators for this study had been involved in the RAND HIS. Again,

### TABLE 6.1. CONCEPTUAL FRAMEWORK FOR THE MEDICAL OUTCOMES STUDY.

| Structure of Care | Process of Care | Outcomes |
|---|---|---|
| *System Characteristics* | *Technical Style* | *Clinical End Points* |
| Organization | Visits | Symptoms & signs |
| Specialty mix | Medications | Laboratory values |
| Financial incentives | Referrals | Death |
| Workload | Test ordering | |
| Access/Convenience | Hospitalizations | *Functional Status* |
| | Expenditures | Physical |
| *Provider Characteristics* | Continuity of care | Mental |
| Age | Coordination | Social |
| Gender | | Role |
| Specialty training | *Interpersonal Style* | |
| Economic incentives | Interpersonal manner | *General Well-Being* |
| Beliefs/Attitudes | Patient participation | Health perceptions |
| Preferences | Counseling | Energy/Fatigue |
| Job satisfaction | Communication level | Pain |
| | | Life satisfaction |
| *Patient Characteristics* | | |
| Age | | *Satisfaction with Care* |
| Gender | | Access |
| Diagnosis/Condition | | Convenience |
| Severity | | Financial coverage |
| Co-morbid conditions | | Quality |
| Health habits | | General |
| Beliefs/Attitudes | | |
| Preferences | | |

*Source:* Adapted from A. R. Tarlov, J. E. Ware, Jr., S. Greenfield, et al., "The Medical Outcomes Study an Application of Methods for Monitoring the Results of Medical Care," *Journal of the American Medical Association* 262 (1989), p. 926.

Ware and colleagues at RAND were central figures in the development of the health outcome measures for the Medical Outcomes Study. Thus, it is not surprising that the MOS measures of functional status, health, and well-being draw heavily on the prior measures developed for the Health Insurance Study.[38]

The self-report measures of HRQL used in the MOS were quite lengthy.[39] However, one of the major methodological advances from this project was the realization that shorter measures might be as effective as the lengthier measures traditionally used in this type of research. While longer measures lead to added precision, they also increase respondent burden and the likelihood of missing data. Furthermore, they are too cumbersome for most clinical settings. An additional conceptual breakthrough was the desirability of a generic HRQL tool that could facilitate the comparison of common diseases across specific dimensions of HRQL. Noteworthy results from this research include the development of the MOS short form, first published as a twenty-item questionnaire[40] and later an expanded version known as the MOS Short Form 36 or the RAND 36-Item Health Survey 1.0.[41] The short forms of the MOS instruments are being widely used in a variety of research and clinical settings to examine health outcomes of care.[42] Furthermore, these measures are being translated for use in multinational studies as well as national studies that include diverse populations.[43] Although very promising, there are limitations to the use of the MOS in quality-of-life research because of the multiple scale or dimension scores, rather than a global score. Work is ongoing, however, to address this issue (J. E. Ware, Jr., personal communication, 1994).

## Efficacy Studies

Quality of life has long been an implied outcome of treatments for a variety of common, chronic medical conditions. For a disease such as rheumatoid arthritis, the subjective assessment of response to anti-inflammatory agents (for example, pain relief, increased mobility) has been critical to the evaluation of new treatments.[44] In the case of antihypertensive treatments, side effects from medications may interfere with compliance and affect the successful control of this clinically silent condition.[45] Cancer treatments are another area where quality-of-life outcomes are salient.[46]

Randomized clinical trials of treatment efficacy are the most compelling studies in which quality-of-life measures have been used. The studies that have been most successful included adequate resources to collect extensive quality-of-life data and used a comprehensive battery of instruments. Recently, there has been a move toward more abbreviated quality-of-life outcome measures for integration into large multicenter trials.[47] In these situations, respondent and staff burden is an important consideration. It is hoped that these shorter forms will be equally sensitive to measurement of differences in quality-of-life outcomes. Many studies are underway currently, and results should be forthcoming in the next few years.

Two examples of the use of quality-of-life measures in efficacy studies illustrate the added value of this outcome to standard end points. In 1986, Bombardier and colleagues reported on the results of a randomized, double-blind, multicenter trial, in which auranofin (an oral gold salt preparation) was compared to placebo in patients with classic or definite rheumatoid arthritis.[48] Treatment was administered over a six-month period during which there was serial evaluation of traditional clinical endpoints (number of tender and swollen joints, grip strength, fifty-foot walk time, duration of morning stiffness) along with administration of an extensive battery of questionnaires designed to assess HRQL (function, pain, global impression, utility, depression, health perception). This trial demonstrated that auranofin therapy was superior to placebo using standard clinical measures, which was confirmed by similar results among the wide array of HRQL measures. The authors comment that although objective clinical benefits were modest in the auranofin-treated group (for example, the reduction in the number of tender and swollen joints), there were meaningful improvements in patients' performance and other outcomes valued in daily life as measured by the HRQL assessments.

This was an important study from the perspective of HRQL assessment, since a variety of independent instruments were used to measure the components of HRQL. For example, three different instruments were used to assess functional status. Although each measure had a slightly different emphasis, the direction of change on each instrument and the comparative results in the two treatment groups were similar. Further evaluation will be necessary to determine which instruments are most sensitive in detecting treatment effects.

In 1986, Croog and colleagues reported the results of a randomized trial that was designed specifically to address the impact of antihypertensive therapy on quality of life.[49] In the opening paragraph of their paper, the authors state, "Physicians who are successful in controlling blood pressure may be unaware of the negative effect that antihypertensive drugs can have on the quality of life on the physical state, emotional well-being, sexual and social functioning, and cognitive acuity of their patients."[50] Furthermore, they note that patients may believe that the side effects of antihypertensive medications are so serious that they are non-compliant, with resulting lack of therapeutic efficacy.

In this multicenter, randomized, double-blind clinical trial, men with mild to moderate essential hypertension were evaluated for the effects of captopril, methyldopa, and propranolol on the quality of life and control of blood pressure. Since all three drugs had been shown to be effective in controlling hypertension, the major question of interest was related to their effects on HRQL. An important additional goal was the evaluation of selected measures for their ability to discriminate the effects of the three medications on the HRQL of patients with hypertension. In this study, HRQL was defined conceptually in five domains: sense of well-being and satisfaction with life, physical state, emotional state, intellectual functioning, and ability to perform in social roles and the degree of satisfaction from these roles. An extensive battery of previously validated measures, as well as some newly created scales, were administered to patients by trained interviewers at a baseline assessment and twenty-four weeks later.

A number of changes in HRQL were observed within each group at twenty-four weeks. Patients treated with captopril had a significant improvement in general well-being (anxiety, positive well-being, and vitality), as well as improvement in work performance and in cognitive functioning, with other HRQL scales remaining unchanged. In contrast, patients receiving methyldopa showed no significant improvement except in cognitive functioning, and they had significant worsening in measures of depression, work performance, sexual dysfunction, physical symptoms, and life satisfaction. Patients receiving propranolol in this study experienced an improvement in cognitive functioning and social participation, but experienced increased sexual dysfunction and physical symptoms.

The degree of change between treatment groups was compared using multivariate analysis. This evaluation revealed significant differences between the captopril and methyldopa groups, and the captopril and propranolol groups, but not between the methyldopa and propranolol groups. The authors observed that there was significantly more worsening or no change in general well-being, physical symptoms, and sexual dysfunction for those patients taking methyldopa or propranolol as compared to patients receiving captopril.

The large sample sizes in this trial allowed detection of very small but significant changes in HRQL, as evaluated by a wide range of measures. Are these differences clinically relevant? The authors support the clinical importance of their findings with two comments. Most of the patients who withdrew from the trial before the second HRQL assessment did so because of adverse effects on HRQL (determined through an exit interview). Secondly, other studies have indicated that even a change of 0.15 SD on scales similar to those used in this study were associated with being laid off or fired from a job, or were predictive of using mental health services.[51] Thus, although the effect size detected in these studies was relatively small, it was related to clinically meaningful events and could thus be interpreted as showing an important change in quality of life.

Perhaps the most important aspect of this study was the observation that different antihypertensive medications vary in their impact on various aspects of HRQL, and that this effect can be successfully evaluated through the use of currently available psychosocial measures. The rigorous design of the study, as well as the use of standardized measures, should encourage similar evaluation of other cardiovascular drugs that may have differing effects on HRQL but similar patterns of efficacy. Beyond the research applications of HRQL assessment, the HRQL profile of various antihypertensive medications may be useful for the practicing clinician, to individualize therapy and promote optimal adherence to the recommended regimen.

These two examples demonstrate that the evaluation of quality-of-life endpoints in efficacy studies is important because they provide an additional outcome that includes the patient perspective. This is most important in therapeutic situations where the toxicity of treatment is high and the benefits may be few. Quality-of-life assessment has been widely adopted by the pharmaceutical industry as a component of the drug approval process.[52] These assessments are also an expanding part of large clinical treatment trials for patients with cancer and HIV infection. We are still in the early phases of experience with HRQL as an outcome in such large-scale and long-term trials.

## Effectiveness Research

The newest aspect of health services research is in the area of effectiveness. In contrast to controlled clinical trials that examine efficacy, effectiveness research examines the outcomes of treatment as they are actually practiced in clinical settings. To this end, the Agency for Health Care Policy and Research has funded a number of patient outcome research teams (PORTs) to investigate common medical treatments and procedures.[53] While this research effort has emphasized literature review of efficacy studies, as well as the examination of practice variations using administrative databases, it has also provided an opportunity to collect quality-of-life outcome data from patients undergoing various procedures. The work of these PORTs is just emerging, and we can expect valuable quality-of-life outcome data from this research in the future.[54]

# Future Research and Policy Issues

To date, HRQL has been used primarily as an outcome in research, with limited application to clinical care and policy making. A number of obstacles and questions remain to be addressed.

- *How can HRQL endpoints be more effectively incorporated in research, clinical care, and policy decisions?* Several recent workshops among health services researchers,[55] sponsored through the NIH and NCI,[56] have emphasized the need for incorporating HRQL endpoints into research and clinical care settings. The technologies, although not as yet perfect, are much more accessible and feasible than just a short time ago. Scannable, user-friendly instruments are available and normative databases are being developed rapidly. Health care consumers and providers would like access to such information.

As has been emphasized by several prominent health services researchers,[57] it is patient outcomes that must drive our policy decisions. Prolonged survival with a poor quality of life may not be desirable to patients. Consumers are anxious to have information about the HRQL impact of new treatments. When there is uncertainty about the efficacy or effectiveness of a treatment or choices among treatments, then HRQL endpoints will take on paramount importance.

Only through a concerted effort to collect HRQL data will this outcome be considered as a primary endpoint. All studies of efficacy and effectiveness must include patient-rated measures of HRQL when there is a potential quality-of-life question. Common core measures should be shared across studies so that relevant comparisons can be made. However, we must not fail to ask critical questions related to new therapies, to better understand their relevance to patients. These measures of HRQL must be considered routine and not exceptional for enough data to materialize. The additional costs of data collection should be borne by funding agencies, insurers, and providers so that the value of new tests or procedures can be fully evaluated.

- *Are HRQL endpoints sufficient to force changes in health policy?* In asking whether HRQL outcomes are sufficient to force changes in health policy, we must consider the reliability and validity of currently available HRQL tools. In addition, we must ask whether statistically significant changes in the evaluation of HRQL are clinically significant. To obtain a more precise evaluation of the quality of our tools, it will be necessary to reference or calibrate our HRQL instruments against known outcomes of clinical importance to patients, purchasers of health care, and health care providers. For this work to proceed, we must invest in the collection of important clinical information along with our HRQL data. Research in HRQL needs to be supported to extrapolate effectively from the HRQL endpoint to decisions on public health policy. Shorter-term management applications include the use of HRQL endpoints and other outcomes and effectiveness research as critical measures in the quality assurance arena.
- *How can the HRQL research agenda be advanced?* Up until recently, HRQL research has been patient focused, with limited attention to HRQL's relationship to the structure and process of care. In a recent paper, Andersen

and his colleagues[58] suggest that it might be fruitful to consider the health services research paradigm when designing quality-of-life studies. Similarly, health services research must more fully account for HRQL outcomes and look beyond issues of access to care and the organization and delivery of care as primary outcomes. Andersen and colleagues propose a more comprehensive and integrated conceptual framework for predicting HRQL outcomes, an extension of the framework for health services research and other health-related research. They note, "The central idea is that the domain of quality-of-life encompasses multiple core structures and processes from other types of health research, all of which can contribute to quality-of-life outcomes."[59] They argue that health services research examines the causal link between medical care delivery (that is, structure and process) and its effect on HRQL outcomes. Therefore, expansion of the conceptual framework to incorporate health services research should enhance the value of quality-of-life research.

Thus, until recently, with the exception of the few studies cited earlier, HRQL has been included infrequently in traditional health services research. The expansion and development of HRQL measurement has emerged primarily from clinical research. What is needed urgently is the careful and appropriate inclusion of HRQL outcomes in traditional health services research. Similarly, researchers in clinical settings who are measuring HRQL should account for the structure and process of care in designing their research and data collection. As suggested by Andersen and his colleagues, "This era of health care reform calls for a paradigm shift, away from the heroic and costly therapeutic measures that extend the quantity of life, to a patient or consumer-focused approach aimed at health promotion and disease prevention, using QOL [quality-of-life] measures as the ultimate criteria for success."[60] As indicated throughout this chapter, the potential for accomplishing this goal is on the horizon.

# Notes

1. P. M. Ellwood, "Shattuck Lecture. Outcomes Management: A Technology of Patient Experience," *New England Journal of Medicine* 318 (1988): 1549–1556, see p. 1550.
2. Ellwood, "Shattuck Lecture. Outcomes Management: A Technology of Patient Experience," see p. 1551.
3. Ellwood, "Shattuck Lecture. Outcomes Management: A Technology of Patient Experience," see p. 1552.
4. A. R. Tarlov, "The Coming Influence of a Social Sciences Perspective on Medical Education," *Academic Medicine* 67 (1992): 724–731.
5. P. A. Ganz, "Quality of Life and the Patient with Cancer: Individual and Policy Implications," *Cancer* 74 (1994): 1445–1452.

6. A. Donabedian, *The Definition of Quality and Approaches to Its Assessment* (Ann Arbor, Mich.: Health Administration Press, 1980).

7. D. L. Patrick and P. Erickson, "Assessing Health-Related Quality of Life for Clinical Decision-Making," in *Quality of Life Assessment: Key issues in the 1990s,* eds. S. R. Walker and R. M. Rosser (Dordrecht: Kluwer, 1993), p. 19.

8. World Health Organization, *Constitution of the World Health Organization, Basic Documents* (Geneva: World Health Organization, 1948).

9. D. A. Tulsky, "An Introduction to Test Theory," *Oncology* 4 (May 1990): 43–48.

10. D. L. Patrick and R. A. Deyo, "Generic and Disease-Specific Measures in Assessing Health Status and Quality of Life," *Medical Care* 27 (1989): S217–S232.

11. I. McDowell and C. Newell, *Measuring Health, A Guide to Rating Scales and Questionnaires* (New York: Oxford University Press, 1987); D. L. Patrick and P. Erickson, *Health Status and Health Policy, Allocating Resources to Health Care* (New York: Oxford University Press, 1993); and B. Spilker (ed.), *Quality of Life Assessments in Clinical Trials* (New York: Raven Press, 1990).

12. C. M. Moinpour, "Quality of Life Assessment in Southwest Oncology Group Trials," *Oncology* 4 (May 1990): 79–89.

13. G. H. Guyatt, M. Townsend, L. B. Berman, and J. L. Keller, "A Comparison of Likert and Visual Analogue Scales for Measuring Change in Function," *Journal of Chronic Diseases* 40 (1987): 1129–1133.

14. I. F. Tannock, "Management of Breast and Prostate Cancer: How Does Quality of Life Enter the Equation?" *Oncology* 4 (May 1990): 149–156.

15. G. H. Guyatt, D. H. Feeny, and D. L. Patrick, "Measuring Health-Related Quality of Life," *Annals of Internal Medicine* 118 (1993): 622–629.

16. J. P. Kassirer and M. Angell, "The Journal's Policy on Cost-Effectiveness Analysis," *New England Journal of Medicine* 331 (1994): 669–670; D. M. Eddy, "Cost-Effectiveness Analysis: Is It Up to the Task?" *Journal of the American Medical Association* 267 (1992): 3342–3348; M. C. Weinstein and W. B. Stason, "Foundations of Cost-Effectiveness Analysis for Health and Medical Practices," *New England Journal of Medicine* 296 (1977): 716; and D. S. Shepard and M. S. Thompson, "First Principles of Cost-Effectiveness Analysis in Health," *Public Health Reports* 94 (1979): 535.

17. T. J. Smith, B. E. Hillner, and C. E. Desch, "Efficacy and Cost-Effectiveness of Cancer Treatment: Rational Allocation of Resources Based on Decision Analysis," *Journal of the National Cancer Institute* 85 (1993): 1460–1474.

18. H. E. Dean, "Political and Ethical Implications of Using Quality of Life as an Outcome Measure," *Seminars in Oncology Nursing* 6 (1990): 303–308.

19. A. Coates, V. Gebski, J. F. Bishop, et al., "Improving the Quality of Life During Chemotherapy for Advanced Breast Cancer," *New England Journal of Medicine* 317 (1987): 1490–1495.

20. P. A. Ganz, C.A.C. Schag, J. J. Lee, et al., "Breast Conservation Versus Mastectomy: Is There a Difference in Psychological Adjustment or Quality of Life in the Year After Surgery?" *Cancer* 69 (1992): 1729–1738.

21. M. S. Litwin, R. D. Hays, A. Fink, P. A. Ganz, B. Leake, G. E. Leach, and R. H. Brook, "Quality of Life Outcomes in Men Treated for Localized Prostate Cancer," *Journal of the American Medical Association* 273 (1995): 129–135.

22. Lester Breslow, "A Quantitative Approach to the World Health Organization Definition of Health: Physical, Mental and Social Well-Being," *International Journal of Epidemiology* 1 (1972): 347–355; and World Health Organization, *Constitution of the World Health Organization, Basic Documents.*

23. N. B. Belloc, L. Breslow, and J. R. Hochstim, "Measurement of Physical Health in a General Population Survey," *American Journal of Epidemiology* 93 (1971): 328–336.

24. P. L. Berkman, "Measurement of Mental Health in a General Population Survey," *American Journal of Epidemiology* 94 (1971): 105–111.

25. N. B. Belloc and L. Breslow, "Relationship of Physical Health Status and Health Practices," *Preventive Medicine* 1 (1972): 409–421.

26. L. Breslow and J. E. Enstrom, "Persistence of Health Habits and Their Relationship to Mortality," *Preventive Medicine* 9 (1980): 469–483.

27. L. Breslow and N. Breslow, "Health Practices and Disability: Some Evidence from Alameda County," *Preventive Medicine* 22 (1993): 86–95.

28. P. Starr, *The Social Transformation of American Medicine* (New York: Basic Books, 1982).

29. R. H. Brook, J. E. Ware, Jr., W. H. Rogers, et al., "Does Free Care Improve Adults' Health? Results from a Randomized Controlled Trial," *New England Journal of Medicine* 309 (1983): 1429–1434; J. Newhouse, W. G. Manning, C. N. Morris, et al., "Some Interim Results from a Controlled Trial of Cost Sharing in Health Insurance," *New England Journal of Medicine* 305 (1981): 1501–1507; and W. G. Manning, A. Leibowitz, G. A. Goldberg, et al., "A Controlled Trial of the Effect of a Prepaid Group Practice on Use of Services," *New England Journal of Medicine* 310 (1984): 1505–1510.

30. J. E. Ware, Jr., "Conceptualizing Disease Impact and Treatment Outcomes," *Cancer* 53, Supplement (1984): 2316–2323.

31. J. E. Ware, Jr., "Conceptualizing Disease Impact and Treatment Outcomes," p. 2317.

32. J. E. Ware, Jr., "Conceptualizing Disease Impact and Treatment Outcomes," p. 2317.

33. World Health Organization, *Constitution of the World Health Organization, Basic Documents.*

34. C. T. Veit and J. E. Ware, Jr., "The Structure of Psychological Distress and Well-Being in General Populations," *Journal of Consulting and Clinical Psychology* 51 (1983): 730–742.

35. Veit and Ware, "The Structure of Psychological Distress and Well-Being in General Populations."

36. M. A. Testa and J. F. Nackley, "Methods for Quality-of-Life Studies," *Annual Review of Public Health* 15 (1994): 535–559.

37. A. R. Tarlov, J. E. Ware, Jr., S. Greenfield, et al., "The Medical Outcomes Study an Application of Methods for Monitoring the Results of Medical Care," *Journal of the American Medical Association* 262 (1989): 925–930.

38. A. L. Stewart and J. E. Ware, Jr. (eds.), *Measuring Functioning and Well-Being: The Medical Outcomes Study Approach* (Durham, N.C.: Duke University Press, 1992).

39. Stewart and Ware, *Measuring Functioning and Well-Being.*

40. A. L. Stewart, R. D. Hays, and J. E. Ware, Jr., "The MOS Short-Form General Health Survey: Reliability and Validity in a Patient Population," *Medical Care* 26 (1988): 724–735; and A. L. Stewart, S. Greenfield, R. D. Hays, et al., "Functional Status and Well-Being of Patients with Chronic Conditions: Results from the Medical Outcomes Study," *Journal of the American Medical Association* 262 (1989): 907–913.

41. J. E. Ware, Jr., and C. D. Sherbourne, "The MOS 36-Item Short-Form Health Survey (SF–36): I. Conceptual Framework and Item Selection," *Medical Care* 30 (1992): 473–483; and R. D. Hays, C. D. Sherbourne, and R. M. Mazel, "The RAND 36-Item Health Survey 1.0," *Health Economics* 2 (1993): 217–227.

42. K. B. Meyer, D. M. Espindle, J. M. DeGiacomo, et al., "Monitoring Dialysis Patients' Health Status," *American Journal of Kidney Diseases* 24 (1994): 267–279; A. M. Jacobson, M. DeGroot, and J. A. Samson, "The Evaluation of Two Measures of Quality of Life in Pa-

tients with Type I and Type II Diabetes," *Diabetes Care* 17 (1994): 267–274; and D. U. Jette and J. Downing, "Health Status of Individuals Entering a Cardiac Rehabilitation Program as Measured by the Medical Outcomes Study 36-Item Short-Form Survey (SF–36)," *Physical Therapy* 74 (1994): 521–527.

43. N. K. Aaronson, C. Acquadro, J. Alonso, et al., "International Quality of Life Assessment (IQOLA) Project," *Quality of Life Research* 1 (1992): 349–351.

44. M. K. Potts, S. A. Mazzuca, and K. D. Brandt, "Views of Patients and Physicians Regarding the Importance of Various Aspects of Arthritis Treatment: Correlations with Health Status and Patient Satisfaction," *Patient Education and Counseling* 8 (1986): 125–134.

45. S. H. Croog, S. Levine, M. A. Testa, et al., "The Effects of Antihypertensive Therapy on the Quality of Life," *New England Journal of Medicine* 314 (1986): 1657–1664; and M. A. Testa, R. B. Anderson, J. F. Nackley, et al., "Quality of Life and Antihypertensive Therapy in Men," *New England Journal of Medicine* 328 (1993): 907–913.

46. Coates, Gebski, Bishop, et al., "Improving the Quality of Life During Chemotherapy for Advanced Breast Cancer"; Ganz, Schag, Lee, et al., "Breast Conservation Versus Mastectomy"; and Litwin, Hays, Fink, Ganz, Leake, Leach, and Brook, "Quality of Life Outcomes in Men Treated for Localized Prostate Cancer."

47. Moinpour, "Quality of Life Assessment in Southwest Oncology Group Trials."

48. C. Bombardier, J. Ware, I. J. Russell, et al., "Auranofin Therapy and Quality of Life in Patients with Rheumatoid Arthritis," *American Journal of Medicine* 81 (1986): 565–578.

49. Croog, Levine, Testa, et al., "The Effects of Antihypertensive Therapy on the Quality of Life."

50. Croog, Levine, Testa, et al., "The Effects of Antihypertensive Therapy on the Quality of Life," p. 1657.

51. Croog, Levine, Testa, et al., "The Effects of Antihypertensive Therapy on the Quality of Life."

52. J. R. Johnson and R. Temple, "Food and Drug Administration Requirements for Approval of New Anticancer Drugs," *Cancer Treatment Reports* 69 (1985): 1155–1157.

53. K. A. Heithoff and K. N. Lohr, *Effectiveness and Outcomes in Health Care,* proceedings of an invitational conference by the Institute of Medicine, Division of Health Care Services (Washington, D.C.: National Academy Press, 1990).

54. H. I. Goldberg and M. A. Cummings (eds.), "Conducting Medical Effectiveness Research: A Report from the Inter-PORT Work Groups," *Medical Care* 32, Supplement (1994): JS1–JS110.

55. K. N. Lohr (ed.), "Advances in Health Status Assessment: Conference Proceedings," *Medical Care* 27, 3 Supplement (1989): S1–S294; and K. N. Lohr (ed.), "Advances in Health Status Assessment: Fostering the Application of Health Status Measures in Clinical Settings," *Medical Care* 30, 5 Supplement (1992): S1–S293.

56. S. G. Nayfield and B. J. Hailey, *Quality of Life Assessment in Cancer Clinical Trials,* Report of the Nayfield workshop, Quality of Life Research in Clinical Trials, held July 16–17, 1990 (Bethesda, Md.: U.S. Department of Health and Human Services, Public Health Service, NIH, 1990); and C. D. Furberg and J. A. Schuttinga, *Quality of Life Assessment: Practice, Problems, Promise,* proceedings of a workshop held October 15–17, 1990 (Bethesda, Md.: U.S. Department of Health and Human Services, Public Health Service, NIH, 1993).

57. Ellwood, "Shattuck Lecture. Outcomes Management: A Technology of Patient Experience."

58. R. M. Andersen, P. L. Davidson, and P. A. Ganz, "Symbiotic Relationships of Quality of Life Health Services, Research and Other Health Research," *Quality of Life Research* 3 (1994): 365–371.

59. Andersen, Davidson, and Ganz, "Symbiotic Relationships of Quality of Life Health Services, Research and Other Health Research," p. 369.

60. Andersen, Davidson, and Ganz, "Symbiotic Relationships of Quality of Life Health Services, Research and Other Health Research," p. 370.

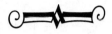

CHAPTER SEVEN

# ENSURING QUALITY OF CARE

Elizabeth A. McGlynn and Robert H. Brook

The fundamental goal of the U.S. health care system is to provide the mix of health services that will optimize the overall health of the population. The key to achieving this goal is to ensure a continued commitment to improving the quality of health services provided. The Institute of Medicine (IOM) has defined quality of care as "the degree to which health services for individuals and populations increase the likelihood of desired health outcomes and are consistent with current professional knowledge."[1] The main purpose of this chapter is to review various methods for assessing quality of care and to summarize some of what is known about current levels of quality in the United States. We begin by considering criteria for selecting topics for quality assessment. Next, we present a conceptual framework useful for organizing evaluations of quality. The definitions, methods, and state of the art in assessing the structure, process, and outcomes of care are then discussed. We consider then how the methods reviewed might be used to assess quality within a single entity (internal) or to compare quality among several entities (external). Finally, we describe some of the strengths and weaknesses of different data sources for evaluating quality. The bottom line of this chapter is that scientifically sound methods exist for assessing quality and that these must be employed systematically in the future to guard against a deterioration in quality that might otherwise occur as an unintended result of organizational and financial changes in the health services system.

# Selecting Topics for Quality Assessment

It is neither feasible nor desirable to examine everything that occurs in the health care system. Quality assessment or monitoring is conducted by selectively examining different dimensions of the health delivery system. There are two possible approaches to selecting topics in order to understand performance quality. The first approach is to examine the health services delivery system without reference to specific clinical problems or treatments. Much of the work that is being done by health plans and hospitals to improve quality (programs such as total quality management or continuous quality improvement) examines systems issues. An example of this approach would be to look at the timeliness with which laboratory test results are received by the physicians who ordered the tests. The second approach is to examine quality from a clinical perspective, focusing on specific health conditions or services and evaluating care delivered to the population of individuals with those health problems or who require particular services. An example of this approach is to examine compliance with specific standards of care such as whether the appropriate medications are used at the right dosages to treat persons with hypertension. In addition, quality can be assessed by a single entity with the intention of improving its own quality (that is, internal quality assessment) or quality can be compared among several similar entities and the information made available for decision making (external quality assessment). This chapter will focus more on the clinical approach than on the systems approach and more on external assessments than on internal assessments. These biases reflect the authors' beliefs that future public expenditures on quality methods should be targeted in these two areas.

# Criteria for Selecting Quality Assessment Areas

The clinical approach to external quality monitoring begins with selecting the health conditions or problems to be included. From the work of the HMO Quality of Care Consortium,[2] five criteria for selecting conditions are recommended:

- The condition is highly prevalent and/or has a significant effect on mortality and morbidity in the population.
- There is reasonable scientific evidence that efficacious or effective interventions exist to prevent a disease from developing (primary prevention), to identify and treat the disease at an early stage (secondary prevention), or to reduce impairment, disability, and suffering associated with having an illness (tertiary prevention).

- Improving the quality of service delivery will enhance the health of the population.
- The recommended interventions are cost effective.
- The recommended interventions are under the control of health plans or providers.

The first criterion emphasizes that quality assessment should focus on those conditions that seriously threaten the health and well-being of the population, as opposed to conditions without serious consequences. From a logistical viewpoint, focusing on conditions that are highly prevalent increases the likelihood of identifying a sufficient number of cases for review so that there is adequate statistical power to draw conclusions.

The second criterion underscores that health plans and providers should be held accountable only for those interventions that are supported by scientific studies or professional consensus. The health care system should not be encouraged to deliver care of uncertain benefit, and systems that have not embraced unproven practices should not be penalized. Many health services provided in this country do not meet these standards; some services may never be subjected to the rigorous evaluation of a randomized trial because of concerns about the ethics of withholding treatment (as would be necessary for a no-treatment control group) or providing a treatment that is believed to be less desirable (as would be necessary to test competing treatments). For these areas, we should rely on studies with less rigorous designs or on consensus opinion. Figure 7.1 shows the distribution of evidence for some common surgical procedures and one medical condition. Among articles that were included in several systematic reviews of the literature, randomized controlled trials represented only a small fraction (4 percent to 11 percent) of the available literature.[3] As scientific knowledge expands, so too will the capacity for scientifically based quality monitoring.

The third criterion suggests quality assessment should target those interventions that have a significant positive impact on the health of the population. This recognizes that one of the potential effects of quality monitoring is to shift health plan resource allocation or physician practice choices to areas that are being evaluated over areas that are not subject to assessment. This should only occur among services for which improved quality will make a positive contribution to the overall health of the population, rather than focusing on improving services that will make only a negligible improvement in health. The greatest potential for improving health occurs with interventions that are highly efficacious or effective and that are frequently underused or misused.

The fourth criterion acknowledges that there are limited resources available for health care today, and as a result, cost must be taken into account in

## FIGURE 7.1. DISTRIBUTION OF RESEARCH ARTICLES REVIEWED BY STRENGTH OF RESEARCH DESIGN.

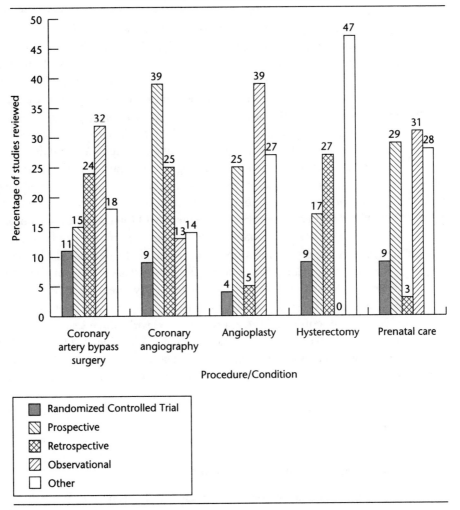

selecting areas for quality assessment. There is limited information available in the literature on the cost-effectiveness of various interventions, but the criterion remains important in the framework for evaluating potential assessment areas. Within a clinical area, there may be several possible ways of evaluating quality. Among interventions for which positive health benefits can be shown, one should also consider whether there are differences among the interventions in the cost-effectiveness of achieving the health benefit. If significant differences exist, the more cost-effective intervention should be selected for quality monitoring.

The final criterion affirms that only those interventions that are under the control of health plans or providers or for which methods exist to control for variation due to nonplan factors should be included. Many primary prevention campaigns (for example, seat belt use) have been most effective in a public health rather than private health context. Initial survival after a myocardial infarction may be more a function of the adequacy of the trauma system in an area than the quality of medical care; after admission, the focal point of responsibility shifts more clearly from the trauma system to the health plan, hospital, or provider. Some interventions may be highly dependent on patient compliance, and this may be difficult to achieve or may vary depending on the characteristics of the enrolled population. For example, return to work after a back injury may be more dependent on workers' compensation benefits than on the quality of care provided.

When we used these criteria with the HMO Quality of Care Consortium to select potential areas for quality-of-care assessment in managed care, we identified thirteen conditions for which measures might be developed.[4] The conditions were low birthweight, childhood infectious diseases, otitis media, childhood asthma, influenza, breast cancer, coronary artery disease, lung cancer and other smoking-related diseases, stroke, diabetes mellitus, medical problems of the frail elderly, hip fracture, and the appropriateness with which common medical and surgical procedures are used. These were areas in which we believed that measurement development was immediately feasible. A secondary list of conditions requiring more methodological development was also identified. It included post-trauma care for accidents and injuries, arthritis, chronic bronchitis and emphysema, and treatment of uncommon serious diseases amenable to intervention (such as meningitis).

## Conceptual Framework for Quality Assessment

A conceptual framework provides a useful mechanism for defining the aspects of care that will be evaluated for each condition in the quality assessment. The most commonly used conceptual framework in quality assessment is the one proposed by Donabedian.[5] He identified three dimensions of quality: structure, process, and outcomes (Figure 7.2). We will organize our review of quality assessment around these three dimensions. In each section, we will provide a definition of the dimension of quality, discuss methods available for assessing that dimension, and summarize what is known about that aspect of quality of care in the U.S. health care system today.

## FIGURE 7.2. CONCEPTUAL FRAMEWORK FOR QUALITY ASSESSMENT.

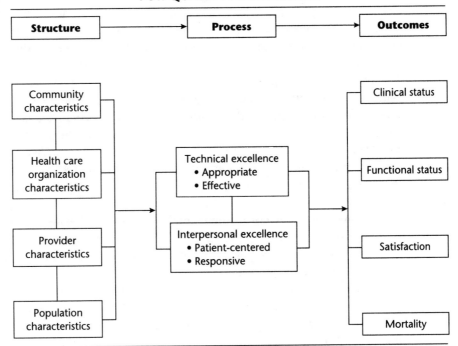

## Structural Quality

*Structural quality* refers to those stable elements of the health care delivery system in a community that facilitate or inhibit access to and provision of services. The elements include community characteristics (such as prevalence of disease), health care organization characteristics (such as number of hospital beds per capita), provider characteristics (such as specialty mix), and population characteristics (such as demographics and insurance coverage). Structural characteristics can be used to describe both the need for health care (prevalence or incidence of disease) and the capacity of the community or health care delivery system to meet those needs (such as the availability of properly trained personnel).

***Methods of Structural Quality Assessment.*** For purposes of quality assessment, we are particularly interested in those elements of structure that predict variations in the processes or outcomes of care and are subject to change. For example, the characteristics of the population residing in a community may predict differences in processes of care or outcomes. Persons without health insurance or who are otherwise economically disadvantaged may experience barriers to accessing the health service system; such barriers might be suggested by comparatively lower utilization rates of necessary services among different populations. In turn, such reductions in utilization might be associated with less favorable outcomes. However, policy makers are unlikely to be able to change the characteristics of the population. The more appropriate focus for quality improvement is on reducing barriers to access either through changes in the availability of insurance or through changes in characteristics of the health services delivery system (for example, the number of public health clinics or the hours of operation for other health providers). Because the relationship between the structure of the health services delivery system and the process or outcomes of care is indirect, structural quality measures are often less useful for policy makers than measures of process quality or outcomes.

Community characteristics represent the context in which the health services delivery system operates and provide one perspective for evaluating the capacity of the service system to respond to community needs. The prevalence of disorders in the community, for example, may be useful in estimating specific community needs. Information about the availability of health resources may be an indicator of the potential for meeting those needs. One common measure of resource availability is the physician-to-population ratio; in 1992 in the United States, there were 204 patient care physicians for every 100,000 persons.[6] However, there is considerable variation across the United States; at the state level, the range is from 380 physicians per 100,000 population in Massachusetts to 146 physicians per 100,000 population in Alaska.[7] The location of the community relative to health resources is another key indicator of the ease with which residents may obtain certain services; inner-city and rural residents, for example, may have to travel longer than those living elsewhere to obtain services. While an evaluation of community characteristics is not generally included in quality assessment, it may be an important precursor to understanding the particular quality challenges likely to be faced in a community.

Health care organization characteristics have been evaluated in terms of the capacity of the organization to provide high-quality services. Various factors including the quality of the physical plant and equipment, ownership, accreditation, staffing patterns, distribution of reimbursement by source of payment, organizational structure, and governance mechanisms have been considered markers of the likelihood that an organization will provide good quality of care. Most of these factors at best can be viewed as facilitating or inhibiting the likelihood of delivering good care; because these factors always appear in combination, it is difficult to evaluate the incremental effect each of these factors might have on quality.

Provider characteristics have been included as explanatory factors in quality assessments, including age (or years in practice), gender, race/ethnicity, medical school attended, location of residency training program, specialty, board certification status, job satisfaction, and method of compensation. Board certification is the professional indicator of quality; additional years of training and an examination are required to become board certified.[8] Various specialty boards are responsible for granting board certification. Overall, about 60 percent of physicians are board certified. The specialties with the highest rates (80 percent and above) of board certification include pediatric cardiology, radiology, gastroenterology, pulmonary disease, and cardiovascular disease. The specialties with the lowest rates (60 percent and below) of board certification include general practice, psychiatry, internal medicine, anesthesiology, and general surgery.

Population characteristics may be useful in predicting the likelihood that an individual will receive high-quality care. Information may be used to identify individuals who are at risk for receiving lower quality of care; in particular, organizations that provide services to individuals at high risk should be aware of the special needs of these populations. Various population characteristics have been examined, including sociodemographics, insurance coverage and type, presence of co-morbid conditions, and functional status.

***What Do We Know About Structural Quality?*** Few structural factors have been found to be associated with significant variations in health outcomes, although they are frequently associated with differences in the process of care. A study of the effect of implementation of the prospective payment system on the quality of care delivered to Medicare beneficiaries, for example, found that patients who were black or from poor neighborhoods or who were admitted to rural hospitals received poorer quality care than other Medicare patients.[9] These differences in quality, however, did not result in higher death rates among patients who were black, Medicaid beneficiaries, or living in the poorest neighborhoods or rural areas. The same study found that higher quality care was delivered in teaching, larger, and more urban hospitals.[10] Mortality rates in the hospitals with the worst quality were four percentage points higher than mortality rates in the hospitals with the best quality. This study illustrates an important application of quality assessment for evaluating the impact of changes in public policies.

The Medical Outcomes Study found that specialty training, payment system, and practice organization had independent effects on resource utilization after controlling for differences in patient case mix.[11] Cardiologists and endocrinologists had higher utilization rates than other specialties; general internists had somewhat higher utilization rates than family physicians. Solo practitioners and those in single specialty groups had 41 percent more hospitalizations than physicians in health maintenance organizations.

However, from a policy perspective it is important to note that variations in resource use generally have not been associated with significant differences in outcomes. A study comparing rates of hospital discharge, readmission, length of stay, and reimbursement for Medicare beneficiaries in two communities with different resource profiles (Boston and New Haven) found significant differences in the use of the hospital but no differences in mortality rates.[12] Another study comparing Massachusetts and California found no relationship between lengths of stay and outcomes (that is, deaths, functional status after discharge, readmission, and patient satisfaction) for Medicare beneficiaries treated for one of six medical and surgical conditions.[13] One conclusion is that substantial reductions in utilization (and thus cost) may be possible without negative effects on health.

Socioeconomic differences (such as education, income, and race) have been shown to predict differences in utilization even when insurance coverage is similar. For example, a comparison of breast and cervical cancer screening in Ontario and the United States found that despite the availability of universal coverage in Ontario, women with less than a high school diploma and those with lower incomes were less likely to receive these two preventive services in both countries.[14] Another study examining predictors of utilization among children with special health care needs found that children who were poor, minorities, living with their mother or someone other than both of their parents, and without health insurance or a regular medical provider were more likely to experience barriers to access and to use fewer services than other children with similar characteristics.[15] The policy implication is that improving care for these populations may require more than a simple reduction of financial barriers.

The structure of health insurance benefits can significantly affect utilization. In the RAND Health Insurance Study, the rate of cost sharing contributed to a 45 percent differential in per-person expenditures between the most and least generous health plans.[16] Reductions in the use of ambulatory services were greater than reductions in the use of hospital services. Despite the dramatic differences in utilization rates, there were few differences in health outcomes for average individuals. Low-income persons in the plan with no cost sharing had somewhat better control of high blood pressure, correction for vision problems, and care for dental problems compared to those in plans with cost sharing.[17] Private policy makers may have used these findings to guide development of plans with much higher cost sharing.

There is some evidence that a relationship exists between the number of procedures done by an individual physician or institution and the outcomes, with higher volume being associated with better outcomes.[18] New York State found that since the cardiac procedures reporting system was introduced, risk-adjusted mortality decreased for both high-volume and low-volume surgeons.[19] For low-volume surgeons (50 or fewer procedures annually), the risk-adjusted mortality rate declined from 7.94 percent in 1989 to 3.20 percent in 1992 (a 60 percent decrease). Among high-volume surgeons (150 procedures or more annually), the risk-adjusted mortality rate declined 34 percent from 3.57 in 1989 to 2.36 in 1992. One of the contributing factors to reductions in unadjusted mortality rates was that 25 percent fewer procedures were being done by low-volume surgeons in 1992 as compared with 1989. The other factors were that low-volume, high-mortality physicians stopped performing surgery in the state and newer low-volume surgeons performed better than average. Policy makers could limit reimbursement for certain procedures to facilities and physicians performing a minimum volume of procedures.

## Process Quality

*Process quality* refers to what occurs in the interaction between a patient and a provider and is generally divided into two aspects: technical excellence and interpersonal excellence. Technical excellence means that the intervention was appropriate (that is, the health benefit to the patient exceeded the health risk by a significant margin) and that it was provided skillfully. Interpersonal excellence means that the intervention was humane and responsive to the preferences of the individual.

For purposes of quality assessment, we are primarily interested in those processes of care that are likely to produce optimal outcomes—either an improvement in health or a reduction in the rate of its decline. The best evidence of the relationship between processes and outcomes comes from randomized clinical trials because such trials can prove conclusively the efficacy of an intervention (that is, the potential to produce desired outcomes under ideal circumstances). Evidence from other scientific methods, while not as conclusive, is often used to demonstrate the importance of a variety of interventions in medical care. The IOM definition of quality emphasizes this relationship between the process of service delivery and outcomes as well as noting the role of professional consensus in defining high-quality processes.

***Methods of Process Quality Assessment.*** We discuss four methods that have been used to evaluate the quality of medical care processes: appropriateness of an intervention, adherence to practice guidelines or professional standards of care, practice profiling, and consumer ratings. These four methods share some features, but we discuss them separately to emphasize different methodological considerations.

*Appropriateness of an intervention* means that for individuals with particular clinical and personal characteristics, the expected health benefit from doing an intervention (such as a diagnostic or therapeutic procedure) exceeds the expected health risks by a sufficient margin that the intervention is worth doing. RAND and UCLA have pioneered a method of assessing the appropriateness with which a variety of interventions are evaluated.[20] The basic method involves five steps:

- *A detailed literature review* is conducted to summarize what is known about the efficacy, utilization, complications, cost, and indications for the subject intervention. Where possible, outcome evidence tables are constructed for clinically homogeneous groups.

- *A preliminary list of indications* is developed for the intervention, categorizing patients in terms of their symptoms, past medical history, results of previous diagnostic tests, and clinically relevant personal characteristics (such as age). The indications list is designed to be detailed enough so that patients within an indication are homogeneous with respect to the clinical appropriateness of performing a procedure; the indications are comprehensive enough so that all persons presenting for the procedure can be categorized.

- *A nine-person multispecialty panel* is assembled to assume responsibility for developing and rating the final set of indications. The panel is selected to be diverse with respect to geographic location, practice style, and other characteristics, and includes both people who perform the procedure and those who do not.

- *The indications are rated* using a modified Delphi process. In the first round, indications are individually rated by panelists, who have the literature review available; the panelists may also recommend changes to the structure of the indications. In the second round, the panel meets face-to-face for a discussion of the results from the first round of ratings and makes final ratings. The indications are rated from 1 to 9 where 1 means that the procedure is very inappropriate for persons with that indication and 9 means that the procedure is very appropriate for persons with that indication. The median panel score is used to determine the appropriateness category for each indication; a median rating of 1–3 is considered inappropriate; 4–6 is equivocal or of uncertain value; 7–9 is appropriate. There is also a requirement that the panelists have a reasonable and statistically determined level of agreement among themselves.

- *The appropriateness of interventions is evaluated;* generally, information is abstracted from the medical record (inpatient or outpatient) because of the level of clinical detail required to assign patients to indications. An alternate approach that has been applied when appropriateness is assessed prospectively is to interview both the patient and the physician.

The reliability and validity of the appropriateness method has been tested. While the results of such evaluations are promising, more work remains to be done.[21] For example, regression analysis performed on indications for patients with chronic stable angina undergoing coronary angiography demonstrated that appropriateness ratings were higher among patients with more severe disease, as well as among patients who failed medical therapy and among patients who had positive findings on noninvasive tests.[22]

The ratings for each indication are the explicit standards by which care is evaluated. The indications can be linked to the quality of scientific evidence and ratings can be updated as knowledge changes. It is also possible to conduct sensitivity analyses that evaluate the importance of different factors in the indication structure with respect to determining appropriateness. For example, in our study of appropriateness of hysterectomy, we found that among women who wanted to maintain fertility, the expert panel required considerable evidence of efforts to find an alternative solution to the presenting problem before the hysterectomy was considered appropriate.[23] Because there are no national averages established for the expected appropriateness of care, most of the comparisons have been made among groups (such as hospitals or managed care organizations) participating in a study.[24]

*Adherence to practice guidelines or professional standards of care* is a method of process quality assessment that evaluates the extent to which care is consistent with professional knowledge either by examining adherence to specific practice guidelines or by evaluating whether care meets certain professional standards. The Agency for Health Care Policy and Research (AHCPR) defines clinical practice guidelines as "systematically developed statements to assist practitioner and patient decisions about appropriate health care for specific clinical conditions."[25] Practice guidelines are often formulated graphically as decision algorithms to reflect the complexity of clinical decision making.

AHCPR has been funding the development of practice guidelines in a variety of areas over the past few years[26] and has recently published a monograph on various methodological approaches to the development of clinical practice guidelines.[27] In addition to the AHCPR practice guidelines program, most specialty societies are developing clinical practice guidelines. For many preventive services (for example, immunizations, Pap smears, mammograms), specialty societies and others have established standards for when these services should be delivered (for example, age of the individual, interval between services). Because of the relative ease of evaluating adherence to preventive service standards, these represent a common basis for quality assessment. One argument that is frequently raised in objection to using the rate of adherence to preventive services recommendations as a marker of quality is the role of patient compliance in seeking such services. Despite this concern, use of preventive services is one of the most common quality indicators reported.

For purposes of quality assessment, it is almost always necessary to translate guidelines into review criteria by establishing operational definitions of adherence and nonadherence to the guidelines as well as definitions for key clinical concepts employed in the guidelines. Many practice guidelines, for example, contain vague clinical terms (such as *mild, moderate,* and *severe*) that must be explicitly defined in order to evaluate whether a particular patient is eligible for a portion of the guidelines and then to assess adherence to the guideline. The performance expectation is generally 100 percent adherence to the guideline, and comparisons are made either among similar groups or to a benchmark.

*Practice profiling* is a method for comparing the patterns of cost, utilization, or quality of processes among providers.[28] The method compares practice patterns to a norm (such as the average of other physicians in the organization) or to a preestablished standard (that is, to a practice guideline). Profiles are generally constructed as a rate of occurrence of some process (such as an office visit, service, surgical procedure, or laboratory test) over a specified period of time for a defined population.[29] What distinguishes profiling from most appropriateness or guideline adherence approaches is that the review is not necessarily conducted specific to a clinical condition but rather may cover a broader range of practice patterns (for example, hospital admission rate). Profiles can be constructed at any level in the health delivery system: nationally, regionally, health plan, specialty, medical group, or individual physician. Profiling is most often used to examine utilization of a variety of services, including hospital admissions, ambulatory visits, laboratory test use, referral patterns, diagnostic test use, or medication prescriptions.

Profiling has been used for internal quality improvement and cost containment more often than for external reporting of performance. One consequence of this is that there are fewer reports in the literature about the results of profiling analyses. There are, however, a few articles that emphasize some of the critical issues that must be addressed if profiling is to be used routinely for quality assessment.[30] Perhaps the most important issue that has arisen is the need for case-mix or severity adjustment (that is, differences in the severity and prevalence of diseases and other characteristics of the populations being compared). The methods for case-mix adjustment, particularly in the ambulatory setting, are in a developmental stage. In addition, much of the clinical information that is typically required for case-mix adjustment cannot be found on claims data; this implies that supplemental data will be required in order to make adequate adjustments. One study of referral patterns found that adjusting for the age and sex distribution of patients in a physician's panel reduced the coefficient of variation in referrals by more than 50 percent.[31] When a case-mix adjustment was applied, 75 percent of physicians identified as outliers under the age and sex adjustment method were no longer classified as outliers. This problem is particularly important to solve for the purpose of external comparisons, but even internal uses of profiling would benefit substantially from improved adjustment methods. For example, the Medical Outcomes Study found that patients of cardiologists were older, had lower functional status and well-being scores, and had more chronic diagnoses than patients of general internists; patients of family practitioners were younger and had better functional status and fewer chronic conditions than patients of general internists.[32] These case-mix characteristics were associated with differences in hospitalization rates, physician visit rates, and rates of prescription drug use. Internal plan comparisons should account for these differences.

The other challenge for profiling is the problem of sample size. There is considerable interest in using profiling techniques to examine the practice patterns of individual physicians. However, one must have an adequate number of observations on each physician in order to determine whether the differences observed are statistically significant. Among other things, this implies that common processes (such as use of screening mammography) will be more suitable for profiling than rarer processes (such as use of adjuvant chemotherapy for breast cancer treatment). Among processes, greater aggregation will be more suitable than less (for example, use of all laboratory tests versus use of a single test). These issues have been pointed out even by proponents of profiling.[33]

*Consumer ratings* are the most appropriate method for evaluating the interpersonal quality of care. Surveys of health plan enrollees are the most common method for eliciting information from individuals about their health care. Two types of information are generally sought: reporting of events and evaluations of care. We discuss reporting of events here and evaluations of care (that is, patient satisfaction) under the outcomes section.

Consumers may be asked to report events such as immunizations, mammography, or cholesterol testing that are indicators of access to care. To the extent that some of these services are obtained outside of the health plan in which the patients are enrolled, such reports can be used to construct an estimate of the proportion of the population receiving certain services regardless of source. Consumer reports are also used to evaluate a variety of access issues such as waiting times for appointments or to see the doctor, distance to the nearest health facility, hours of operation, ability to see the provider you want to see, and other similar questions regarding consumers' experiences trying to obtain services. Consumers may also report on what the physician did during an encounter (such as explain options, provide requested information, or counsel about health habits). Patients' ability to report on events varies with the time frame (a shorter time span produces more reliable information) and the type of event (invasive events such as surgery may be more memorable than health promotion counseling).

**What Do We Know About Process Quality?** It is beyond the scope of this chapter to summarize all of the literature regarding process quality. We will, however, provide some examples of what is known about process quality from published studies that have used one of the four methods we have discussed.

*Appropriateness.* Figure 7.3 illustrates the results of various studies of appropriateness that have been conducted over the past ten to fifteen years.[34] Overall, the proportion of procedures judged to be inappropriate ranges from 2 percent (coronary artery bypass graft surgery, cataract) to 32 percent (carotid endarterectomy). The proportion of procedures judged to be of uncertain clinical value ranges from 7 percent (coronary artery bypass graft surgery) to 38 percent (percutaneous transluminal coronary angioplasty). Combining these estimates of inappropriate and uncertain care suggests that about one-third of the procedures performed in this country are of questionable health benefit relative to their risks.

There is little evidence to suggest that a relationship exists between the rates at which procedures are done and the appropriateness of care. A study examining geographical variations in the rates of use of coronary angiography, carotid endarterectomy, and upper gastrointestinal tract endoscopy and the appropriateness with which those procedures were used found that the rates of inappropriate use were similar among high- and low-use sites.[35] Another study failed to find a relationship between rates of hospital admission in a community and the appropriateness of those admissions.[36] The considerably higher rates of use for coronary angiography and coronary artery bypass graft surgery in the United States as compared to Canada were also not found to be associated with differences in the appropriateness with which the procedures were performed.[37]

We have also found little evidence to suggest that economic incentives have an influence on appropriateness. For example, in the Trent region of the United Kingdom, the proportion of inappropriate coronary angiographies was similar to rates found in the United States and varied among centers within the region.[38] In Israel, where physicians are salaried, the proportion of inappropriate or uncertain cholecystectomies ranged from 17 percent to 36 percent.[39] The findings for managed care organizations within the United States are consistent with these international findings. The proportion of hysterectomies judged to be inappro-

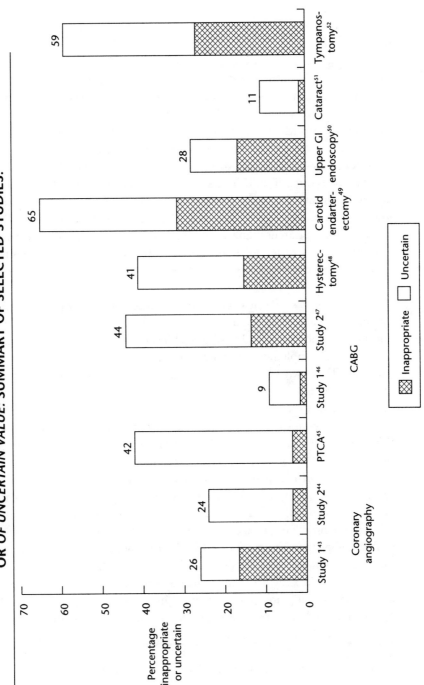

**FIGURE 7.3. PROPORTION OF PROCEDURES JUDGED EITHER *CLINICALLY INAPPROPRIATE* OR *OF UNCERTAIN VALUE*: SUMMARY OF SELECTED STUDIES.**

priate among seven managed care organizations ranged from 10 percent to 27 percent. In the RAND Health Insurance Study, while hospitalization rates were lower in the managed care organization as compared to fee-for-service, reductions occurred in both discretionary and nondiscretionary admissions.[40] Reductions in utilization in response to cost containment concerns may occur in ways that are not clinically sensible. For example, limitations on the number of paid prescriptions in a Medicaid program reduced the overall number of prescriptions filled by 30 percent, but these reductions occurred among effective and essential medications as well as among those with limited effectiveness.[41] The lower rates of cardiac procedures found in Canada as compared to the United States are achieved almost exclusively through providing these procedures at significantly lower rates to persons age 65 and older.[42] The key policy implication to be drawn from the appropriateness literature is that resource allocation strategies must incorporate clinical criteria if resources are to be spent in a way that has the greatest health benefits.

*Adherence to Guidelines.*  Because guidelines are a relatively new phenomenon, there are few systematic studies of adherence to guidelines. Perhaps the most important consistent finding from studies of guideline adherence is that there is substantial variability in compliance with guidelines or treatment recommendations among providers. Further, when guidelines are first promulgated, adherence tends to be fairly low overall.

A recent review of the effect of guidelines on clinical practice found that fifty-five of the fifty-nine evaluations reviewed detected a significant improvement in the process of care.[43] The rates of adherence reported in these studies were frequently well below 50 percent even after implementation of the guidelines.

In a study of the quality of prenatal care, we examined adherence to thirty-seven process quality criteria based on medical record reviews at six managed care organizations.[44] We found significant variations in compliance with the criteria among the organizations, although the rates of adherence were considerably higher than many reported in the review article cited earlier. The proportion of women in each of the six health plans that received seven routine screening tests in early pregnancy ranged from 64 percent to 95 percent with an average across all plans of 82 percent. On average, about 84 percent of these women received other recommended routine prenatal care; the range was from 78 percent to 87 percent. The adherence to criteria covering care for specific problems encountered in pregnancy was considerably lower; overall, 70 percent of women received recommended care, and the range was from 54 percent to 77 percent.

The recently released pilot study of managed care performance on the Health Plan Employer Data and Information Set (HEDIS) quality indicators found considerable variation among participating plans in adherence to provision of a set of preventive services.[45] For example, the average proportion of children receiving all childhood vaccinations among the twenty-one participating plans was 79 percent, but the range was from 60 to 91 percent. Cholesterol screening was received by 67 percent of eligible persons (that is, those who were continuously enrolled for five years) among all health plans, with a range from 34 to 87 percent. Mammograms were received by 71 percent of women in these health plans, and the range was from 43 to 83 percent. One of the few chronic disease indicators illustrated even lower rates of compliance. Annual diabetic retinal screening was received by 47 percent of enrolled diabetics, but the range was from 12 to 58 percent.

Although not as systematic as an examination of guidelines, another indicator of process quality is the use of best practices for certain conditions. For example, thrombolytic therapy has been shown to substantially improve the chances of survival among individuals who have suffered a myocardial infarction.[46] An evaluation of the use of thrombolytic therapy found that about 18 percent of patients with a myocardial infarction received thrombolytic therapy and that the proportion receiving this drug declined with age—despite evidence of increased efficacy with older persons.[47] Similar results have been reported for use of antidepressants. Only 20 percent to 30 percent of general medical patients with depression are prescribed antidepressant medications—and 30 percent of those with prescriptions are receiving a subtherapeutic dosage.[48] Minor tranquilizers are often used to treat depression[49] despite the lack of evidence for efficacy.[50] The quality of medication use among ethnic minority patients is even lower than that found for white patients.[51] Greater attention to the use of best practices through monitoring adherence to guidelines should substantially improve the quality of health care processes.

*Practice Profiling.* The framework for practice profiling comes from the literature reporting significant variations in the use of a variety of common medical and surgical procedures over the last two decades. Variations have been documented among countries, regions of the same country, within states, and between cities in the same state or region. For example, rates of prostatectomy are 35 percent higher in the Midwest than the West and hysterectomy rates are 80 percent higher in the Midwest than in the Northeast.[52] Similar results have been reported for hip and knee replacement and diagnostic procedures such as CT scan and ultrasound. A comparison of two communities in the same region found that the rates of use of a variety of common medical procedures ranged from 127 per 1,000 population in New Haven to 214 per 1,000 population in Boston. The same study found that rates of use of various surgical procedures ranged from 62 per 1,000 in New Haven to 86 per 1,000 in Boston.[53]

A study designed to illustrate the use of practice profiling as a cost containment tool compared the patterns of resource use between physicians providing care to Medicare beneficiaries in Oregon and Florida.[54] The study found that Florida physicians used more resources on average than Oregon physicians; the results were consistent across specialties and practice types. Considerable variation within each state was found. The authors acknowledge that at the individual physician level, profiling is best used to screen for potential problems rather than to draw firm conclusions.

*Consumer Reports.* There is evidence that consumers are able to report accurately many experiences in the health service system. One study, for example, found that consumers accurately reported 80 percent to 94 percent of history and physical elements that were performed during a health examination.[55] That study found some variation by patient characteristics; elderly and less educated consumers were less accurate in their reporting of events. Another study comparing various data collection methods found that patients and physicians agreed 96 percent of the time on what tests had been ordered, 94 percent of the time on what treatments were discussed, and 88 percent on patient education.[56] A more recent study, however, found somewhat lower rates of agreement among audio tapes, physician notes in the medical record, and patient reports of health promotion activities (regarding smoking, alcohol use, and blood pressure).[57] The authors concluded that when audio tapes are used as the gold standard, the medical record tends to underestimate the frequency of health promotion counseling (on smoking and alcohol use) and patient reports tend to overestimate the frequency of this activity. For reporting on whether blood pressure was taken, both the medical record and patient reports are quite accurate.

The 1988 National Maternal and Infant Health Survey relied on patient reports to assess adherence to recommendations from the Public Health Service's Expert Panel on the Content of Prenatal Care. Only 56 percent of respondents indicated that they had received all six of the procedures recommended by the panel in the first two visits (blood pressure measurement, urine test, blood test, weight and height measurement, pelvic examination, and pregnancy history).[58] Only 32 percent of respondents said they had received any counseling in all seven of the recommended areas (nutrition, vitamin use, smoking cessation, alcohol use, drug use, breast-feeding, and maternal weight gain). This study found that women receiving care from private offices were significantly less likely to receive the full range of services than women receiving their care from publicly funded clinics.

## Assessing Outcomes

*Outcomes* can be defined as the intermediate or ultimate results of efforts to prevent, diagnose, and treat various health problems encountered by the population. Outcomes are seen by many as the bottom-line measure of the effectiveness of the health care delivery system. A wide range of potential dimensions can be included in the broad category of outcomes. In Figure 7.2, for example, we list clinical status, functional status, consumer satisfaction, and mortality to illustrate a few possible outcomes.

Clinical status refers to biologic, physiologic, and symptom-based aspects of health. These are the outcomes that are generally of interest to physicians because they are most directly amenable to treatment. Functional status captures multiple dimensions including physical, mental, role, and social functioning. Assessments of functional status typically ask respondents to indicate the frequency or extent to which physical or mental disorders interfere with their ability to perform their usual activities. Functional status is of greatest interest to consumers because it represents how changes in clinical status affect everyday life. Consumer satisfaction assesses the extent to which experiences in the health service system were consistent with expectations and were acceptable to those receiving care.

There are two key challenges in using outcome assessments for evaluating the quality of care. Both of these challenges reflect the fact that the outcomes we observe are produced through the interaction of a variety of factors both in and out of the health service delivery system. First, to use outcomes to make externally valid comparisons among health plans or providers, adequate methods must be employed to control for differences in the severity of illness or the health profile of the populations being compared. A familiar example of an initial failure to do this was the release by the Health Care Financing Administration (HCFA) of hospital mortality data. Initially, the data were not adjusted for differences in the severity of illness for patients; not surprisingly, some of the hospitals that had the worst performance records were those serving the sickest patients (for example, hospices for the terminally ill).[59] While there is still considerable controversy as to whether the severity adjustments introduced by HCFA subsequent to the initial release were adequate, the addition of severity adjustments substantially improved the discriminant validity of the model.[60]

The second key challenge for the use of outcomes data is the issue of attribution, that is, determining the extent to which the health plan or physician that is currently being evaluated is responsible for the observed outcomes. Health outcomes are affected by a variety of factors, not all of which can be modified by the health delivery system. Because these factors may be distributed differently among populations enrolled in health plans or those seeking care from primary care physicians, these external effects must be controlled for in statistical analyses in order to understand the extent to which variations in the quality of care are contributing to the observed variations in outcomes. For interventions that take place over a long period of time (as in chronic disease care), outcomes observed in the current time period may be the result of actions taken (or not taken) much earlier in the course of illness—and those actions might not have been under the purview of the physicians or health plan currently responsible for treating the patient. To the extent that individuals change health plans frequently, discontinuities in service may further contribute to a less-than-optimal course of treatment. Who bears the responsibility for these complex series of events remains an open question for debate.

## Methods of Outcome Assessment

We will consider three approaches to outcome assessment that have been used to evaluate the quality of care delivered: condition-specific, generic, and sentinel events or adverse outcomes.

*Condition-Specific.* This approach, sometimes referred to as a tracer condition approach, examines the outcomes for individuals who have a particular diagnosis (for example, hypertension). The outcomes for condition-specific approaches may emphasize clinical status (as with blood pressure control for hypertension), although disease-specific measures of functional status should also be assessed. For example, for prostate cancer, treatment assessments should include incontinence, impotence, and bowel function. The advantage of condition-specific outcome assessment from a quality perspective is that it may most closely reflect a link to the processes of care delivered. Thus if one health plan has an unusually high proportion of individuals with hypertension whose blood pressures are outside the controlled range, one might reasonably conclude that the plan has problems in the management of the disease. The difficulty with condition-specific approaches to quality assessment is that they require substantial investment in developing methods across a sufficiently wide range of diseases to provide a picture of the overall quality of care delivered in a health plan.

One of the things we do not know is the extent to which quality is consistent from condition to condition within a health plan. We hypothesize that even within health plans there is variability in outcomes by condition; some plans may have good outcomes for adult chronic diseases and be less successful in achieving good outcomes for chronic disease in childhood. One study of quality at the hospital level found that the relative rates of complications were similar within institutions, but there was less correlation between medical and surgical cases.[61] The other difficulty in the context of today's information systems is that one may not be able to identify individuals who have particular health problems so that population-based outcome assessments can be conducted.

**Generic.** The generic approach examines outcomes that can be assessed on all individuals, regardless of their health problems. Mortality, general functional status, and patient satisfaction outcomes are most commonly assessed in generic approaches. The advantage to the generic approach is that it can be applied across the entire population enrolled in a health plan or seeing a particular physician. The difficulty with this approach is that research has provided considerably less understanding of the link between what is done in the medical care system and the resulting generic outcomes among the population. There is reason to believe that other factors (such as education and socioeconomic status) enter into determining these outcomes. Further, the need to control for variations in severity and case-mix of a population when making comparisons of generic outcomes is extremely important—and no reliable methods for doing this currently exist.

Patient satisfaction may be the most commonly evaluated generic outcome at the health plan level. Patient satisfaction measures consumers' attitudes about the quality and acceptability of care. A recent review of measures being used in health plans identified a variety of dimensions that are currently being assessed: overall, interpersonal, communication and information giving, timeliness, intention to recommend or use plan again, technical quality, time spent with providers, access and availability, outcomes, choice and continuity, financial aspects and billing, and physical environment.[62] Patient satisfaction is an important predictor of certain patient behaviors such as the likelihood of changing health plans[63] or physicians,[64] and compliance with recommended medical therapy.[65]

**Sentinel or Adverse Events.** This approach identifies some event (usually an adverse outcome) likely to be associated with poor quality of care and tracks the frequency with which such events occur. Some examples of adverse outcomes include mortality, early readmission to a hospital, complications of a surgical procedure, nosocomial infections (those incurred in the hospital), suicide, adverse drug reaction (especially drug-drug interactions), and very low birthweight births. Sentinel events can be useful for identifying potential problems, but it is almost always necessary to conduct further assessments before concluding whether an adverse event was preventable or not. The frequency with which adverse events occur will affect their practicality for quality assessments. Events that occur rarely are less useful for quality monitoring because it is more difficult to determine whether differences are statistically significant.

## What Do We Know About Outcomes?

As with the literature on process quality, it is beyond the scope of this chapter to summarize everything that is known about the outcomes of care. Rather, we provide examples of some of the important findings from the published literature. It should be noted that the three categories of outcomes studies—condition-specific, generic, and adverse events—are not mutually exclusive. For example, mortality is an outcome measure that can be applied in any of these contexts; however, each approach provides a different type of insight into variations in the quality of care.

*Condition-Specific Outcomes.* There is evidence that appropriate monitoring of outcomes can contribute to improvements in the quality and outcomes of care. Perhaps one of the leading examples of this comes from New York State's Cardiac Surgery Reporting System, administered by the New York State Department of Health. Since 1989, hospitals have voluntarily reported data to this system on all open heart surgeries. A clinical database is used to identify preoperative risk factors for coronary artery bypass graft surgery (CABG); these factors are used to estimate and predict risk-adjusted mortality rates for each hospital and surgeon performing CABG in the state. Performance is evaluated by comparing the predicted rates to the actual mortality rates, and the results are made public. Since the system was implemented in 1989, the risk-adjusted mortality rate has declined from 4.17 percent to 2.45 percent—a 41 percent decrease.[66] The policy lesson is encouraging—making severity-adjusted outcomes data publicly available can lead to improved health outcomes.

When evaluating outcomes associated with a particular health plan or provider, it may be useful to examine the overall context in which changes are occurring. For example, mortality due to heart disease has been falling for the past two decades, so improvements in outcomes for heart disease might be part of a general national trend. A recent study examining changes in outcomes of acute myocardial infarction (AMI) among the elderly between 1987 and 1990 found that, in the month following the AMI, mortality decreased from 26 percent to 23 percent; in the year following the AMI, mortality declined from 40 percent to 36 percent.[67] The authors indicate that only a portion of the improvement in outcomes can be attributed to changes in treatment, such as the use of thrombolytic therapy.

Condition-specific outcomes may be used to compare the results of different treatment approaches or for different groups of patients. One study examined the outcomes for Medicare patients undergoing lung resection for lung cancer. The authors found that perioperative mortality was 7.4 percent, while one-year postoperative survival was 69 percent and two-year survival was 54 percent.[68] Survival following surgery was lower for men, older persons, and those who had pneumonectomy rather than a lesser procedure. A study examining clinical outcomes (such as mortality or recurrent infarctions) for men and women treated with thrombolytic therapy after an acute myocardial infarction found that women had worse outcomes than men. Some of the difference was attributable to baseline clinical status (that is, the women were older and had a higher prevalence of co-morbid conditions), but further investigation of sex-related differences in outcome is recommended.[69]

Although mortality is one of the most common outcome measures used, it is a rather blunt instrument for examining variations in quality. Another approach is to examine variations in clinical status variables (for example, glycemic control for diabetics, blood pressure control for hypertensives). A study of diabetes outcomes in the United Kingdom, for example, found that gender (male), years since diagnosis, and characteristics of the practice setting (larger, better equipped, dietician on team, physician specialized in diabetes treatment) were significantly related to better glycemic control.[70] Factors such as age, social class, life-style, attitudes, satisfaction, and knowledge were not correlated with glycemic control.

Condition-specific examinations of quality can also be conducted using symptoms rather than diagnoses. A study comparing access and outcomes of care for Medicare beneficiaries enrolled in HMOs versus fee-for-service who reported having either joint pain or chest pain found that although there were differences in access to care for these patient groups, there were no significant differences in elimination of symptoms. Even so, enrollees with joint pain reported less improvement in symptoms. (HMO enrollees with joint pain had better access to care than fee-for-service enrollees, but HMO enrollees with chest pain had somewhat less access, and HMO enrollees with either symptom were less likely to see a specialist, receive follow-up care, or have their progress monitored.)[71]

Condition-specific measures may also be used for evaluating the quality of comprehensive programs such as community-oriented primary care. A study examining the effectiveness of this approach for control of hypertension found that hypertensive adults treated in the community-oriented primary care model were more likely to have their hypertension under control.[72] While improved control was greatest for men and blacks, all age and racial groups demonstrated improved outcomes in the model program as compared to other sources of care.

*Generic Outcomes.* A summary article examining the efficiency and effectiveness of generic occurrence screening for hospital-based quality assessment concluded that this method is relatively inefficient because of high error rates; sensitivity was estimated to be 70 to 80 percent but specificity ranged from 22 to 73 percent.[73] Effectiveness of the method was limited by lack of interrater reliability among peer reviewers. The authors propose that condition-specific outcome measures be used rather than generic approaches.

Functional outcomes may be used to assess the effect of a policy change. The Medicaid Demonstration Project in Hennepin County, Minnesota, randomly assigned clients with chronic mental illnesses to prepaid plans or to usual (fee-for-service) care. Some of the generic outcome measures used to evaluate the effects of prepaid care on these clients included general health status, physical functioning, social functioning, and community function. The authors found no consistent evidence that enrolling chronically mentally ill clients in prepaid care resulted in worse outcomes in the short run.[74]

Patient satisfaction has been used to compare different systems of care, particularly HMOs and indemnity insurance, but the conclusions from this work are mixed. A recent review of the literature on HMO performance indicates that HMO enrollees tended to be less satisfied with perceived quality of care and patient-physician interactions but were more satisfied with many other aspects of their care, including financial aspects, than patients in indemnity plans.[75] Results from the Medical Outcomes Study indicate that financial access was rated highest in prepaid systems; organizational access, continuity, and accountability were rated highest in indemnity systems; and coordination and comprehensiveness were rated lowest in HMOs.[76] Another review of patient satisfaction with outpatient care indicated that compared to patients in traditional indemnity insurance, patients in HMOs were less satisfied with care overall, access, interpersonal aspects, continuity, and availability of appointments; they were more satisfied with waiting times in physicians' offices and similarly satisfied with technical aspects of care.[77]

*Sentinel or Adverse Events Outcomes.* A study examining variations among hospitals in the frequency of adverse events (defined as injuries due to medical treatment) found that primary teaching hospitals had significantly higher rates of adverse events (4.1 percent versus 3.2 percent on average) and rural hospitals had significantly lower rates (1 percent).[78] The proportion of adverse events due to negligence was lower among primary teaching hospitals (10.7 percent) versus nonteaching hospitals (26.9 percent) and among for-profit hospitals (9.5 percent) versus nonprofit hospitals (25.2 percent) and was significantly higher among hospitals serving predominantly minority populations (37 percent) versus hospitals with fewer than 15 percent minority admissions (21.1 percent).

An example of the potential for using readmission rates as an indicator of quality in the United Kingdom found that readmission rates peaked early in the month following discharge and were considerably lower among surgical specialties as compared with medical specialties (for example, general surgery was 4.1 percent compared with 15.1 percent for geriatric medicine).[79] Readmission patterns did vary with the age and sex of the patient, indicating that standardization for these factors is important.

Complications of care are often used as a generic indicator of adverse outcomes. One study, for example, examined complications in trauma care to evaluate whether the adverse outcomes were the result of provider process errors or patient disease-related events. Complications were a common outcome for trauma cases, with 83 percent of patients experiencing at least one complication. However, 27 percent of the complications were due to provider-related factors, and of those, 23 percent (or 6 percent of all complications) were judged to be a quality problem.[80] Complications of revascularization procedures (death, renal impairment, myocardial infarction) were also used to assess the quality of care delivered to Medicare patients in sixteen hospitals. The study found substantial variation in complications among the hospitals studied; risk-adjustment changed the quality ranking of hospitals performing coronary artery bypass graft surgery but did not significantly change the quality rankings of hospitals performing angioplasty.[81] The authors conclude that when sample sizes are small, adverse outcome measures may be more sensitive than mortality alone for detecting differences in quality.

Adverse events may be used to evaluate the consequences of a policy change. For example, when Massachusetts made health coverage available to uninsured low-income pregnant women, there was interest in whether this would contribute to a statewide reduction in low-birthweight births. During the time period when benefits were expanded for low-income women, however, the rates of adequate prenatal care (that is, care initiated before the third trimester or more than four total visits) declined statewide for women in all insurance categories (Medicare, uninsured, and privately insured). The overall effect was that the improved benefits for low-income women did not result in a decrease in low-birthweight births in the state. One policy lesson is that changes in insurance coverage alone may not significantly improve use of specific services and the outcomes associated with those services.[82]

A study in the twelve Veterans Affairs hospitals found that lower quality of care significantly increased the risk of early hospital readmission ($p < 0.05$) for patients with diabetes, chronic obstructive lung disease, or heart failure.[83] Patients with diabetes and heart failure are at increased risk of readmission because of a failure to adhere to discharge readiness criteria. Patients with chronic obstructive lung disease were at increased risk for readmission because of poor quality workup at admission.

## Uses of Quality Assessments

What are the implications of this review of different approaches to quality assessment for the appropriate uses of these tools and methods? The conclusions differ somewhat depending on the intended audience for the quality assessment. We consider the benefits of these various approaches for use internally, within a health plan, versus externally, for making comparisons among health plans or providers practicing in different systems.

### Internal

The purpose of an internal quality assessment is to identify factors in a single delivery system that might be contributing to substandard performance on quality measures. Internal quality assessment efforts today are an integral part of quality improvement activities such as total quality management or continuous quality improvement. Generally, quality improvement activities involve multidisciplinary teams that start with a problem (for example, low childhood immunization rates) and, through a variety of techniques developed in manufacturing and other industries, attempt to uncover the causes of a failure to achieve performance at the level of best practices within the industry. As discussed earlier in this chapter, much of the quality improvement work undertaken in hospitals and health plans today focuses on systems issues—how information and patients move through the complex organizations. Many quality problems occur because of a failure in communications or data transfer from one part of the organization to another, such as getting laboratory results back to the ordering physician in a timely manner or coordinating care delivery for individuals with complex medical problems.

The focus of internal quality assessment is typically on the process and outcome methods discussed earlier. Within process assessments, adherence to guidelines, practice profiling, and consumer ratings are all used. The standard for comparison is either historical (that is, this year compared to last year within the same plan or clinic or group of physicians) or best practices within the industry. In general, however, the goal is to improve performance over time so while the best practices may define the goal, improvement in historical trends is the objective.

For outcome assessments, there tends to be greater focus on generic and adverse events approaches than on condition-specific approaches. This to some extent reflects the systems orientation of quality improvement activities. For internal assessments, the requirements for case-mix control are substantially lower, especially when examining historical trends, because there are unlikely to be large changes in the characteristics of the population within the time frames used for these activities.

Perhaps the most important factor limiting greater intensity of internal quality improvement activities is the availability of clinically valid data. As information systems increase in their coverage of activities and in the sophistication of their retrieval capacities, opportunities for expanding quality improvement activities will also expand. The competitive markets are likely to witness dramatic changes (for either good or bad in terms of quality) as health plans, hospitals, and medical groups strive to maintain market share.

## External

The purpose of external quality assessment is to make information about quality available to consumers and purchasers to inform their choices among health plans, hospitals, and physicians. There has been a considerable increase in the attempt to use quality assessments for making external comparisons among health plans and physicians. Health insurance purchasers, particularly large employers, have been one of the groups demanding greater accountability for the health care dollar. The development of consumer report cards reflects a belief that individual purchasers require more systematic information about quality in order to make choices among health plans. These efforts are critical to ensuring that information about quality will be available to make comparisons of the cost of care meaningful. We have previously outlined some principles for selecting quality assessment measures for external purposes:[84]

- The methods should be population-based, that is, they should take into account everyone who could benefit from care regardless of whether such services are used.
- The methods should focus on all dimensions of the delivery system rather than on a single setting because of differences among plans in the way care is organized.
- Potential quality problems arising from either overuse or underuse of services should be evaluated.

- The methods should control for differences in the populations enrolled and for factors extraneous to the health delivery system that influence the processes or outcomes of care.

The appropriateness and adherence to guidelines methods meet these criteria and for this reason are the preferred approaches to process quality evaluation. We have recently begun applying the appropriateness methodology to the investigation of underuse.[85] We believe that currently most outcome measures are unsuitable for external comparisons because inadequate methods exist for case-mix adjustment; examinations of the prevalence of preventable adverse events offer one potential outcome approach.[86] Of course, patient satisfaction measures remain an important tool for external comparisons.

The future use of external assessments will be determined by two key factors. The first is the availability of a common set of assessment tools that allow fair comparisons to be made. These tools must either be developed and placed in the public domain, or a consensus must be reached on a proprietary tool that everyone will use. We prefer the first approach. Second, the cost of conducting and producing external assessments must be included in the cost of doing business. Without these factors, the future for comprehensive external assessments is limited.

## Data Sources for Evaluating Quality

For most of these methods, there are some common questions regarding the best source of data for evaluating care. The three sources that are most commonly used are claims or administrative data, medical record data, and consumer surveys.

### Administrative

Administrative data are frequently the preferred source for information about health system performance because they already exist and thus represent a potentially less expensive data resource. Administrative data offer perhaps the best source of information about utilization patterns (such as hospitalization or outpatient visits), prescriptions filled, laboratory tests conducted, and similar billable events. They are also useful for tracking expenditures on care. Administrative data, however, are unlikely to provide information about clinical or functional status, quality of life, adverse events that occur outside the health care system, and satisfaction with care.

## Medical Records

Medical records are an excellent source of information about the technical aspects of care delivery. The medical record is the best source of information for most measures of clinical status and the content of care (such as medications prescribed, test results, and history). Some medical records will contain information about functioning, particularly if the patient is experiencing functional deficits related to treatment interventions (for example, medication side effects). Adverse events that occur in the medical care system will be recorded in the medical record. The medical record is not a very good source of information about other aspects of functioning, quality of life, adverse events outside the medical system (for example, incarceration of a person with a mental disorder), satisfaction, and expenditures.

## Surveys

Surveys of individuals are an excellent source of information about outcomes from the perspective of the individual. In particular, surveys are used to assess functional status, quality of life, and satisfaction. Surveys may also be useful for identifying certain adverse events, particularly those outside the health care system. Surveys are generally considered less accurate for evaluating clinical status and technical processes of care.

## Evidence from the Literature

It is somewhat unusual for the results of internal quality assessments to be published; thus, this section discusses the suitability of the three data sources for external comparisons. Many of the conclusions will apply to internal uses. A comparison of the results for ranking hospitals on risk-adjusted adverse outcomes of coronary artery bypass graft surgery using administrative versus clinical data found that the correlations between rankings based on administrative data and rankings based on clinical data were insignificant.[87] Using only the clinical database, the correlation between rankings based on mortality and major complications was significant—but the correlation between major complications and any complication was negative and insignificant. The authors conclude that administrative data are not adequate for assessing quality of care and that the results based on clinical data will depend on the outcomes selected. Another study evaluating the use of administrative data to screen hospitals for quality improvement actions by Medicare's Peer Review Organizations confirmed the finding that different hospitals were identified for quality review depending on whether the screen was based on mortality rates or complication rates.[88]

A comparison in New York state of clinical versus administrative databases for predicting an individual patient's risk of in-hospital mortality following CABG surgery and for assessing the risk-adjusted mortality rate for CABG procedures for a hospital found that the clinical database was better than the administrative database at predicting case-specific mortality and that the correlations between risk-adjusted hospital mortality rates using the two data systems were moderately high.[89] Much of the difference in the two systems was accounted for by three clinical factors—ejection fraction, reoperation, and greater than 90 percent narrowing of the left main trunk.

An examination of a different set of databases (from Duke University, Minneapolis-St. Paul, the state of California, and the province of Manitoba, Canada) came to the conclusion that clinical databases were superior to administrative data for estimating the relative risk of short-term mortality from coronary artery bypass graft surgery.[90] Much of the difference between the databases is due to incomplete or incorrect coding in administrative databases. An evaluation of the accuracy of Medicare's hospital claims data indicated that while progress had been made between 1977 and 1985, considerable variability existed in the accuracy of diagnosis coding across all major surgical procedures examined.[91] An examination of the agreement between clinical and administrative databases on twelve prognostic indicators for patients with ischemic heart disease found that agreement ranged from 83 percent for the diagnosis of diabetes to 9 percent for the diagnosis of unstable angina.[92] The claims database failed to identify more than half of the patients who were identified in the clinical database as having prognostically important conditions. The authors concluded that claims data were inadequate for identifying clinical subgroups of patients and for performing risk-adjustment that is necessary for comparing hospitals based on outcome data. Because a truly comprehensive quality monitoring system will have to incorporate all of these data sources, efforts must be made to improve the ease with which clinical data are obtained as well as the accuracy with which diagnosis and procedure data are coded in administrative data systems.

## Conclusions

Over the next decade, as policy makers design mechanisms for controlling rising health care costs and the structure of the delivery system continues to change, the need to measure, monitor, and report on the quality of care will only become more important. We have demonstrated in this chapter that a variety of methods exist for systematically evaluating the quality of care. Quality is a multidimensional topic, and efforts to understand how quality is changing with the dynamics of organization and financing in the health delivery system must include both technical and interpersonal excellence in the process of care as well as the full range of outcomes of care—clinical, functional, satisfaction, and life expectancy. While the field of quality assessment stands ready to make a substantial contribution to providing purchasers of health care with the information necessary to make informed choices among health plans, physicians, and hospitals, considerable methodological and logistical work remains to be done to bring quality monitoring into the mainstream of such decision making. Better methods must be developed for adjusting the results of quality assessment for differences in the severity and other characteristics of populations whose care is being evaluated. Improved techniques must be designed to effectively disseminate information on quality to different audiences.

As systems are developed to monitor and publicly report on the quality of care delivered in different health plans and by different providers, more efficient methods for obtaining the data necessary to conduct these activities must be designed. An adequate quality monitoring system will require data from administrative, clinical, and consumer sources; a single data source will never be adequate to inform the multidimensional quality concerns that have been discussed in this chapter. Administrative data have been used extensively for quality assessment because of easy availability; the results from these efforts are of questionable validity, and it is unlikely that administrative data will ever be completely satisfactory for these purposes. In addition to improving administrative data, over the next decade detailed clinical and consumer data must also be made routinely available for quality monitoring.

The U.S. health care system will continue to face the challenge of balancing its three competing goals—containing health care costs, improving access to care, and enhancing the quality of care. As health reform efforts continue in the private sector, at the state level, and perhaps even at the federal level, quality cannot be left behind. The incentives in current cost containment mechanisms pose a direct challenge to quality; without an adequate system for assessing the value of the health care product, quality of care—the dimension in which this country takes greatest pride—may be severely undermined.

## Notes

1. Kathleen N. Lohr (ed.), *Medicare: A Strategy for Quality Assurance*, vol. 1 (Washington, D.C.: National Academy Press, 1990), p. 4.
2. Albert L. Siu, Elizabeth A. McGlynn, Mark H. Beers, et al., *Choosing Quality-of-Care Measures Based on the Expected Impact of Improved Quality of Care for the Major Causes of Mortality and Morbidity*, RAND Pub. No. JR–03 (Santa Monica, Calif.: RAND, 1992).
3. Lucian L. Leape, Lee H. Hilborne, James P. Kahan, et al., *Coronary Artery Bypass Graft: A Literature Review and Ratings of Appropriateness and Necessity*, RAND Pub. No. JRA–02 (Santa Mon-

ica, Calif.: RAND, 1991); Steven J. Bernstein, Marianne Laouri, Lee H. Hilborne, et al., *Coronary Angiography: A Literature Review and Ratings of Appropriateness and Necessity*, RAND Pub. No. JRA–03 (Santa Monica, Calif.: RAND, 1992); Lee H. Hilborne, Lucian L. Leape, James P. Kahan, et al., *Percutaneous Transluminal Coronary Angioplasty: A Literature Review and Ratings of Appropriateness and Necessity*, RAND Pub. No. JRA–01 (Santa Monica, Calif.: RAND, 1991); Steven J. Bernstein, Elizabeth A. McGlynn, Caren J. Kamberg, et al., *Hysterectomy: A Literature Review and Ratings of Appropriateness*, RAND Pub. No. JR–04 (Santa Monica, Calif.: RAND, 1992); and Paul J. Murata, Elizabeth A. McGlynn, Albert L. Siu, and Robert H. Brook, *Prenatal Care: A Literature Review and Quality Assessment Criteria*, RAND Pub. No. JR–05 (Santa Monica, Calif.: RAND, 1992).

4. Siu, McGlynn, Beers, et al., *Choosing Quality-of-Care Measures*.

5. Avedis Donabedian, *Explorations in Quality Assessment and Monitoring;* vol. 1: *The Definition of Quality and Approaches to its Assessment* (Ann Arbor, Mich.: Health Administration Press, 1980).

6. American Medical Association, *Physician Characteristics and Distribution in the U.S.* (Chicago: American Medical Association, 1993).

7. American Medical Association, *Physician Characteristics*.

8. American Medical Association, *Physician Characteristics*.

9. Katherine L. Kahn, Marjorie L. Pearson, Ellen R. Harrison, et al., "Health Care for Black and Poor Hospitalized Medicare Patients," *Journal of the American Medical Association* 271 (1993): 1169–1174.

10. Emmett B. Keeler, Lisa V. Rubenstein, Katherine L. Kahn, et al., "Hospital Characteristics and Quality of Care," *JAMA* 268 (1992): 1709–1714.

11. Sheldon Greenfield, Eugene C. Nelson, Michael Zubkoff, et al., "Variations in Resource Utilization Among Medical Specialties and Systems of Care: Results from the Medical Outcomes Study," *JAMA* 267 (1992): 1624–1630.

12. John E. Wennberg, Jean L. Freeman, Roxanne M. Shelton, and Thomas A. Bubolz, "Hospital Use and Mortality Among Medicare Beneficiaries in Boston and New Haven," *New England Journal of Medicine* 321 (1989): 1168–1173.

13. Paul D. Cleary, Sheldon Greenfield, Albert G. Mulley, et al., "Variations in Length of Stay and Outcomes for Six Medical and Surgical Conditions in Massachusetts and California," *JAMA* 266 (1991): 73–79.

14. Steven J. Katz and Timothy P. Hofer, "Socioeconomic Disparities in Preventive Care Persist Despite Universal Coverage: Breast and Cervical Cancer Screening in Ontario and the United States," *JAMA* 272 (1994): 530–534.

15. Lu Ann Aday, Eun Sul Lee, Bill Spears, et al., "Health Insurance and Utilization of Medical Care for Children with Special Health Care Needs," *Medical Care* 31 (1993): 1013–1026.

16. Joseph P. Newhouse and the Insurance Experiment Group, *Free for All? Lessons Learned from the RAND Health Insurance Experiment* (Cambridge, Mass.: Harvard University Press, 1993).

17. Robert H. Brook, John E. Ware, Jr., William H. Rogers, et al., "Does Free Care Improve Adults' Health? Results from a Randomized Controlled Trial," *New England Journal of Medicine* 309 (1983): 1426–1434.

18. Harold S. Luft, Sandra S. Hunt, and Susan C. Maerki, "The Volume-Outcome Relationship: Practice-Makes-Perfect or Selective-Referral Patterns?" *Health Services Research* 22 (June 1987): 157–182.

19. Edward L. Hannan, Albert L. Siu, Dinesh Kumar, et al., "The Decline in Coronary Artery Bypass Graft Surgery Mortality in New York State: The Role of Surgeon Volume," *JAMA* 273 (1995): 209–213.

20. Robert H. Brook, "The RAND/UCLA Appropriateness Method," in *Clinical Practice Guideline Development: Methodology Perspectives,* AHCPR Pub. No. 95–0009, eds. Kathleen A. McCormick, Steven R. Moore, and Randie A. Siegel (Rockville, Md.: U.S. Department of Health and Human Services, Public Health Service, Agency for Health Care Policy and Research, November 1994), pp. 59–70; and Robert H. Brook, Mark R. Chassin, Arlene Fink, et al., "A Method for the Detailed Assessment of the Appropriateness of Medical Technologies," *International Journal of Technology Assessment* 2 (1986): 53–63.

21. Robert H. Brook, "The RAND/UCLA Appropriateness Method," pp. 59–70.

22. Mark R. Chassin, Jacqueline Kosecoff, and R. E. Park, "Does Inappropriate Use Explain Geographic Variations in the Use of Health Care Services? A Study of Three Procedures," *JAMA* 258 (1987): 2533–2537; and Lucian L. Leape, Elizabeth A. McGlynn, C. David Naylor, et al., *Coronary Angiography: Ratings of Appropriateness and Necessity by a Canadian Panel,* RAND Pub. No. MR–129–CWF/PCT (Santa Monica, Calif.: RAND, 1993).

23. Bernstein, McGlynn, Kamberg, et al., *Hysterectomy: A Literature Review.*

24. Lucian L. Leape, Lee H. Hilborne, Rolla Edward Park, et al., "The Appropriateness of Use of Coronary Artery Bypass Graft Surgery in New York State," *JAMA* 269 (1993): 753–760; and Steven J. Bernstein, Elizabeth A. McGlynn, Albert L. Siu, et al., "The Appropriateness of Hysterectomy: A Comparison of Care in Seven Health Plans," *JAMA* 269 (1993): 2398–2402.

25. Urinary Incontinence Guideline Panel, *Urinary Incontinence in Adults: Clinical Practical Guidelines,* AHCPR Pub. No. 92–0038 (Rockville, Md.: U.S. Department of Health and Human Services, Public Health Service, Agency for Health Care Policy and Research, March 1992), p. ii.

26. As of this writing, guidelines had been developed for acute pain management for operative or medical procedures and trauma; urinary incontinence in adults; prediction, prevention, and treatment of pressure ulcers in adults; management of functional impairment due to cataracts in adults; detection, diagnosis, and treatment of major depression in primary care; screening, diagnosis, management, and counseling regarding sickle cell disease in newborns and infants; evaluation and management of early HIV infection; diagnosis and treatment of benign prostatic hyperplasia; management of cancer pain; diagnosis and management of unstable angina; evaluation and care of patients with left-ventricular systolic dysfunction; otitis media with effusion in young children; and acute low back problems in adults.

27. Kathleen A. McCormick, Steven R. Moore, and Randie A. Siegel (eds.), *Clinical Practice Guideline Development: Methodology Perspectives,* AHCPR Pub. No. 95–0009 (Rockville, Md.: U.S. Department of Health and Human Services, Public Health Service, Agency for Health Care Policy and Research, November 1994).

28. Roz Diane Lasker, David W. Shapiro, and Anthony M. Tucker, "Realizing the Potential of Practice Pattern Profiling," *Inquiry* 29 (1992): 287–297.

29. Lasker, Shapiro, and Tucker, "Realizing the Potential of Practice Pattern Profiling."

30. H. Gilbert Welch, Mark E. Miller, and W. Pete Welch, "Physician Profiling: An Analysis of Inpatient Practice Patterns in Florida and Oregon," *New England Journal of Medicine* 330 (1994): 607–612; Susanne Salem-Schatz, Gordon Moore, Malcolm Rucker, and Steven D. Pearson, "The Case for Case-Mix Adjustment in Practice Profiling: When Good Apples Look Bad," *JAMA* 272 (1994): 871–874; Barbara J. McNeil, Sarah H. Pedersen, and Constantine Gatsonis, "Current Issues in Profiling Quality of Care," *Inquiry* 29 (1992): 298–307; and Lasker, Shapiro, and Tucker, "Realizing the Potential of Practice Pattern Profiling."

31. Salem-Schatz, Moore, Rucker, and Pearson, "The Case for Case-Mix Adjustment."

32. Richard L. Kravitz, Sheldon Greenfield, William Rogers, et al., "Differences in the Mix of Patients Among Medical Specialties and Systems of Care: Results from the Medical Outcomes Study," *JAMA* 267 (1992): 1617–1623.

33. McNeil, Pedersen, and Gatsonis, "Current Issues in Profiling"; and Welch, Miller, and Welch, "Physician Profiling."

34. Mark R. Chassin, Jacqueline Kosecoff, David H. Solomon, and Robert H. Brook, "How Coronary Angiography Is Used: Clinical Determinants of Appropriateness," *JAMA* 258 (1987): 2543–2547; Steven J. Bernstein, Lee H. Hilborne, Lucian L. Leape, et al., "The Appropriateness of Use of Coronary Angiography in New York State," *JAMA* 269 (1993): 766–769; Lee H. Hilborne, Lucian L. Leape, Steven J. Bernstein, et al., "The Appropriateness of Use of Percutaneous Transluminal Coronary Angioplasty in New York State," *JAMA* 269 (1993): 761–765; Leape, Hilborne, Park, et al., "The Appropriateness of Use of Coronary Artery Bypass Graft Surgery in New York State"; Constance Monroe Winslow, Jacqueline B. Kosecoff, Mark Chassin, et al., "The Appropriateness of Performing Coronary Artery Bypass Surgery," *JAMA* 260 (1988): 505–509; Bernstein, McGlynn, Siu, et al., "The Appropriateness of Hysterectomy"; Constance M. Winslow, David H. Solomon, Mark R. Chassin, et al., "The Appropriateness of Carotid Endarterectomy," *New England Journal of Medicine* 318 (1988): 721–727; Chassin, Kosecoff, and Park, "Does Inappropriate Use Explain Geographic Variations?"; Personal communication from Paul Lee, M.D., April 27, 1995; and Lawrence C. Kleinman, Jacqueline Kosecoff, Robert W. Dubois, and Robert H. Brook, "The Medical Appropriateness of Tympanostomy Tubes Proposed for Children Younger Than 16 Years in the United States," *JAMA* 271 (1994): 1250–1255.

35. Chassin, Kosecoff, and Park, "Does Inappropriate Use Explain Geographic Variations?"

36. Albert L. Siu, Arleen Leibowitz, and Robert H. Brook, "Use of the Hospital in a Randomized Trial of Prepaid Care," *JAMA* 259 (1988): 1343–1346.

37. Elizabeth A. McGlynn, C. David Naylor, Geoffrey M. Anderson, et al., "Comparison of the Appropriateness of Coronary Angiography and Coronary Artery Bypass Graft Surgery Between Canada and New York State," *JAMA* 272 (1994): 934–940.

38. David Gray, John R. Hampton, Steven J. Bernstein, et al., "Clinical Practice: Audit of Coronary Angiography and Bypass Surgery," *Lancet* 335 (1990): 1317–1320.

39. Dina Pilpel, Gerald M. Fraser, Jacqueline Kosecoff, et al., "Regional Differences in Appropriateness of Cholecystectomy in a Prepaid Health Insurance System," *Public Health Reviews* 20 (1992/93): 61–74.

40. Albert L. Siu, Frank A. Sonnenberg, Willard G. Manning, et al., "Inappropriate Use of Hospitals in a Randomized Trial of Health Insurance Plans," *New England Journal of Medicine* 315 (1986): 1259–1266.

41. Stephen M. Soumerai, Jerry Avorn, Dennis Ross-Degnan, and Steven Gortmaker, "Payment Restrictions for Prescription Drugs Under Medicaid: Effects on Therapy, Cost, and Equity," *New England Journal of Medicine* 317 (1987): 550–556.

42. Geoffrey M. Anderson, Kevin Grumbach, Harold S. Luft, et al., "Use of Coronary Artery Bypass Surgery in the United States and Canada," *JAMA* 269 (1993): 1661–1666.

43. Jeremy M. Grimshaw and Ian T. Russell, "Effect of Clinical Guidelines on Medical Practice: A Systematic Review of Rigorous Evaluations," *Lancet* 342 (1993): 1317–1322.

44. Paul J. Murata, Elizabeth A. McGlynn, Albert L. Siu, et al., "Quality Measures for Pre-natal Care: A Comparison of Care in Six Health Care Plans," *Archives of Family Medicine* 3 (1994): 41–49.

45. National Committee on Quality Assurance, *Report Card Pilot Project* (Washington, D.C.: National Committee on Quality Assurance, 1995).

46. Andrew J. Doorey, Eric L. Michelson, and Eric J. Topol, "Thrombolytic Therapy of Acute Myocardial Infarction: Keeping the Unfulfilled Promises," *JAMA* 268 (1992): 3108–3114.

47. Chris L. Pashos, Sharon-Lise T. Normand, Jeffrey B. Garfinkle, et al., "Trends in the Use of Drug Therapies in Patients with Acute Myocardial Infarction: 1988 to 1992," *Journal of the American College of Cardiology* 23 (1994): 1023–1030.

48. Kenneth B. Wells, Wayne Katon, Bill Rogers, and Patti Camp, "Use of Minor Tranquilizers and Antidepressant Medications by Depressed Outpatients: Results from the Medical Outcomes Study," *American Journal of Psychiatry* 151 (1994): 694–700; and Wayne Katon, Michael Von Koeff, Elizabeth Lin, et al., "Adequacy and Duration of Antidepressant Treatment in Primary Care," *Medical Care* 30 (1992): 67–76.

49. Mark Olfson and Gerald L. Klerman, "Trends in the Prescription of Psychotropic Medications: The Role of Physician Specialty," *Medical Care* 31 (1993): 559–564; and Wells, Katon, Rogers, and Camp, "Use of Minor Tranquilizers."

50. Depression Guideline Panel, *Depression in Primary Care;* vol. 2: *Treatment of Major Depression, Clinical Practice Guideline Number 5,* AHCPR Pub. No. 93–0551 (Rockville, Md.: U.S. Department of Health and Human Services, Public Health Service, Agency for Health Care Policy and Research, 1993).

51. Wells, Katon, Rogers, and Camp, "Use of Minor Tranquilizers."

52. Edmund J. Graves, "Detailed Diagnoses and Procedures, National Hospital Discharge Survey, 1990," in *Vital and Health Statistics,* DHHS Pub. No. (PHS) 92–1774, 13 (Hyattsville, Md.: National Center for Health Statistics, 1992).

53. Wennberg, Freeman, Shelton, and Bubolz, "Hospital Use and Mortality Among Medicare Beneficiaries."

54. Welch, Miller, and Welch, "Physician Profiling."

55. Allyson Ross Davies and John E. Ware, Jr., "Involving Consumers in Quality of Care Assessment," *Health Affairs* 7 (Spring 1988): 33–48.

56. Barbara Gerbert and William A. Hargreaves, "Measuring Physician Behavior," *Medical Care* 24 (1986): 838–847.

57. Andrew Wilson and Paul McDonald, "Comparison of Patient Questionnaire, Medical Record, and Audio Tape in Assessment of Health Promotion in General Practice Consultations," *British Medical Journal* 309 (1994): 1483–1485.

58. Michael D. Kogan, Greg R. Alexander, Milton Kotelchuck, et al., "Comparing Mothers' Reports on the Content of Prenatal Care Received with Recommended National Guidelines for Care," *Public Health Reports* 109 (1994): 637–646.

59. Donald M. Berwick and Donald L. Wald, "Hospital Leaders' Opinions of the HCFA Mortality Data," *JAMA* 263 (1990): 247–249.

60. Steven T. Fleming, Lanis L. Hicks, and R. Clifton Bailey, "Interpreting the Health Care Financing Administration's Mortality Statistics," *Medical Care* 33 (1995): 186–201.

61. Lisa I. Iezzoni, Jennifer Daley, Timothy Heeren, et al., "Using Administrative Data to Screen Hospitals for High Complication Rates," *Inquiry* 31 (1994): 40–55.

62. Marsha Gold and Judith Woolridge, "Plan-Based Surveys of Satisfaction with Access and Quality of Care: Review and Critique," paper delivered at Consumer Survey Information in a Reformed Health Care System conference, co-sponsored by the Agency for Health Care Policy and Research and the Robert Wood Johnson Foundation, September 1994).

63. Davies and Ware, "Involving Consumers."

64. M. Susan Marquis, Allyson R. Davies, and John E. Ware, Jr., "Patient Satisfaction and Change in Medical Care Provider: A Longitudinal Study," *Medical Care* 21 (1983): 821–829.

65. John E. Ware, Jr., Mary K. Snyder, W. Russell Wright, and Allyson Ross Davies, "Defining and Measuring Patient Satisfaction with Medical Care," *Evaluation and Program Planning* 6 (1983): 247–263; and Cathy Donald Sherbourne, Ron D. Hays, Lynn Ordway, et al., "Antecedents of Adherence to Medical Recommendations: Results from the Medical Outcomes Study," *Journal of Behavioral Medicine* 15 (1992): 447–468.

66. Edward L. Hannan, Harold Kilburn, Michael Racz, et al., "Improving the Outcomes of Coronary Artery Bypass Surgery in New York State," *JAMA* 271 (1994): 761–766.

67. Chris L. Pashos, Joseph P. Newhouse, and Barbara J. McNeil, "Temporal Changes in the Care and Outcomes of Elderly Patients with Acute Myocardial Infarction, 1987 Through 1990," *JAMA* 270 (1993): 1832–1836.

68. Jeffrey Whittle, Earl P. Steinberg, Gerard F. Anderson, and Robert Herbert, "Use of Medicare Claims Data to Evaluate Outcomes in Elderly Patients Undergoing Lung Resection for Lung Cancer," *Chest* (1991): 729–734.

69. Richard C. Becker, Michael Terrin, Richard Ross, et al., "Comparison of Clinical Outcomes for Women and Men After Acute Myocardial Infarction," *Annals of Internal Medicine* 120 (1994): 638–645.

70. Mike Pringle, Carol Stewart-Evans, Carol Coupland, et al., "Influences on Control in Diabetes Mellitus: Patient, Doctor, Practice, or Delivery of Care?" *BMJ* 306 (1993): 630–634.

71. Delores G. Clement, Sheldon M. Retchin, Randall S. Brown, and MeriBeth H. Stegall, "Access and Outcomes of Elderly Patients Enrolled in Managed Care," *JAMA* 271 (1994): 1487–1492.

72. Patrick J. O'Connor, Edward H. Wagner, and David S. Strogatz, "Hypertension Control in a Rural community: An Assessment of Community-Oriented Primary Care," *Journal of Family Practice* 30 (1990): 420–424.

73. Paul J. Sanzaro and Don H. Mills, "A Critique of the Use of Generic Screening in Quality Assessment," *JAMA* 265 (1991): 1977–1981.

74. Nicole Lurie, Ira S. Moscovice, Michael Finch, et al., "Does Capitation Affect the Health of the Chronically Mentally Ill? Results from a Randomized Trial," *JAMA* 267 (1992): 3300–3304.

75. Robert H. Miller and Harold S. Luft, "Managed Care Plan Performance Since 1980: A Literature Analysis," *JAMA* 271 (1994): 1512–1519.

76. Dana G. Safran, Alvin R. Tarlov, and William H. Rogers, "Primary Care Performance in Fee-for-Service and Prepaid Health Care Systems: Results from the Medical Outcomes Study," *JAMA* 271 (1994): 1579–1586.

77. Donald A. Barr, "The Effects of Organizational Structure on Primary Care Outcomes Under Managed Care," *Annals of Internal Medicine* 122 (1995): 353–359.

78. Troyen A. Brennan, Liesi E. Hebert, Nan M. Laird, et al., "Hospital Characteristics Associated with Adverse Events and Substandard Care," *JAMA* 265 (1991): 3265–3269.

79. Mike Chambers and Aileen Clarke, "Measuring Readmission Rates," *BMJ* 301 (1990): 1134–1136.

80. D. B. Hoyt, P. Hollingsworth-Fridlund, R. J. Winchell, et al., "Analysis of Recurrent Process Errors Leading to Provider-Related Complications on an Organized Trauma Service: Directions for Care Improvement," *Journal of Trauma* 36 (1994): 377–384.

81. Arthur J. Hartz, Evelyn M. Kuhn, Kenneth L. Kayser, et al., "Assessing Providers of Coronary Revascularization: A Method for Peer Review Organizations," *American Journal of Public Health* 82 (1992): 1631–1640.

82. Jennifer S. Haas, I. Steven Udvarhelyi, Carl N. Morris, and Arnold M. Epstein, "The Effect of Providing Health Coverage to Poor Uninsured Pregnant Women in Massachusetts," *JAMA* 269 (1993): 87–91.

83. Carol M. Ashton, David H. Kuykendall, Michael L. Johnson, et al., "The Association Between the Quality of Inpatient Care and Early Readmission," *Annals of Internal Medicine* 122 (1995): 415–421.

84. Albert L. Siu, Elizabeth A. McGlynn, Hal Morgenstern, and Robert H. Brook, "A Fair Approach to Comparing Quality of Care," *Health Affairs* (Spring 1991): 62–75.

85. David M. Carlisle, Barbara D. Leake, and Martin F. Shapiro, "Racial and Ethnic Differences in the Use of Invasive Cardiac Procedures Among Cardiac Patients in Los Angeles County, 1986 Through 1988," *AJPH* 85 (1995): 352–56.

86. Robert W. Dubois and Robert H. Brook, "Preventable Deaths: Who, How Often, and Why?" *Annals of Internal Medicine* 109 (1988): 582–589.

87. Arthur J. Hartz and Evelyn M. Kuhn, "Comparing Hospitals That Perform Coronary Artery Bypass Surgery: The Effect of Outcome Measures and Data Sources," *AJPH* 84 (1994): 1609–1614.

88. Iezzoni, Daley, Heeren, et al., "Using Administrative Data."

89. Edward J. Hannan, Harold Kilburn, Jr., Michael L. Lindsey, and Rudy Lewis, "Clinical Versus Administrative Data Bases for CABG Surgery: Does It Matter?" *Medical Care* 30 (1992): 892–907.

90. Patrick S. Romano, Leslie L. Roos, Harold S. Luft, et al., "A Comparison of Administrative Versus Clinical Data: Coronary Artery Bypass Surgery as an Example," *Journal of Clinical Epidemiology* 47 (1994): 249–260.

91. Elliott S. Fisher, Fredrick S. Whaley, Mark Krushat, et al., "The Accuracy of Medicare's Hospital Claims Data: Progress Has Been Made, but Problems Remain," *AJPH* 82 (1992): 243–248.

92. James G. Jollis, Marek Ancukiewicz, Elizabeth R. DeLong, et al., "Discordance of Databases Designed for Claims Payment Versus Clinical Information Systems: Implications for Outcomes Research," *Annals of Internal Medicine* 119 (1993): 844–850.

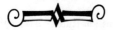

CHAPTER EIGHT

# LONG-TERM CARE AND THE ELDERLY

Steven P. Wallace, Emily K. Abel, and Pamela Stefanowicz

The health service needs of people in the United States have changed dramatically during the past century as a result of the shift from acute to chronic conditions and an increasing life expectancy. In 1900, the major health problems stemmed from acute infectious diseases such as typhoid, smallpox, and dysentery. People usually recovered or died rapidly from those diseases. By midcentury, three chronic conditions alone—heart disease, cancer, and stroke—accounted for over 50 percent of deaths; today, chronic illnesses are the predominant cause of death.[1] Reductions in acute illnesses have contributed to a historic increase in life expectancy, from 47 years in 1900 to 75.3 years in 1989. Because the birthrate also is falling, elderly people constitute a growing segment of the population. By 2035, one in five U.S. residents (sixty-seven million people) will be age sixty-five and over.[2] Disabilities can affect people of any age, but the rate increases with age. Only 2.4 percent of people under sixty-five need any assistance with daily activities, compared to almost half of those eighty-five and over.[3] People with chronic illnesses frequently experience disabilities and require assistance over extended periods.

Long-term care is the set of health and social services delivered over a sustained period to people who have lost (or never acquired) some capacity for personal care; ideally, it enables recipients to live with as much independence and dignity as possible.[4] Provided in institutional, community, and home settings, long-term care encompasses a wide array of services ranging from rehabilitation and nursing care to assistance with such daily activities as walking, bathing, cooking, and managing money. The care can be furnished either by paid providers (formal care) or by unpaid family and friends (informal care), or a combination of the two. Long-term care differs from most topics discussed in this volume because it includes social as well as medical services.

This chapter reviews the recent literature on long-term care, showing how financial considerations have framed the dominant policy debates and research agenda. Policy makers frequently view nursing homes as low-cost alternatives to hospitals and consider community services and family care as less expensive substitutes for nursing homes. Both policy makers and researchers tend to ignore the diversity among older people as well as the problems faced by low-income women who serve as caregivers in both paid and unpaid capacities.

## Nursing Homes

The term *nursing home* covers a wide variety of institutions including *skilled nursing facilities,* which offer twenty-four-hour nursing care, and *residential care facilities,* which provide some personal care but no licensed nursing care. Public policy first encouraged the establishment of private nursing homes in 1935, when Old Age Assistance (public aid for low-income elderly; part of the Social Security Act) specifically barred residents of public alms houses or similar facilities from receiving this aid. The federal government provided funds directly for the construction of nursing homes in the 1950s in an attempt to solve a hospital bed shortage and to save money by discharging hospital patients to a less intensive level of care. Public funding of nursing homes expanded dramatically after the passage of Medicare and Medicaid in 1965, leading to a rapid growth in the number of facilities. Both programs defined nursing homes as predominantly medical institutions, emphasizing the nursing over the home.[5] The reimbursement formula encouraged for-profit enterprises; three-quarters of free-standing nursing homes now are profit making.[6]

Although most older people assume that Medicare covers nursing home stays,[7] Medicare accounts for only 8.8 percent of total nursing home expenditures. The program pays for one hundred days of posthospital recovery care in a nursing home; it provides no coverage for custodial care. Medicaid, by contrast, pays for custodial as well as skilled nursing care and has thus become the primary funding source. It finances 51.7 percent of all nursing home expenditures and represents approximately 83 percent of the total $43.6 billion government expenditure on nursing homes.[8] While about 40 percent of nursing home users enter facilities paying privately, many of them become eligible for Medicaid after spending down or depleting their resources. The annual cost of a nursing home stay in 1993 was $37,000, a sum that exceeded the incomes of four-fifths of elderly people.[9] Nursing home spend-down has attracted policy attention because those who spend down account for a significant proportion of Medicaid nursing home costs and because the phenomenon demonstrates the catastrophic costs of long-term care.[10]

Nursing homes dominate long-term care spending. The rapid and unexpected rise in government expenditures for nursing homes during the 1960s and 1970s contributed to the policy focus on containing costs. Research has distinguished two types of nursing home users: those with short stays, typical of posthospital use, and those with longer stays, typical of more custodial use.[11] The long-stay residents consume most nursing home funds.[12] Research in this area has been used extensively in developing private long-term care insurance.[13]

Other research has concentrated on designing, implementing, and evaluating alternative reimbursement methods.[14] Studies suggest that although various techniques, especially prospective payment, have slowed increasing costs, they also have reduced access for Medicaid patients and limited the supply of beds below needed levels.[15] To discourage nursing homes from taking only the least disabled (and least expensive) Medicaid patients, some states have tried reimbursement formulas that pay more for the care of the most disabled. But this system may have the unintended consequence of reducing access for those needing only custodial care. One group of researchers concluded that reimbursements often reflect state budget balances and overall states resources more than the actual costs of providing nursing home care or improving quality.[16]

Although economic issues dominate research and policy, widespread concern about the treatment of nursing home residents (especially after highly publicized scandals) has kept some attention on quality-of-care issues. The definition of quality has changed over the years. Initially, regulations defined quality in terms of such structural features as conforming to fire and safety codes. Regulations then began to include measures of process, such as whether bedbound patients are repositioned frequently enough to prevent pressure sores. Most recently, federal nursing home regulations have broadened to cover some outcome measures, such as changes in functional status and psychosocial well-being as indicators of quality.[17] Some researchers have shown how nursing homes can reduce accidental falls, urinary incontinence, decubitus ulcers, and the use of physical restraints and psychotropic drugs.[18] Others have examined quality differences between for-profit and not-for-profit nursing homes, finding that the latter generally provide better care.[19] Studies documenting the high use of chemical and physical restraints, inadequate supervision of care by physicians and professional nurses, and the poor quality of life in many institutions helped inform the detailed language in the 1987 federal Omnibus Budget Reconciliation Act (OBRA) on nursing home quality.

OBRA included national standards for the training of nursing home aides, the presence of social work staff, and the delivery of medical care in nursing homes,[20] but poor quality facilities remain common.[21]

## Community-Based Services

For many, long-term care conjures up the image of bedridden elderly residents in nursing homes. But most older people with functional limitations remain at home, often receiving assistance from family and friends as well as community agencies. Community-based services include adult day care, transportation services, and congregate meals. Home care includes home-delivered meals, visiting nurses, home health aides who can provide basic help from bathing to housework, and homemakers or chore workers who assist with housecleaning as well as personal care. We refer to both in- and out-of-home services as *community-based services* in this chapter.

Public funding for community-based services is limited. Medicare emphasizes medically oriented home care, not the social support services many people need to live independently in the community. Recipients must be homebound, under the care of a physician, and in need of part-time or intermittent skilled nursing or physical or speech therapy.[22] The experimental Social Health Maintenance Organizations (SHMOs), which combine the prepaid, at-risk features of regular HMOs with a $6,500 to $12,000 chronic care benefit, offer an exception to these Medicare restrictions. However, continuing difficulties in controlling costs, as well as failure to coordinate acute and chronic medical services,[23] make it unlikely that SHMOs will represent a major expansion of long-term care under Medicare.

Medicaid, unlike Medicare, does not limit community-based services to post-acute care. The government's concern with reducing Medicaid nursing home spending encouraged the expansion of Medicaid coverage for community-based services. Legislation passed in 1981 gave states the option of applying for waivers from existing Medicaid rules in order to provide case management, personal care, respite care, and adult day care.[24] Regulations sought to ensure that such services substituted for, and cost less than, nursing home placement. Largely as a result of these waivers, Medicaid spending on community-based services doubled between 1989 and 1993. Nevertheless, just 5 percent of Medicaid's $191 billion budget is spent on community-based services, while 33 percent is spent on nursing homes.[25]

Two other major programs that fund services for elderly people in the community are Title III of the Older Americans Act and the Social Services Block Grant. Both have fixed annual budgets that are substantially smaller than the amount spent by Medicaid on community-based services and thus may run out of money before the end of the year and refuse to accept new clients. Moreover, the amount of assistance provided to each recipient tends to be even smaller than that furnished by Medicaid programs.[26]

The policy focus on cost containment has shaped the direction of research on community care. A major policy concern has been to develop methods of targeting community-based services. A series of channeling demonstration projects in the early 1980s provided a range of community services in an attempt to evaluate the money saved by keeping disabled elderly people out of nursing homes. Evaluators concluded that some highly disabled clients would not have entered institutions even without access to the community services.[27] Thus, although community-based services are usually cheaper than nursing home care for an individual, total costs tend to be higher because more persons are served by community-based care than would have been served by nursing homes. These findings, coupled with rising Medicaid costs, have stimulated research on identifying clients at imminent risk of institutionalization or those inappropriately placed in nursing homes so that community services can be targeted to them alone.[28] Drawing primarily on the Andersen model of health services utilization,[29] researchers have identified characteristics of elderly people that increase the probability of nursing home placement—increased age, poorer health status, increased functional impairment, being white, living alone, and not owning a home.[30]

Another body of research addresses the policy concern that publicly funded care not substitute for care provided without charge by family and friends. Such a concern is based on the premise that formal and informal (unpaid) services are interchangeable and that an hour of paid care results in one less hour of care by family members. Most studies of the intersection of formal and informal services focus exclusively on the allocation of tasks between family caregivers and formal providers. Most family members, however, conceptualize caregiving as a complex relationship, not simply as a set of discrete tasks. It is thus unsurprising that researchers consistently find that formal services supplement rather than supplant informal care.[31]

A similar line of research arises from a fear that large numbers of elderly people will come out of the woodwork to use new services because community-based services like household cleaning, unlike nursing homes, are believed to lack built-in limitations on consumption. Although the potential pool of clients of community-based services is vast, a critical issue for some community agencies is recruiting clientele, not controlling intake.[32] Some elderly people postpone accepting assistance until they are extremely disabled in order to maintain a sense of independence.[33] Having absorbed a value system that glorifies self-sufficiency, they may be unable to rely on others even when very needy. Some elderly people also may cling to housekeeping chores as a way of separating themselves from their more severely impaired counterparts. As Alan Sager comments, "The notion of a horde of greedy old people and lazy family members anxious to soak up new public benefits appears to be more a projection by a few wealthy legislators accustomed to domestic and hotel and restaurant service than it is a realistic image of our nation's elderly citizens."[34]

Moreover, one person's latent demand is another's unmet need.[35] Those who fear that the expansion of community services will open the floodgates implicitly acknowledge that the elderly are drastically underserved. Only 36 percent of the 5.6 million functionally impaired elderly people living in the community receive any formal care.[36] More than half of those with the severest disabilities receive no formal help.[37]

Policy on the quality of existing community-based care is at least fifteen years behind similar nursing home policy. Several organizations, such as the Joint Commission on the Accreditation of Health Care Organizations, have developed voluntary accreditation standards for some types of community care, but research that defines quality in community settings and develops a methodology for measuring quality is just beginning.[38]

## Variations in the Need for Formal Services

As the previous two sections have shown, the research and policy focus on financial considerations has overshadowed public health concerns such as equity, adequacy, and quality. Understanding variations by race/ethnicity, gender, and class can help identify critical research and policy issues that previously have received inadequate attention.

The elderly population is becoming increasingly African American, Latino, Native American, and Asian American. These groups constituted approximately 14 percent of the elderly population in 1990 and are expected to represent approximately 33 percent by 2050.[39] Thus, programs aimed at the types and levels of functional disabilities of elderly whites may become less appropriate. Elderly African Americans have the highest age-adjusted rates of death and functional limitations, caused in part by higher rates of hypertension, diabetes, circulatory problems, and arthritis. Elderly African Americans also are more likely to rate their health as fair or poor.[40] Research on the functional disabilities of Latinos is inconsistent. Some studies show that Latinos have fewer disabilities than all other groups, some report similar levels, and some find higher levels. Older Latinos have lower death rates than whites overall, but have higher death rates from diabetes, accidents, and chronic liver disease.[41] Asian American elderly generally have functional limitations and health status similar to those of white elderly. Aggregate data, however, mask the increasing diversity within Asian American communities. Some Asian American groups, especially recent immigrants, have long-term care needs that differ dramatically from those of whites.[42]

Women constitute 60 percent of the elderly population and 72 percent of those eighty-five and over. Women at every age experience more functional limitations than men. Women also have a disproportionate need for formal long-term care because many live by themselves. Eighty percent of elderly people living alone are women; 42 percent of all elderly women and 53 percent of those seventy-five and over live alone.[43]

Class also influences the need for long-term care. Research on aging in the United States generally focuses on income (a point-in-time measure of cash flow) rather than class (a long-term position in the economic stratification system that also includes assets and occupational position). Research outside the United States suggests that class position has a direct impact on health status, independent of access to health care. A Swedish study of people eighty-five and over reported that former blue-collar workers are twice as likely as former white-collar workers to experience limitations in activities of daily living.[44] In the United States, functional limitations are highest among elderly people with relatively low incomes, even after controlling for age and race.[45]

Race/ethnicity, gender, and class interact, intensifying the need for long-term care and aggravating access barriers. The disability rate is highest among African American women, being about 50 percent higher than that among white males.[46] And those with the greatest need for long-term care have the least ability to pay for it. In 1992, elderly men's median income was $14,548 while elderly women's was $8,189. The median income for white men sixty-five and over was $15,276, two and one-half times more than that of elderly African American and Latina women—$6,220 and $5,968, respectively.[47] This results in approximately 80 percent of African American elderly people entering nursing homes on Medicaid, compared to under 40 percent of whites.[48] The term *multiple jeopardy* has been used to describe this cumulative disadvantage of age, race, gender, and class in regard to health, income, and other life situations.[49]

## Variations in the Use of Long-Term Care

Policy makers and the media tend to inaccurately consider the elderly as a homogeneous group. Examining the variations by gender, race, and class in the use of long-term care services highlights some of the problems faced by segments of the older population in obtaining equitable access to needed services.

## Gender

Women are much more likely to enter nursing homes than men; 70 percent of nursing home residents are women, and women have a 50 percent higher chance than men of using a nursing home at some point in their lives.[50] The imbalance in nursing home utilization occurs not only because women have greater disabilities but also because they frequently outlive their husbands and thus lack the social support needed to stay at home.[51] The cruel irony is that after lifetimes of caring for others, many women are bereft of essential support when they are most in need. Policy makers and researchers rarely address the social and economic policies responsible for the predominance of women in nursing homes. It is unclear to what extent women are especially likely to suffer from the inadequacies of community services.

## Race/Ethnicity

As early as 1980, the U.S. Commission on Civil Rights argued that racial differences in the utilization rates of nursing homes *might* indicate access barriers. In 1990, 25.8 percent of whites age eighty-five and over were in nursing homes, compared to 16.7 percent of African Americans, 11.0 percent of Latinos, and 12.1 percent of Asian Americans.[52] Differences persist even after controlling for other predictors of nursing home use.[53]

The relatively little research on the relation between race/ethnicity and the utilization of community services is contradictory. Some studies have found minority elderly people use community-based care at the same or even higher rates compared to whites after controlling for need and resources. Different national data sets on disabled African Americans and Latinos found the prevalence of paid in-home assistance of these two groups to be similar to that of whites.[54] Still other studies indicate that African Americans are more likely than whites to use Medicare's home health benefit and adult day care.[55] However, research using different data finds that African Americans and Latinos are less likely to use community-based services than whites and that those who use such services receive fewer hours of assistance.[56]

One limitation of these studies is that the survey instruments may not capture the higher levels of need of community-dwelling minority elderly persons. The sickest and most disabled whites are more likely to be found in nursing homes. A study of both institutionalized and community-dwelling older persons concluded that disabled elderly African Americans were less likely than whites to receive paid help.[57]

Several reasons could account for the racial and ethnic differences in long-term care utilization.[58] Some studies suggest that minority elderly people are less knowledgeable than whites about the types and functions of many community-based services, others suggest that nursing homes have discriminatory admissions policies, and still others suggest that health professionals are less likely to refer minority elderly people to formal services.[59]

## Class

Some observers argue that social policy for older persons in the United States creates a two-class system. Low-income elderly rely on Medicaid and other poverty programs while the better-off benefit from tax preferences and universal programs such as Medicare. Poverty programs are the most vulnerable to cuts because their constituency lacks political and economic clout.[60]

Specific research on class factors in long-term care is sparse and primarily deals with the problems faced by Medicaid recipients. Some evidence suggests that many nursing homes discriminate against Medicaid patients. High occupancy rates (averaging 95 percent nationwide) enable nursing homes to be choosy about admissions. Because the Medicaid reimbursement rate is lower than the amount nursing homes charge private-pay residents, facilities prefer clients who can pay out-of-pocket.[61] Hospital discharge planners in California estimate that Medicaid patients are four to seven times more difficult to place in nursing homes than are privately funded patients.[62]

The quality of life of Medicaid nursing home residents appears to be especially poor. Medicaid recipients tend to be relegated to institutions that according to some measures offer the worst care.[63] Even within one facility, residents relying on Medicaid sometimes receive less care than private-pay residents. And Medicaid does not pay for incidentals such as laundering private clothes or making phone calls. All such expenses must come from the $30 to $70 per month (varying by state) that Medicaid recipients are allowed to keep.[64]

Class also affects the distribution of community-based services. Because most people who receive such care pay privately, utilization varies directly with income. Not surprisingly, people with higher incomes spend far more than others on care. Moreover, self-pay clients receive more hours of home health care than those who rely on public funds.[65] Although Medicaid increases access to community-based services, 71 percent of noninstitutionalized older persons with poverty-level incomes do not receive Medicaid.[66] Other elderly people, called tweeners, have incomes just above the poverty level and therefore do not quality for Medicaid but are too poor to pay privately for services.[67]

Recent developments have accentuated the class bias of noninstitutional care, especially home health care. First, the deregulation and cost containment measures of the 1980s eased Medicare restrictions on proprietary home health agencies. By 1992, 38 percent of home health agencies were proprietary, and they served approximately one-quarter of all patients.[68] For-profit agencies seek out the best paying (that is, privately insured) patients, leaving other patients for non-profit and government agencies.[69] Second, large multihospital systems looking for a relatively inexpensive way to expand have been eager to acquire home health agencies. Third, for-profit chains have grown, with the thirty largest accounting for 27 percent of all home health agency offices. These changes have increased the competitiveness of the home health care system, putting agencies under growing pressure to generate revenue by focusing on the most remunerative patients and the best-paid services, decreasing access for those whose care is less profitable.[70] Little research has attempted to determine if the quality of care varies by type of payment or ownership or affiliation of the home health agency.

The greatest class differences may lie in services provided outside the bounds of established organizations. Although most studies ignore the vast network of helpers recruited through ad hoc, informal arrangements, some evidence suggests that disabled elderly people rely disproportionately on this type of assistance.[71] Abel's study of fifty-one predominately white middle-class women caring for elderly parents found that just fifteen used services from a community agency, but twenty-eight hired helpers who were unaffiliated with formal agencies. Nine of the unaffiliated home care aides worked forty hours a week, and sixteen provided around-the-clock care.[72] The help provided by such workers typically is not included in government statistics; however, it constitutes a major source of assistance to the affluent that is not available to others.

## Private-Sector Financing Initiatives

The inequities in long-term care may become even more apparent if initiatives to rely more on private-sector financing win increased support. Such initiatives take two forms. Some, such as home equity conversions and individual medical accounts, seek to promote private saving, which can then be used to finance long-term care. Others attempt to bring individuals together to pool the risks of paying for long-term care; these mechanisms include private long-term care insurance and continuing-care retirement communities.[73]

Advocates of such programs argue that the growing segment of the elderly population that is sufficiently well-off to be able to pay for long-term care should not rely on limited government funds.[74] Critics charge that the expansion of the private sector would sharpen the divide between rich and poor. Most private-sector approaches are beyond the reach of low- and middle-income elderly people. Many elderly have neither enough equity in their homes to pay for extended long-term care, nor enough income to pay for comprehensive private long-term care insurance.[75] A high-option long-term care insurance policy, for example, costs approximately $2,525 annually at age sixty-five and $7,675 at age seventy-nine.[76] Entry fees for continuing-care retirement communities range from $50,000 to $100,000; monthly fees start at $575.[77] Increased private financing may also dissolve whatever popular support public programs currently enjoy. Walter Leutz writes: "This could clearly lead to a two-class system of care, which would be rationalized by arguments that blame elderly victims for not insuring. It would not be uncommon to hear the argument that those who don't plan for the future don't deserve such a generous program, and so on into the all-too-familiar pattern."[78]

Although public policy supports privatization, the rhetoric of family love and responsibility does not extend to the very wealthy, who can afford to purchase on their own the supportive services policy makers would deny to others.

## Informal Care

Research provides overwhelming evidence to refute the enduring myth that families abandon their elderly relatives. Shanas[79] was one of the first scholars to show that elderly people remain in close contact with surviving kin. More recent studies demonstrate that this contact translates into assistance during times of crisis. Researchers consistently report that families deliver 70 to 80 percent of long-term care.[80] One study estimated that family members provided over twenty-seven million days of care each week to disabled elderly people in 1982.[81] Informal care clearly is the bedrock on which the long-term care system is built.

Research on informal care often focuses on the impact of caregiving on family members. Studies have found that caregivers experience a range of physical, emotional, social, and financial problems. In many cases, caregiving responsibilities ignite family conflicts, impose financial strains, and encroach on both paid employment and leisure activities.[82] Researchers repeatedly report that caregivers experience stress because they perceive their responsibilities to be burdensome. Numerous studies also examine the mental and physical health outcomes of stress.[83]

Because stress has critical implications for public health, researchers have attempted to identify caregivers most at risk. They have correlated caregiver strain with factors such as the recipient's type of impairment; the level of support available to caregivers; the amount of care they deliver; the quality of the relationship between caregiver and recipient; and various caregiver characteristics such as age, gender, race and ethnicity, marital status, employment status, and income.[84] Investigators also have assessed the reduction of stress associated with a variety of interventions, including programs such as respite care, counseling services, caregiver support groups, educational and training programs, and assorted in-home supportive services.[85]

Although these studies have provided useful information for practitioners, the focus on stress seriously restricts our understanding of the experience of caring for a disabled elderly person. Because studies assume that hardships are converted automatically into strain, they ignore a range of other possible responses. Thus, researchers have rarely examined whether a strong sense of affiliation and attachment simultaneously imbues caregiving with meaning and purpose. Moreover, although stress research has a number of practical applications, it also may limit the range of policies discussed. Stress often results from social structures,[86] but it is a property of individuals. Consequently, most remedies, such as stress management, education, and counseling programs focus exclusively on personal change,[87] reflecting the policy agenda of increasing the adaptive capabilities of family and friends. Even such remedies as respite care and supportive services, which seek to alter the context within which care is delivered, tend to focus on individuals. That focus diverts attention from structural reforms that would make care for the dependent population more just and humane.

In addition, because evaluators typically view interventions primarily as stress-reduction mechanisms, they ignore other benefits these programs provide.[88] One observer has argued that because studies consistently find home care services do not reduce stress, public expenditures on these services cannot be justified.[89] The critical question for evaluators, however, is not whether various programs make caregivers feel better about themselves but whether the programs can improve the quality of caregivers' lives and minimize the sacrifices caregiving requires. By using stress reduction as the only outcome measure, we reinforce the belief that our main concern should be to help caregivers adjust to their unavoidable burdens.

It also is important to challenge the instrumentalist view, which underlies much research on caregiving. Many studies report that the timing of nursing home placement is related more to the intensification of caregiver stress than to changes in the condition of the care recipient[90] and recommend measures to alleviate the stress of family members. But they do so to prolong family caregiving for its cost savings to the government, not to promote the well-being of caregivers as an end in itself.

## Class and Gender

Care for the elderly continues to be allocated on the basis of gender. Women represent 72 percent of all caregivers and 77 percent of children providing care.

Because the elderly turn first to their spouses when they become ill, we might expect spousal caregiving to be divided equally along gender lines. But partly because women tend to marry men who are older than themselves and to live longer than men, a majority (64 percent) of the spouses providing care are women. Daughters are more likely than sons to live with dependent parents and to serve as the primary caregivers.[91] Sons and daughters also assume responsibility for very different chores. Sons are more likely to assist parents with routine household maintenance and repairs, while daughters are far more likely to help with indoor household chores and personal care.[92] This gender division of labor may help to explain why caregiving has different consequences for sons and daughters. Sons take responsibility for tasks they can perform whenever they choose. Daughters, however, often assume responsibilities that keep them on call twenty-four hours a day. Other studies suggest that husbands and wives also assume different caregiving responsibilities. One study of spousal caregivers of elderly people with dementia found that wives were more concerned about treating their spouses with dignity and more willing to respond to their changing needs than husbands were.[93]

Low-income women face special problems in rendering care. They cannot afford special medical equipment and supplies, remodel their homes to adapt to their relatives' disabilities, or buy out of their obligations by hiring other women. The working poor tend to have jobs with rigid schedules and lack leverage to demand special consideration. They thus may suffer greater penalties if they phone disabled relatives from work or take time off to help them during the working day. Female caregivers employed as operatives and laborers are more likely than those employed in professional or managerial positions or in clerical or sales positions to take time off without pay; on the other hand, female caregivers who hold clerical or sales positions and, to a lesser extent, those in professional or managerial positions are more likely than operatives and laborers to rearrange their schedules.[94]

Although a growing literature identifies who the caregivers are in minority communities, few studies to date examine how race and ethnicity affect the caregiving experience.

The intense involvement of many family members in caregiving work suggests that they are not simply responding to external pressures. Nevertheless, long-term care policies create the framework within which the experience of caregiving unfolds. The decisions caregivers make are not solely private choices. Because publicly funded services are not universally available, many women lack the power to control the intrusions of caregiving in their lives and lack the power to hand over responsibilities that become too great.

## Workers in the Long-Term Care System

Paid as well as unpaid carers suffer from the failure to fund long-term care adequately. Nursing homes, home health agencies, and the elderly themselves seek to save money by keeping wages low. In New York City, 99 percent of home care workers are women, 70 percent are African American, 26 percent are Latina, and almost half (46 percent) are immigrants. A high proportion are single mothers with three or four children. They typically earn less than $5,000 a year. Eighty percent cannot afford adequate housing, and 35 percent often cannot buy enough food for their families.[95] Home care work also is characterized by inadequate supervision and training and few opportunities for advancement.[96] National studies of nursing home assistants show that they receive poor wages and few benefits and, in large metropolitan areas, are overwhelmingly women of color and immigrants.[97] One qualitative study found that even though most assistants took extra jobs to make ends meet, staff conversations centered "on not having enough money for rent or transportation or children's necessities."[98]

Most research on home care workers addresses the concerns of home health agencies regarding training, supervision, and especially retention of workers.[99] The high turnover rate of nursing home assistants, estimated to be 40 percent to 75 percent annually, has led to a similar focus in the nursing home literature.[100] The research focuses on factors that could be changed at the level of individual nursing homes, such as the daily organization of work.[101]

Some studies report that nursing home assistants enjoy helping and caring for patients but that rules and regulations designed to protect patients' rights, ensure quality, and promote efficiency frustrate their efforts. Racial/ethnic differences between workers, administrators, and patients further undermine positive relationships.[102] The racial, ethnic, and class composition of the home care labor force similarly creates serious problems. Many workers complain that they are treated like maids, asked to perform tasks they consider inappropriate and demeaning. They also report that they have difficulty overcoming the distrust of some clients.[103]

## Conclusion

Long-term care differs fundamentally from acute care for elderly people. It includes social as well as medical services. It is provided overwhelmingly by family and friends. It is financed primarily by a means-tested program for the poor (Medicaid) rather than by a universal public insurance program (Medicare). And out-of-pocket payments represent a very high proportion of its funding.

Although demographic changes contribute to the growing need for long-term care, economic pressures have determined the shape of the system. Both policy and research consistently emphasize cost containment rather than quality, equity, or adequacy. Nursing homes have been viewed as cost-effective alternatives to hospitals, and community-based services have been supported as cost-effective alternatives to nursing homes. Growing public expenditures on community-based services lead to an increased interest in narrow targeting mechanisms.

The most critical policy and research issue is how we can provide adequate high-quality long-term care services in an equitable manner to a growing and diverse older population. Assuring quality requires a proactive research and policy agenda to identify critical indicators of quality and provide appropriate incentives for providers. Equity requires that research and policy take into account variation in the needs and resources of different racial/ethnic groups, genders, and classes. The limited financial resources of many older persons, especially among racial/ethnic minorities, widows, and the working class, create a need for a universal Medicare type of social insurance.

## Notes

1. John B. McKinlay, Sonja M. McKinlay, and Robert Beaglehole, "Trends in Death and Disease and the Contribution of Medical Measures," in *Handbook of Medical Sociology*, eds. Howard E. Freeman and Sol Levine (Englewood Cliffs, N.J.: Prentice Hall, 1989), pp. 14–15.

2. Cynthia M. Taeuber and Jessie Allen, "Women in Our Aging Society: The Demographic Outlook," in *Women on the Front Lines: Meeting the Challenge of an Aging America,* eds. Jessie Allen and Alan Pifer (Washington, D.C.: Urban Institute Press, 1993), pp. 11–45.

3. Cynthia Taeuber, *Sixty-Five Plus in America,* U.S. Bureau of the Census, Current Population Reports, Special Studies, P23–178 (Washington, D.C.: U.S. Government Printing Office, 1992), p. 3–12.

4. Rosalie A. Kane and Robert L. Kane, *Long-Term Care: Principles, Programs, and Policies* (New York: Springer, 1987), p. 4.

5. Committee on Nursing Home Regulation, Institute of Medicine, *Improving the Quality of Care in Nursing Homes* (Washington, D.C.: National Academy Press, 1986).

6. William E. Aaronson, Jacqueline S. Zinn, and Michael D. Rosko, "Do For-Profit and Not-for-Profit Nursing Homes Behave Differently?" *Gerontologist* 34 (December 1994): 775–786.

7. R. L. Associates, *The American Public Views Long-Term Care* (Princeton, N.J.: R. L. Associates, 1987).

8. Katherine R. Levit, Arthur L. Sensenig, et al. "National Health Expenditures, 1993," *Health Care Financing Review* 16 (Fall 1994): 247–294.

9. Pepper Commission, U.S. Bipartisan Commission on Comprehensive Health Care, *A Call for Action* (Washington, D.C.: U.S. Government Printing Office, 1990); and Joshua M. Wiener, Laurel H. Illston, and Raymond J. Hanley, *Sharing the Burden: Strategies for Public and Private Long-term Care Insurance* (Washington, D.C.: Brookings Institution, 1994).

10. E. Kathleen Adams, Mark R. Meiners, and Brian O. Burwell, "Asset Spend-Down in Nursing Homes," *Medical Care* 31 (January 1993): 1–23.

11. Korbin Liu, Timothy McBride, and Teresa Coughlin, "Risk of Entering Nursing Homes for Long Versus Short Stays," *Medical Care* 32 (1994): 315–327.

12. Peter Kemper, Brenda C. Spillman, and Christopher M. Murtaugh, "A Lifetime Perspective on Proposals for Financing Nursing Home Care," *Inquiry* 28 (1991): 333–344.

13. Marc A. Cohen, Nanda Kumar, and Stanley S. Wallack, "Long-Term Care Insurance and Medicaid," *Health Affairs* 13 (1994): 127–139.

14. Robert E. Schlenker, "Comparison of Medicaid Nursing Home Payment Systems," *Health Care Financing Review* 13 (Fall 1991): 93–109.

15. Andrew F. Coburn, Richard Fortinsky, Catherine McGuire, and Thomas P. McDonald, "Effect of Prospective Reimbursement on Nursing Home Costs," *Health Services Research* 28 (April 1993): 45–68; and James H. Swan, Charlene Harrington, Leslie Grant, John Luehrs, and Steve Preston, "Trends in Medicaid Nursing Home Reimbursement: 1978–89," *Health Care Financing Review* 14 (Summer 1993): 111–132.

16. Marjorie Abend-Wein, "Medicaid's Effect on the Elderly: How Reimbursement Policy Affects Priorities in the Nursing Home," *Journal of Applied Gerontology* 10 (March 1991): 71–87; and Kenneth E. Thorpe, Paul J. Gertler, and Paula Goldman, "The Resource Utilization Group System: Its Effect on Nursing Home Case Mix and Costs," *Inquiry* 28 (Winter 1991): 357–365.

17. Catherine Hawes, John N. Morris, Charles D. Phillips, et al., "Reliability Estimates for the Minimum Data Set for Nursing Home Resident Assessment and Care Screening (MDS)," *Gerontologist* 35 (April 1995): 172–178.

18. Perry Starer and Leslie S. Libow, "Medical Care of the Elderly in the Nursing Home," *Journal of General Internal Medicine* 7 (May-June 1992): 350–362.

19. Aaronson, Zinn, and Rosko, "Do For-Profit and Not-for-Profit Nursing Homes Behave Differently?"

20. Rebecca Elon and L. Gregory Pawlson, "The Impact of OBRA on Medical Practice within Nursing Facilities," *Journal of the American Geriatrics Society* 40 (September 1994): 958–963.

21. "Nursing Homes: A Special Investigative Report," *Consumer Reports,* 60 (August 1995): 518–528.

22. Elizabeth Mauser and Nancy A. Miller, "A Profile of Home Health Users in 1992," *Health Care Financing Review* 16 (Fall 1994): 17–34.

23. Charlene Harrington, Marty Lynch, and Robert J. Newcomer, "Medical Services in Social Health Maintenance Organizations," *Gerontologist* 33 (December 1993): 790–800; and Charlene Harrington and Robert J. Newcomer, "Social Health Maintenance Organizations' Service Use and Costs, 1985–89," *Health Care Financing Review* 12 (Spring 1991): 37–52.

24. U.S. General Accounting Office, *Long-Term-Care Case Management: State Experiences and Implications for Federal Policy,* GAO/HRD–93–52 (Washington, D.C.: U.S. General Accounting Office, 1993).

25. U.S. General Accounting Office, *Long-Term-Care Case Management: State Experiences and Implications for Federal Policy.*

26. Steven P. Wallace, "The No Care Zone: Availability, Accessibility, and Acceptability in Community-Based Long-Term Care," *Gerontologist* 30 (1990): 254–261; and Carroll L. Estes, James H. Swan, and Associates, *The Long-Term Care Crisis: Elders Trapped in the No-Care Zone* (Newbury Park, Calif.: Sage, 1993).

27. William G. Weissert, Cynthia M. Cready, and James E. Pawelak, "The Past and Future of Home- and Community-Based Long Term Care," *Milbank Quarterly* 66 (1988): 309–388.

28. Dana Gelb Safran, John D. Graham, and J. Scott Osberg, "Social Supports as a Determinant of Community-based Care Utilization Among Rehabilitation Patients," *Health Services Research* 28 (1994): 729–750.

29. Ronald M. Andersen, "Revisiting the Behavioral Model and Access to Medical Care: Does It Matter?" *Journal of Health and Social Behavior* 36 (March 1995): 1–10.

30. Alan M. Jette, Sharon Tennstedt, and Sybil Crawford, "How Does Formal and Informal Community Care Affect Nursing Home Use?" *Journals of Gerontology: Social Sciences* 50B (January 1995): S4–S12; William D. Spector and Peter Kemper, "Disability and Cognitive Impairment Criteria: Targeting Those Who Need the Most Home Care," *Gerontologist* 34 (October 1994): 640–651; and Stephanie McFall and Baila H. Miller, "Caregiver Burden and Nursing Home Admission of Frail Elderly Persons," *Journal of Gerontology: Social Sciences* 47 (1992): S73–S79.

31. Linda S. Noelker and David M. Bass, "Home Care for Elderly Persons: Linkages Between Formal and Informal Caregivers," *Journal of Gerontology: Social Sciences* 44 (1989): S63–S70; and Sharon L. Tennstedt, S. L. Crawford, and John B. McKinlay, "Is Family Care on the Decline? A Longitudinal Investigation of the Substitution of Formal Long-Term Care Services for Informal Care, *Milbank Quarterly* 71 (1993): 601–624.

32. William G. Weissert, "Seven Reasons Why It Is So Difficult to Make Community-Based Long-Term Care Cost-Effective," *Health Services Research* 20 (1985): 423–433.

33. Wallace, "The No Care Zone."

34. Alan Sager, "A Proposal for Promoting More Adequate Long-Term Care for the Elderly," *Gerontologist* 23 (1983): 13–17, p. 15.

35. See Chai R. Feldblum, "Home Health Care for the Elderly: Programs, Problems, and Potentials," *Harvard Journal on Legislation* 22 (1985): 193–254.

36. Pamela Farley Short and Joel Leon, *Use of Home and Community Services by Persons Ages 65 and Older with Functional Difficulties,* National Medical Expenditure Survey Research Findings 5, AHCPR (Rockville, Md.: Public Health Service, 1990); and Thomas Prohaska, Robin Mermelstein, Baila Miller, and Susan Jack, "Functional Status and Living Arrangements," in *Health Data on Older Americans: United States, 1992,* eds. Joan F. Van Nostrand, Sylvia E. Furner, and Richard Suzman (Hyattsville, Md.: National Center for Health Statistics, 1993), pp. 23–39.

37. Agency for Health Care Policy and Research, *The Elderly with Functional Difficulties: Characteristics of Users of Home and Community Services,* AHCPR Pub. No. 92–0112 (Rockville, Md.: Public Health Service, July 1992), pp. 1–3.

38. Rosalie A. Kane, Robert L. Kane, Laurel H. Illston, and Nancy N. Eustis, "Perspectives on Home Care Quality," *Health Care Financing Review* 16 (Fall 1994): 69–89.

39. Taeuber and Allen, "Women in Our Aging Society."

40. Karen Smith Blesch and Sylvia E. Furner, "Health of Older Black Americans," in *Health Data on Older Americans: United States, 1992,* eds. Joan F. Van Nostrand, Sylvia E. Furner, and Richard Suzman (Hyattsville, Md.: U.S. Department of Health and Human Services, 1993), pp. 229–273.

41. Steven P. Wallace and Chin-Yin Lew-Ting, "Getting By at Home: Community-Based Long-Term Care of Latino Elders," *Western Journal of Medicine* 157 (September 1992): 337–344.

42. Sora Park-Tanjasiri, Steven P. Wallace, and Kazve Shibata, "Picture Imperfect: Hidden Problems Among Asian Pacific Islander Elderly," *Gerontologist,* 35 (December 1995): 753–760.

43. Taeuber, *Sixty-Five Plus in America,* pp. 2–7, 3–13, 6–4 to 6–7.

44. Marti G. Parker, Mats Thorslund, and Olle Lundberg, "Physical Function and Social Class Among Swedish Oldest Old," *Journal of Gerontology: Social Sciences* 49 (July 1994): S196–S201.

45. James S. House, James M. Lepkowski, Ann M. Kinney, Richard P. Mero, Ronald C. Kessler, and A. Regula Herzog, "The Social Stratification of Aging and Health," *Journal of Health and Social Behavior* 35 (September 1994): 213–234.

46. Taeuber and Allen, "Women in Our Aging Society," p. 34.

47. U.S. Bureau of the Census, Current Population Reports, Series P60–184, *Money Income of Households, Families, and Persons in the United States* (Washington, D.C.: U.S. Government Printing Office, 1993), pp. 100–107.

48. Esther Hing, *The National Nursing Home Survey: 1985 Summary for the United States* (Hyattsville, Md.: National Center for Health Statistics, 1989).

49. Kyriakos S. Markides, "Minority Aging," in *Aging in Society: Selected Reviews of Recent Research,* eds. Matilda White Riley, Beth B. Hess, and Kathleen Bond (Hillsdale, N.J.: Erlbaum, 1983), pp. 115–137.

50. Steven E. Feinleib, Peter J. Cunningham, and Pamela Farley Short, "Use of Nursing and Personal Care Homes by the Civilian Population, 1987," in *National Medical Expenditure Survey Research Findings 23* (Rockville, Md.: Public Health Service, Agency for Health Care Policy and Research, 1994); and Christopher M. Murtaugh, Peter Kemper, and Brenda C. Spillman, "The Risk of Nursing Home Use in Later Life," *Medical Care* 28 (October 1990): 952–962.

51. Murtaugh, Kemper, and Spillman, "The Risk of Nursing Home Use."

52. JoAnne Damron-Rodriguez, Steven P. Wallace, and Raynard Kington, "Service Utilization and Minority Elderly: Appropriateness, Accessibility and Acceptability," *Gerontology and Geriatrics Education* 15 (1994): 45–64.

53. Vernon L. Greene and Jan I. Ondrich, "Risk Factors for Nursing Home Admissions and Exits: A Discrete-Time Hazard Function Approach," *Journal of Gerontology: Social Sciences* 45 (1990): S250–S258; Linda Liska Belgrave, May L. Wykle, and Jung M. Choi, "Health, Double Jeopardy, and Culture: The Use of Institutionalization by African-Americans," *Gerontologist* 33 (June 1993): 379–385; and Steven P. Wallace, Lené Levy-Storms, Ronald M. Andersen, Raynard Kington, and Kevin Campbell, *Minority Elderly Access to LTC,* Final Report to the Agency for Health Care Policy and Research, DHHS, AHCPR Grant R03 HS07672 (Los Angeles, Calif.: UCLA School of Public Health, 1995).

54. Baila Miller, Stephanie McFall, and Richard T. Campbell, "Changes in Sources of Community Long-Term Care Among African American and White Frail Older Persons," *Journal of Gerontology: Social Sciences* 49 (January 1994): S14-S24; and Steven P. Wallace, Lené Levy-Storms, and Linda R. Ferguson, "Access to Paid In-Home Assistance Among Disabled Elderly People: Do Latinos Differ from Non-Latino Whites?" *American Journal of Public Health* 85 (July 1995): 970–975.

55. Mauser and Miller, "Profile of Home Health Users"; and Steven P. Wallace, Judy Snyder, Georgia Walker, and Stanley Ingman, "Racial Differences Among Users of Long-Term Care: The Case of Adult Day Care," *Research on Aging* 14 (December 1992): 471–495.

56. Peter Kemper, "The Use of Formal and Informal Home Care by the Disabled Elderly," *Health Services Research* 27 (October 1992): 421–451; David M. Bass and Linda S. Noelker, "The Influence of Family Caregivers on Elders' Use of In-Home Services: An Expanded Conceptual Framework," *Journal of Health and Social Behavior* 28 (1987): 184–196; and Vernon L. Greene and D. Monahan, "Comparative Utilization of Community-Based Long-

Term Care Services by Hispanic and Anglo Elderly in a Case Management System," *Journal of Gerontology: Social Sciences* 39 (1984): S730–S735.

57. Wallace, Levy-Storms, Andersen, Kington, and Campbell, *Minority Elderly Access to LTC.*

58. Charles M. Barresi and Geeta Menon, "Diversity in Black Family Caregiving," in *Black Aged: Understanding Diversity and Service Needs,* eds. Zev Harel, Edward A. McKinney, and Michael Williams (Newbury Park, Calif.: Sage, in cooperation with the National Council on the Aging, 1990), pp. 221–235; and Susie Ann Spence and Charles R. Atherton, "The Black Elderly and the Social Service Delivery System: A Study of Factors Influencing the Use of Community-Based Services, *Journal of Gerontological Social Work* 16 (1991): 19–35.

59. Douglas Holmes, Jeanne Teresi, and Monica Holmes, "Differences Among Black, Hispanic, and White People in Knowledge About Long-Term Care Services," *Health Care Financing Review* 5 (1985): 51–67; David Falcone and Robert Broyles, "Access to Long-Term Care: Race as a Barrier," *Journal of Health, Politics, Policy, and Law* 19 (1995): 583–595; and Steven P. Wallace, "The Political Economy of Health Care for Elderly Blacks," *International Journal of Health Services* 20 (1990): 665–680.

60. Carroll L. Estes, "The Politics of Ageing in America," *Ageing and Society* 6 (1986): 121–134; and Madonna Harrington Meyer, "Gender, Race, and the Distribution of Social Assistance: Medicaid Use Among the Frail Elderly," *Gender and Society* 8 (March 1994): 8–28.

61. Susan L. Ettner, "Do Elderly Medicaid Patients Experience Reduced Access to Nursing Home Care," *Journal of Health Economics* 12 (October 1993): 259–280; Robert J. Buchanan, Peter Madel, and Dan Persons, "Medicaid Payment Policies for Nursing Home Care: A National Survey," *Health Care Financing Review* 13 (Fall 1991): 55–72; and Committee on Nursing Home Regulation, *Improving the Quality of Care in Nursing Homes.*

62. Lewin and Associates, *An Evaluation of the Medi-Cal Program's System for Establishing Reimbursement Rates for Nursing Homes* (Submitted to the Office of the Auditor General, State of California, 1987).

63. Alice M. Rivlin and Joshua M. Wiener, *Caring for the Disabled Elderly: Who Will Pay?* (Washington, D.C.: Brookings Institution, 1988).

64. Meyer, "Gender, Race, and the Distribution of Social Assistance"; and Estes, Swan, and Associates, *The Long-Term Care Crisis,* pp. 139–140.

65. Korbin Liu, Kenneth G. Manton, and B. Marzetta Liu, "Home Care Expenses for the Disabled Elderly," *Health Care Financing Review* 7 (1985): 51–58; and Nancy M. Kane, "The Home Care Crisis of the Nineties," *Gerontologist* 29 (1989): 24–31, p. 27.

66. U.S. Select Committee on Aging, *Aging America: Trends and Projections* (Washington, D.C.: U.S. Department of Health and Human Services, 1991).

67. Karen C. Holden and Timothy M. Smeeding, "The Poor, the Rich, and the Insecure Elderly Caught In Between," *Milbank Quarterly* 68 (1990): 191–219.

68. Estes, Swan, and Associates, *The Long-Term Care Crisis;* Genevieve Strahan, *Advance Data,* Overview of Home Health and Hospice Care Patients; preliminary data from the 1992 National Home and Hospice Care Survey. No. 235. (Washington, D.C.: National Center for Health Statistics, 1993); and Marion Merrell Dow, *Managed Care Digest: Long Term Care Edition* (Kansas City, Mo.: Marion Merrell Dow, 1993).

69. Estes, Swan, and Associates, *The Long-Term Care Crisis;* and Marion Merrell Dow, *Managed Care Digest.*

70. Marion Merrell Dow, *Managed Care Digest.*

71. Elaine M. Brody and Claire B. Schoonover, "Patterns of Parent Care When Adult Daughters Work and When They Do Not," *Gerontologist* 26 (1986): 372–381.

72. Emily K. Abel, *Who Cares for the Elderly? Public Policy and the Experiences of Adult Daughters* (Philadelphia: Temple University Press, 1991).

73. See Rivlin and Wiener, *Caring for the Disabled Elderly.*

74. Rita Ricardo-Campbell, "Aging and the Private Sector," *Generations* 12 (Spring 1988): 19–22; and Task Force on Long-Term Health Care Policies, *Report to Congress and the Secretary* (Washington, D.C.: U.S. Government Printing Office, 1987).

75. Walter N. Leutz, "Long-Term Care for the Elderly: Public Dreams and Private Realities," *Inquiry* 23 (1986): 134–140

76. Wiener, Illston, and Hanley, *Sharing the Burden.*

77. Leutz, "Long-Term Care for the Elderly"; and Stephen M. Golant, *Housing America's Elderly* (Newbury Park, Calif.: Sage, 1992).

78. Leutz, "Long-Term Care for the Elderly," p. 139.

79. Ethel Shanas, "The Family as a Social Support System in Old Age," *Gerontologist* 19 (1979): 169–174.

80. Robyn Stone, Gail Lee Cafferata, and Judith Sangl, "Caregivers of the Frail Elderly: A National Profile," *Gerontologist* 27 (1987): 616–625; and Rivlin and Wiener, *Caring for the Disabled Elderly.*

81. Cited in Raymond J. Hanley, Joshua M. Wiener, and Katherine M. Harris, "Will Paid Home Care Erode Informal Support?" *Journal of Health, Politics, Policy, and Law* 16 (1991): 507–521.

82. Abel, *Who Cares for the Elderly?*

83. William E. Haley, Ellen G. Levine, S. Lane Brown, Jack W. Berry, and Glenn H. Hughes, "Psychological, Social, and Health Consequences of Caring for a Relative with Senile Dementia," *Journal of the American Geriatrics Society* 35 (1987): 405–411; Richard Schulz, "Theoretical Perspectives on Caregiving: Concepts, Variables, and Methods," in *Aging and Caregiving: Theory, Research, and Policy,* eds. David E. Biegel and Arthur Blum (Newbury Park, Calif.: Sage, 1990), pp. 27–52; Tennstedt, "Is Family Care on the Decline?"; and Linda K. George and Lisa P. Gwyther, "Caregiver Well-Being: A Multidimensional Examination of Family Caregivers of Demented Adults," *Gerontologist* 26 (1986): 253–259.

84. Valerie A. Braithwaite, *Bound to Care* (Sydney: Allen and Unwin, 1990); Amy Horowitz, "Sons and Daughters to Older Parents: Differences in Role Performance and Consequences," *Gerontologist* 25 (1985): 612–17; and Marcia G. Ory, T. Franklin Williams, Marian Emr, Barry Lebowitz, Peter Rabins, Jeffrey Salloway, Teresa Sluss-Radbaugh, Eliza Wolff, and Steven Zarit, "Families, Informal Supports, and Alzheimer's Disease: Current Research and Future Agendas," *Research on Aging* 7 (1985): 623–644.

85. Greene and Monahan, "Comparative Utilization of Community-based Long-Term Care Services"; William E. Haley, S. Lane Brown, and Ellen G. Levine, "Experimental Evaluation of the Effectiveness of Group Intervention for Dementia Caregivers," *Gerontologist* 27 (1987): 376–382; M. Powell Lawton, Elaine Brody, and Avalie R. Saperstein, "A Controlled Study of Respite Service for Caregivers of Alzheimer's Patients," *Gerontologist* 29 (1989): 8–16; Rhonda J. V. Montgomery and Edgar F. Borgatta, *Family Support Project,* Final Report to the Administration on Aging (Seattle: University of Washington, Institute on Aging/Long-Term Care Center, 1985); Ronald W. Toseland, Charles M. Rossiter, and Mark S. Labrecque, "The Effectiveness of Peer-Led and Professionally-Led Groups to Support Family Caregivers," *Gerontologist* 29 (1989): 465–471; and Steven H. Zarit, Cheri R. An-

thony, and Mary Boutsclis, "Interventions with Caregivers of Dementia Patients: A Comparison of Two Approaches," *Psychology and Aging* 2 (1987): 225–232.

86. See Leonard I. Pearlin, "The Sociological Study of Stress," *Journal of Health and Social Behavior* 30 (1989): 241–256.

87. Allan Young, "The Discourse on Stress and the Reproduction of Conventional Knowledge," *Social Science and Medicine* 14B (1980): 133–146.

88. Haley, Brown, and Levine, "Experimental Evaluation of the Effectiveness of Group Intervention."

89. James J. Callahan, Jr., "Play It Again Sam—There Is No Impact," *Gerontologist* 29 (1989): 5–6.

90. See Horowitz, "Sons and Daughters to Older Parents."

91. Douglas A. Wolf and Beth J. Soldo, "The Households of Older Unmarried Women: Micro-Decision Models of Shared Living Arrangements," paper presented at the Annual Meeting of the Population Association of America, San Francisco, 1986; and Stone, Cafferata, and Sangl, "Caregivers of the Frail Elderly."

92. Raymond T. Coward and Eleanor Rathbone-McCuan, "Illuminating the Relative Role of Adult Sons and Daughters in the Long-Term Care of Their Parents," paper presented at the Professional Symposium of the National Association of Social Workers, Chicago, November 1985; and Susan A. Stephens and Jon B. Christianson, *Informal Care of the Elderly* (Lexington, Mass.: Lexington Books, 1986).

93. Baila Miller, "Gender Differences in Spouse Management of the Caregiver Roles," in *Circles of Care: Work and Identity in Women's Lives*, eds. Emily K. Abel and Margaret K. Nelson (Albany: State University of New York Press, 1990), pp. 92–104.

94. Subcommittee on Human Services of the Select Committee on Aging, House of Representatives, *Exploding the Myths: Caregiving in America* (Washington, D.C.: 100th Congress, 1st Session, Comm. Pub. No. 99–611, 1987).

95. Rebecca Donovan, "'We Care for the Most Important People in Your Life': Home Care Workers in New York City," *Women's Studies Quarterly* 17 (1989): 56–65.

96. Margaret A. MacAdam, "Supply of Aides Working with the Elderly: What Do We Know from the Research?" in *Challenges and Innovations in Homecare*, eds. Joanne Handy and Charlotte K. Schuerman (San Francisco: American Society on Aging, 1994), pp. 43–48; and Reiko Hayashi, John W. Gibson, and Richard A. Weatherley, "Working Conditions in Home Care: A Survey of Washington State's Home Care Workers," *Home Health Care Services Quarterly* 14 (1994): 37–48.

97. Alice Quinlan, *Chronic Care Workers: Crisis Among Paid Caregivers of the Elderly* (Washington, D.C.: Older Women's League, 1988).

98. Timothy Diamond, *Making Gray Gold: Narratives of Nursing Home Care* (Chicago: University of Chicago Press, 1992), pp. 44–45.

99. Nola Aalberts, "The Outlook for Home Health Paraprofessionals," *Caring* 7 (May 1988): 20–23; Penny Hollander Feldman, Alice M. Sapienza, and Nancy M. Kane, *Who Cares for Them? Workers in the Home Care Industry* (New York: Greenwood Press, 1990); and Nancy Gilbert, "Home Care Worker Resignations: A Study of the Major Contributing Factors," *Home Health Care Services Quarterly* 12 (1991): 69–84.

100. See Nancy Foner, *The Caregiving Dilemma: Work in an American Nursing Home* (Berkeley: University of California Press, 1994); F. Theodore Helmer, Shirley F. Olson, and Richard I. Heim, "Strategies for Nurse Aide Job Satisfaction," *Journal of Long Term Care Administration* 21 (Summer 1993): 10–14; and Lois Grau, Barbara Chandler, Brenda Burton, and Doreen

Kolditz, "Institutional Loyalty and Job Satisfaction Among Nurse Aides in Nursing Homes," *Journal of Aging and Health* 3 (February 1991): 47–65.

101. Barbara Bowers and Marion Becker, "Nurse's Aides in Nursing Homes: The Relationship Between Organization and Quality," *Gerontologist* 32 (June 1992): 360–366.

102. Foner, *The Caregiving Dilemma;* and Diamond, *Making Gray Gold.*

103. Pamela Stefanowicz, "Home Care for the Frail Elderly: Implications of the Worker/Client Relationship for Quality," paper presented at the Annual Meeting of the Gerontological Society of America, Atlanta, Ga., 1994.

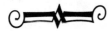

CHAPTER NINE

# AIDS IN TRANSITION

## Challenges for Health Services and Public Health

William E. Cunningham, Christy L. Beaudin,
and Christopher J. Panarites

The emerging epidemic of acquired immune deficiency syndrome (AIDS) presents a myriad of challenges to the health care system. Because the human immunodeficiency virus (HIV) is contagious, chronically disabling, and fatal, it increasingly forces health care policy makers, planners, and administrators to reevaluate the organization, delivery, and financing of services. Issues of particular concern include the following:

- Almost half a million people in the United States have been diagnosed with AIDS, and over half of them have already died.
- Medical care for a person infected with HIV costs over $100,000 between diagnosis of infection and death, much of it concentrated in the relatively brief period after a diagnosis of AIDS.
- Compared to the general population, people with AIDS are more likely to rely on Medicaid or to have no insurance at all. They are thus relatively unlikely to make use of outpatient medical services.
- Nonfinancial as well as financial barriers to access differentially impede the care of the poor, women, children, minorities, and drug users. Quality of care received by these growing segments of the HIV+ population may also vary.

The course of the illness is now characterized by gradual decline in the physical, cognitive, and emotional function and well-being health domains, requiring a continuum of chronic care—emergency care, primary care, housing and supervised living, mental health and social support, nonmedical services, and hospice care. As a result, the new emphasis in HIV/AIDS quality assessment is based on measuring outcomes such as disease-specific parameters of quality of life and illness severity.

Health services providers and researchers need to understand the needs of persons infected with HIV, as well as the accessibility and costs of care and quality of services. First, important characteristics of changing epidemiology and treatment patterns of AIDS should be understood in the context of real-life health care delivery. Second, better measures of access, costs, and quality need to be developed and applied in well-designed studies. At the same time, diverse subpopulations and service systems should be examined more rigorously. Third, these issues need to be examined not only within the arena of formal medical services, but more broadly within the continuum of care from prevention to community-based health and psychosocial services. Fourth, the policy implications and research needs for management, planning, and program administration in health services need to be considered. Developing an agenda for resolving these conflicts within the context of long-range planning is paramount. In this chapter, existing knowledge about critical issues of HIV/AIDS will be discussed. The purpose is to provide a framework for addressing the challenges that HIV disease represents for development of health policy, planning, and program implementation. Approaches to critical policy problems will be suggested, and the crucial areas for new investigation will be identified in order to guide future HIV/AIDS health policy.

## Changes in the Epidemiology and Treatment of HIV/AIDS

AIDS is a chronic disease, characterized by the progressive failure of the immune system and the development of opportunistic infections and malignancies. HIV is an unusual type of virus (a retrovirus) that causes immune suppression leading to AIDS. Individuals infected with HIV develop antibodies within a short period of time but may exhibit no symptoms for many years. Typically, the immune system weakens gradually and the blood level of CD4 cells (a type of white blood cell known as a T-helper/inducer lymphocyte) declines from a normal level of 1200–1400/mm$^3$. Persons with few CD4 cells are prone to opportunistic infections. Symptoms such as persistent fevers, night sweats, and weight loss begin to occur more frequently when the CD4 count drops below 500/mm. It is unclear whether all persons with asymptomatic HIV infection and CD4 count above 200/mm will eventually go on to develop AIDS.[1] However, once immune dysfunction becomes advanced and AIDS complications develop, mortality generally occurs within two years.[2] In addition to the CD4 lymphocyte count, the presence of AIDS-defining clinical diseases, age of onset, and HIV exposure category affect survival time. The development of AIDS is estimated to occur at eleven years on average from time of HIV infection.[3]

As noted earlier, 476,899 people in the United States were diagnosed with AIDS as of June 30, 1995; worldwide, 985,119 estimated AIDS cases had been reported.[4] In addition, 243,423 U.S. deaths from AIDS have occurred, for a case-fatality rate of 61 percent. The majority of deaths occurred in the age group from twenty-five to forty-four; AIDS is now the leading cause of death in this age group. Table 9.1 shows comparative AIDS data by sex, ethnicity, exposure category, and geographical region.

Currently, it is estimated that 1 to 1.5 million persons in the United States are infected with HIV, including a growing number of women and persons of color. A substantial portion of these persons are unaware of their underlying HIV infection. Many cases of HIV infection remain unreported. Some do not meet the Centers for Disease Control (CDC) definition of AIDS, while other cases are in states that have no reporting requirements. The accuracy of diagnosing and reporting HIV infection varies by geographical location and affected population.[5] The growth of the HIV/AIDS epidemic is, however, in large part due to changes in the modes of transmission and the sociodemographic characteristics of the groups in which the epidemic is growing fastest.[6]

Widely recognized risk factors for the transmission of HIV include male-to-male sexual contact, male-to-female sexual contact, injection drug use (IDU), blood product exposure, and perinatal transmission from mother-to-infant (during pregnancy, delivery, or possibly breast-feeding). Contrary to public perception, the rate of increase in HIV transmission is slower among whites and homosexuals than among communities of color and heterosexuals.[7] Frequently, individuals are exposed through multiple infection routes, and so the actual mode of HIV transmission may be unclear.

## Treatment

The main types of treatment include medications to combat loss of immune function and to prevent specific disease complications. The most widely used drugs are antiretrovirals that slow the progress of HIV infection. These include zidovudine

## TABLE 9.1. CUMULATIVE AIDS CASES IN THE UNITED STATES THROUGH JUNE 1995.

| Category | Number (476,899) | Percentage |
|---|---|---|
| Gender | | |
| Male | 408,874 | 86 |
| Female | 68,021 | 13 |
| Unknown | 4 | <1 |
| Ethnicity | | |
| White, not Hispanic | 228,644 | 48 |
| Black, not Hispanic | 160,148 | 34 |
| Hispanic | 82,910 | 17 |
| Asian/Pacific Islander | 3,265 | 1 |
| American Indian/Alaska Native | 1,202 | <1 |
| Exposure | | |
| Adult ($n$ = 470,288) | | |
| Men who have sex with men | 244,235 | 52 |
| Injection drug use | 118,694 | 25 |
| Men who have sex with men and inject drugs | 31,024 | 7 |
| Hemophilia/coagulation disorder | 3,872 | 1 |
| Heterosexual contact | 35,683 | 8 |
| Blood transfusion, blood components or tissue | 7,128 | 2 |
| Other/risk not reported or identified | 29,652 | 6 |
| Pediatric ($n$ = 6,611) | | |
| Hemophilia/coagulation disorder | 226 | 3 |
| Mother with/at risk for HIV infection | 5,925 | 90 |
| Blood transfusion, blood components or tissue | 359 | 5 |
| Other/risk not reported or identified | 101 | 2 |
| Residence by census area | | |
| Metropolitan areas with populations >500,000 | 403,626 | 85 |
| Metropolitan areas with 50,000 to 500,000 | 46,042 | 10 |
| Nonmetropolitan areas | 25,109 | 5 |
| Unknown area of residence | 2,122 | <1 |

*Source:* Data for this table taken from *HIV AIDS Surveillance Report 7,* 1 (1995). Data are for fifty states, the District of Columbia, and four U.S. territories.

(ZDV/AZT), didanosine (ddI), and zalcitabibe or dideoxycitidine (ddC). Oral antibiotics are frequently used to prevent a common pneumonia (*Pneumocystis carinii* or PCP) that develops in persons with AIDS.[8] Most clinical services are directed toward monitoring for immune function decline, the development of specific HIV complications (for example, wasting syndrome, parasitic diarrhea, and candidiasis), and the reduction of treatment side effects. This monitoring involves use of the full range of medical services from radiology to laboratory tests. Ongoing monitoring is even more important as concomitant infectious diseases (such as tuberculosis and hepatitis) and HIV reinfection are becoming more common.

In the absence of a cure from traditional medical treatment, many people with HIV/AIDS may also use alternative medicine to combat compromised immunity and opportunistic infections. Alternative therapies fall into four primary groups: nonconventional drug treatment, nutrition and diet modification (vitamins, minerals, and herbs), acupuncture and chiropractic treatment, and psychospiritual intervention. Estimates of the incidence of alternative therapy usage range from 29 percent to 42 percent of AIDS patients surveyed.[9]

## Challenges for Health Services

Investigators are beginning to shed light on important characteristics of persons with HIV/AIDS who utilize health care services. Available information on population and system characteristics and how they determine access to medical care, costs, and quality of services are important considerations.

### Access to Care

As HIV disease progresses, many persons experience disability and unemployment and rely on public entitlement and private disability programs for income maintenance and health care benefits. These include Social Security Disability Income (SSDI) and Supplemental Security Income (SSI), administered by the Social Security Administration. Medicare and Medicaid become primary payers for health care with the onset of disability and depletion of personal funds.

Medicaid is the primary payer for HIV/AIDS health care. Medicaid covered more than 40 percent of health services for persons with AIDS in 1991.[10] In 1992, most hospitals were paid according to diagnosis-related groups (DRGs) or prospective per diem payments for Medicare and Medicaid patients. Many states also limit coverage for the number of inpatient hospital days per year. This policy created financial risks for providers as the average length of stay and the number of admissions were higher than average for those with AIDS-related illnesses.[11] In a study of New York Medicaid patients, groups of more seriously ill people with

AIDS demanded more health care services, particularly during diagnosis and mid-illness intervals.[12]

The lack of insurance and underinsurance represent formidable financial barriers to HIV/AIDS care. Persons with HIV/AIDS are more likely than the general population to be uninsured or to have Medicaid insurance.[13] As in the general population, the uninsured and those without a regular source of outpatient care are less likely to utilize outpatient medical services.[14] Even among the insured, substantial disparities in access persist due to disability from HIV/AIDS disease, loss of employment, and social stigma resulting in the loss of private insurance coverage—which, if provided at all, is generally at a less generous level.[15] Others may be reluctant to use their private insurance because of concerns about confidentiality and threats to employment.

The groups in which the epidemic is spreading most rapidly tend to experience poverty and lack of insurance, and make the least effective use of ambulatory services. For example, compared with gays and bisexuals, injection drug users (IDUs) have lower rates of private medical insurance, fewer outpatient medical visits, and lower income. Disadvantaged groups (minorities, women, IDUs, the poor) often have difficulty with access to continuous care and do not receive needed treatment.[16] Stability and continuity of care are particularly important for persons with HIV infection. One potential consequence of discontinuity is greater use of hospital emergency departments for nonemergency medical services. Inadequate access is often cited as the reason for inappropriate use of emergency care and services.[17]

Expanded measures of access are needed. Measures include structural factors affecting access, such as distance to care, transportation problems, insurance arrangements, and time delays in obtaining various services, as well as problems people may perceive when trying to obtain services.[18] Language, literacy, homelessness, and substance abuse problems may contribute to the barriers faced by certain groups. These access problems may also influence the use of costly services, as well as health outcomes and patient satisfaction. Access to care in HIV/AIDS should be examined in light of health care costs, as well as quality of care.

## Costs

The best current estimate of medical care costs is $119,000 per person expended from diagnosis of HIV until death, with $69,000 of that expended after a diagnosis of AIDS.[19] The forecast for the cumulative cost of treating all HIV+ individuals nationally is an increase from $10.3 billion in 1992 to $15.2 billion in 1995.[20]

The majority of direct AIDS care costs (73 percent to 82 percent) is due to hospital utilization. It is estimated that nearly 30 percent of AIDS patients are uninsured and that the eighteen cities with the largest AIDS caseloads lose more than $400 per day in hospital costs.[21] However, recent national estimates of the lifetime costs of AIDS are lower than previous estimates. This change is attributed to lower lifetime hospitalization rates nationally and a recent national shift toward a larger proportion of AIDS deaths outside the hospital.[22] Another study in Massachusetts also showed decreasing costs of AIDS care, due to shorter lengths of stay and lower hospital resource use.[23] A critical issue in estimating the cost of AIDS care is the stage and severity of the disease. Sicker patients require more therapy, resulting in greater costs.[24]

In summary, available data suggest that HIV/AIDS patients from groups with lower socioeconomic status and less access to care use costlier sources of care for longer durations. In addition, the variation in estimates of AIDS care costs by region, subpopulation, and provider-type raises the concern that these variations in costs are due to variations in provider quality. Hence, the costs of HIV/AIDS care should be examined in the context of quality as well.

## Quality

Recently, the emphasis in HIV/AIDS quality-of-care assessment has moved from traditional measures of structure and processes of care to outcomes measurement, particularly health-related quality of life (HRQL). Moreover, disease-specific parameters of quality of life and illness severity have emerged as important considerations. HRQL refers to how well an individual functions in daily life and his or her perceived well-being. It is conceptualized as encompassing physical, mental, and social function and well-being.[25] By contrast, most of the clinical research on HIV disease has focused on mortality or physiologic indexes to evaluate treatment efficacy.

HRQL outcomes are especially important in studies of HIV disease due to the nature of its chronic debilitating course, the multiplicity of potential interventions for the disease, and the controversies regarding timing and usefulness of some of these interventions. HRQL is perhaps the most important consideration in the delivery of medical care to persons with HIV, particularly in light of the modest impact of current treatments on survival.[26] Substantial evidence for the reliability and validity of several HRQL measures for patients with HIV/AIDS is accumulating from AIDS clinical trials[27] and observational studies.[28]

***Patient Satisfaction.*** Satisfaction is an important indicator of the quality of care and adequacy of services. Patient dissatisfaction has been shown in general populations to predict utilization, continuity of care, provider transition, adherence to treatment, delays in obtaining treatment, and health outcomes.[29] In a study of persons with AIDS, Stein and his colleagues found that IDUs, the uninsured, and public hospital patients were less satisfied with the technical and interpersonal care they received as well as with their access to care.[30]

***Standards and Guidelines.*** Standards for optimal care of HIV disease are difficult to construct because much of the variation in care is medically reasonable. However, medically unreasonable variations in care can be identified. A useful approach for identifying quality problems is to use available literature and expert opinion to determine the appropriateness and necessity of specific treatments for well-defined groups of patients. Despite wide variations in HIV/AIDS care, inadequate use of a few tests (such as CD4 count) and treatments (such as PCP prophylaxis) could constitute poor quality, including the failure to provide necessary care and the provision of inappropriate care.[31] Health policy research groups such as the RAND Corporation are developing the expertise to convert guidelines into explicit quality review criteria. Although guidelines for acute care such as hospitalization are less available, existing guidelines for chronic care are generally applicable. In the future, review criteria for chronic care will be combined with the outcome data producing meaningful comparisons of quality of care across a range of health care and social service systems.

# Toward a Comprehensive Continuum of Care

Persons with HIV/AIDS often present themselves to health care delivery systems in need of immediate acute care services. However, the course of the illness is now more commonly characterized by a gradual decline in physical, cognitive, and emotional function and well-being, which may require primary care, supportive care, housing, supervised living, home health care, and hospice services.[32] Intermittent episodes of severe complications sometimes represent specific disease complications or less definitive symptoms. Longer periods of relative quiescence eventually give way to subtle declines in functioning and the loss of ability to perform usual daily activities without assistance.[33] As a result, people living with AIDS need a wide array of personal and social services to support community-based living in the least restrictive setting.

Providing a continuum of care is the ideal. What the continuum consists of is open to debate and is shaped by the availability of financial resources supporting these programs. The continuum can encompass the following elements:

- Outreach and case finding
- Primary, secondary, and tertiary prevention

- Primary, secondary, and tertiary health care
- Coordination of long-term care, primary care, therapy, nonmedical services, public benefits, and insurance
- Legal services

Combining medical and nonmedical services may be the best approach to providing a continuum of care on a community level. As public and private payers search for cost-effective ways to provide quality care, the focus has shifted from hospital care to integrating key services such as prevention, mental health, legal, and dental services.

## Prevention and Education

Controlling the AIDS epidemic will depend on education and public health strategies to reduce high-risk behaviors. Groups with increasing incidence rates are targeted for intervention—men who have sex with men, IDUs, adolescents, and certain ethnic groups. Education and outreach have been major approaches to risk reduction, however controversy continues to mount around condom education in schools and needle-exchange programs.

Testing and reporting are considered key to monitoring HIV/AIDS, but practices vary across the United States (as shown in Table 9.2). There are many licensed tests for the clinical diagnosis of HIV infection, the most common being the enzyme-linked immunosorbent assay test. The Public Health Service has provided guidelines for counseling and testing, which promote individual behavioral changes, targeting the reduction of risk of HIV transmission among uninfected and infected persons.[34] In addition to reducing further transmission, timely medical care is promoted in the guidelines.

Partner notification, while potentially beneficial in promoting risk reduction and prevention of HIV, is not systematically addressed across states. Most states have voluntary programs and are not required to reveal the identity of the person infected. Additionally, notification is not possible if the index case has had anonymous sex partners, and it may be inefficient in populations with high HIV infection rates.[35]

## Mental Health and Social Support

In the beginning of the AIDS epidemic, many community-based organizations, such as the Shanti Foundation, were created to help with the grief associated with death and dying from AIDS. As more people with HIV became long-term survivors, mental health services and formal or informal support networks have become more important for the individual and his or her family, friends, and extended social support network. Depression in HIV+ clinic populations ranges

## TABLE 9.2. HIV TESTING AND REPORTING REQUIREMENTS IN THE UNITED STATES AND DISTRICT OF COLUMBIA.

| No Requirements | Strictly Anonymous (Demographics Only) | Anonymous with Names Reported in Specific Situations[a] | Names with Opportunities for Anonymous Testing | Names Only |
|---|---|---|---|---|
| Alaska | Florida | California | Arizona | Alabama |
| District of Columbia | Georgia | Delaware | Arkansas | Idaho |
| Louisiana | Hawaii | Oregon | Colorado | Minnesota |
| Massachusetts | Illinois | Tennessee | Connecticut[b] | North Dakota |
| Nebraska | Iowa | | Indiana | South Carolina |
| New Mexico | Kansas | | Kentucky | South Dakota |
| Pennsylvania | Maine | | Michigan | |
| Vermont | Maryland | | Mississippi | |
| | Montana | | Missouri | |
| | Nevada | | New Jersey | |
| | New Hampshire | | North Carolina | |
| | New York | | Ohio | |
| | Rhode Island | | Oklahoma | |
| | Texas | | Utah | |
| | Washington | | Virginia | |
| | | | West Virginia | |
| | | | Wisconsin | |
| | | | Wyoming | |

[a]For example, blood bank donations.

[b]Requires combined reporting of HIV and tuberculosis.

*Source:* The George Washington University Intergovernmental Project, AIDS Policy Center, Washington, D.C., January 1992.

from 15 percent to 30 percent, and anxiety disorders may be even more common. Effective treatment of these psychiatric disorders can improve functioning.[36]

Social support has been shown to benefit HRQL.[37] In HIV populations, the perceived availability of social support has been shown to be related to lowered hopelessness and depression and to increased feelings of psychological well-being.[38] Social resources are also important influences on service use. Persons with more social services available to them were less likely to use formal mental health services.[39] Social support can be key in facilitating access to necessary services by helping to overcome disruptions of health care due to unemployment and financial problems.

## Oral Health and Dental Services

Oral manifestations such as candida, mouth ulcers, and gum disease are common in HIV disease. The occurrence of oral lesions is important for disease prognosis. Dental care has been reported to be the most commonly needed service.[40] HIV-infected patients have substantial dental care needs, but they have difficulty accessing dental services. In 1988, only 31 percent of U.S. dental care providers were willing to treat AIDS patients.[41] In the United States, 52 percent of persons reported a need for dental care; IDUs and low-income patients were most likely to perceive a need for dental care.

## Nonmedical Services

Few studies have assessed the need for nonmedical health-related and social services. These services have been traditionally provided by AIDS service organizations such as Gay Men's Health Care Crisis in New York, AIDS Project Los Angeles, and the San Francisco AIDS Foundation. Nonmedical services can include meals, food banks or pantries, residential facilities, buddies, transportation, child care, public benefits counseling, and respite care. In a multisite study of 907 HIV+ persons, high levels of need were identified for mental health services, housing, entitlement programs, and transportation.[42] Unmet needs were highest for housing, transportation, mental health services, and access to entitlement programs. Evaluation data about nonmedical services are important in determining the level of unmet needs among persons with HIV/AIDS.

The number of persons who provide home care to people with HIV/AIDS has increased. This trend suggests the need to focus on the development of more home and community-based services. While there are no national estimates of the number of HIV+ persons using home care services, data from the 1991 AIDS Costs, Services and Utilization Survey (ACSUS) indicate that nearly half of the respondents with AIDS relied on informal home care and a quarter used some type of formal care during a three-month reference period.[43] It is not clear under what circumstances home care services may substitute for or complement more expensive inpatient services although there is some evidence that its use decreases overall costs.[44] As the population with HIV changes, however, the availability of informal home care (that provided by friends and family) may decrease, threatening the adequacy of the formal home care system.

## Legal Issues

People with HIV/AIDS have faced complex legal problems. Preparing wills, powers of attorney, and living wills are a few of the main concerns. Health insurance is another area of concern for those infected with HIV. As with other costly chronic conditions, insurance companies have denied benefits to HIV+ individuals based on policies about preexisting conditions. Insurance companies increasingly require HIV antibody testing of insurance applicants—and deny policies to those testing positive. Litigation has been the common avenue to resolve eligibility for health insurance benefits.[45]

# Organizing Comprehensive Care and Services

The organization and delivery of appropriate coordinated HIV/AIDS services involves several components. An adequate distribution of direct medical care providers is needed. Increasingly, providers must be able to function effectively within the structure of managed care plans. Finally, the use of case management is favored as a constructive cost-effective approach to organizing and integrating HIV/AIDS care.

## Providers

Up to three-quarters of primary care physicians in the United States have cared for an HIV+ patient, but national data on the distribution of current providers and the amount of care they provide are lacking. Understanding current HIV care requires understanding both the sites and types of providers. Costs, access, and quality of care depend not only on patient characteristics but also those of the providers. As the HIV epidemic spreads into new populations, it also is reaching new providers. Accurate assessments of present and future care require representative samples of all types of health care providers. Current data are limited to small numbers of institutional centers or highly identified AIDS practices, such as those involved in centrally funded research efforts.

## Managed Care

HIV/AIDS treatment is provided in an increasingly wide array of settings, including those that incorporate managed care practices. While most people in the United States receive their health coverage through private insurance companies and managed care organizations, the number of persons with AIDS covered by private plans has decreased over time.[46] Private insurers have reduced their coverage of HIV-infected persons because of the fear of high-cost individuals, partially as a result of highly inflated estimates placing the average cost of an AIDS case at $147,000.[47] Thus, persons with HIV find it virtually impossible to purchase individual policies. Strategies to reduce provider risk also include tighter underwriting guidelines, use of HIV testing for enrollment, and denying insurance to those with a history of sexually transmitted diseases.[48]

Some states are experimenting with capitated arrangements and managed care as a way to provide better access to care for Medicaid recipients. In these arrangements, providers are at risk for the costs of care, creating an incentive to limit costly treatment and procedures. Very little is known about the impact on costs and quality of care when reimbursement for AIDS is capitated. Even with Medicaid's shortcomings, some have advocated an expansion of Medicaid eligibility to address the problem of financing of care for HIV/AIDS.[49]

## Case Management

Addressing problems of access, cost, and quality of HIV/AIDS care in medical and community-based settings may reduce service fragmentation and provide more comprehensive services. Case management has often been suggested as a strategy for coordinating care. There are many definitions of case management; however, most approaches include core activities—intake and assessment, a comprehensive, multidisciplinary care plan, referrals to services, monitoring of care, modification of care plans based on current problems, and client advocacy.[50] For many, case management may offer community-based alternatives to hospitalization and may thus be both more cost effective and more humane. Use of home services such as intravenous antibiotics and total parenteral nutrition may save 30 percent to 50 percent of hospital costs.[51]

Case management has been found to contribute to longevity between HIV diagnosis and death and between first hospitalization and death.[52] A mixed model of case management, which combines AIDS risk-reduction education and modified service brokerage, has been suggested as an approach that might have greater impact with higher-risk groups (such as IDUs and cocaine abusers) in assessment and timely response to immediate client need.[53] More research is needed to evaluate the effects of case management on cost, access, and quality. Information about case management and patterns of care for HIV/AIDS are needed by policy makers and managers who are attempting to reduce reliance on costly inpatient care.

## Research Needs and Policy Implications

The medical, social, and epidemiological realities of HIV/AIDS have forced researchers and policy makers to reconsider priorities in developing their agendas for the future. Resource allocation decisions may be shaped by political will and the changing sociodemographics and needs of persons infected by HIV and living with AIDS. The implications are immense for health services research, program development and implementation, and public- and private-sector policy.

## AIDS Health Services Research

The initial interest in HIV/AIDS research was primarily clinical and not far-reaching. As the problem of AIDS grew in scope, research efforts expanded. Public and private organizations funding and performing research now include the American Foundation for AIDS Research (AmFAR), the Robert Wood Johnson Foundation, the Agency for Health Care Policy and Research (AHCPR), the Centers for Disease Control and Prevention, and the Health Resources and Services Administration. Although health services researchers have responded to the AIDS epidemic with an array of studies, these studies have invariably been based in large metropolitan areas using purposive and convenience sampling.

Several studies nearing completion may provide relevant starting points for developing coherent HIV/AIDS health policy, as well as for guiding program development, implementation, and evaluation. However, many existing studies are substantially limited in one or more features of design, implementation, measurement, and analytic procedures. In general, HIV/AIDS population-based studies are limited by coverage error, sampling error, measurement error, and nonresponse error. Each of these types of errors contributes to differences between the true population value of the variable and the estimate derived from the particular study.[54]

Another concern affecting comparability of studies is the definition of AIDS and its use in defining populations for health services research. Since the epidemic began in the early 1980s, the understanding of the disease has changed. Consequently, clinical criteria have redefined what constitutes a case of AIDS. In turn, surveillance findings have been influenced. Misreporting and underreporting of HIV/AIDS are likely affected by changing case definitions, the most recent CDC definition being implemented in 1993. The immunosuppressed conditions now known as HIV and AIDS have been referred to as GRID, AIDS-related complex (ARC), Simian AIDS, lesser AIDS, symptomatic and asymptomatic HIV, frank AIDS, or full-blown AIDS.[55] The changing case definitions need to be acknowledged in research and planning, particularly when temporal changes are considered.

Future studies should evaluate specific access problems encountered in seeking specific services and levels of care. Furthermore, data are needed about various health delivery systems (public, private, and teaching) and financing mechanisms (admixtures of prepaid and fee-for-service, levels of deductibles and co-payments) that provide care for economically and ethnically diverse populations with HIV/AIDS. Future studies should examine how the satisfaction of HIV+ persons relates to subsequent utilization of services and to outcomes; the extent of the need for and availability of services across the entire range of HIV+ persons; the degree to which those needs are being met; barriers to, satisfaction with, and costs of such care; and how to provide need-sensitive care for diverse populations.

Costs associated with AIDS have been assessed in three ways—evaluating costs of inpatient care, estimating annual costs of care, and examining lifetime costs associated with care.[56] These have provided limited data about the true costs of care. Valid estimates on the cost of providing care to subpopulations infected with HIV, the medical and nonmedical services that are used and needed by these populations, and how that care is financed are critical for the formulation of resource allocation policies. Yet this knowledge is limited by the existing body of research, as well as by the evolving changes of HIV/AIDS epidemiology and treatment. The course of the epidemic is changing in a number of ways that affect cost and use of services: the demographic composition of the infected population, the geographical areas where the disease is being treated, the length of survival after HIV or AIDS diagnosis, the range of available treatments, the provider's experience and skill in giving care, and the financing and organization of delivery systems where care is received. Although detailed cost studies in particular regions and populations may be useful to local policy and planning, coherent national policy requires nationally representative data. Much available cost information is based on subpopulations, such as persons with advanced HIV infection who meet the criteria for AIDS, or IDUs, or gay and bisexual men.[57]

Few analyses have examined the full spectrum of costs, including the indirect costs of AIDS. Longitudinal data are needed to allow changes in costs and use for a given person to be tracked over time. Even the largest study, ACSUS, may provide biased estimates of use and costs because it includes only large metropolitan areas and mostly very large providers of care. However, methods for cost measurement, such as determining unit cost of services, are becoming more commonplace in determining the costs of AIDS care.[58]

## AIDS Policy in Transition

The HIV/AIDS epidemic has moved away from its initial epicenters to much broader communities of the socially and economically disadvantaged. Concurrently, the range of medical treatments for HIV and AIDS complications has grown. The settings in which these treatments are administered are increasingly diverse, including those incorporating managed care principles, such as health maintenance organizations (HMOs). Despite these developments, public policy decisions related to HIV/AIDS have thus far relied primarily on studies that utilize convenience samples of the earliest affected cohort—Caucasian males with sexual contact as the identified mode of exposure. Information currently used to guide public policy and other decisions concerning HIV/AIDS is incomplete and potentially misguiding.

HIV/AIDS is only one of many public health problems and social issues that confront the United States as it moves into the twenty-first century. The initial impetus for action has diminished as the epidemic enters its second decade and AIDS activists either burn out or succumb to the virus. Within the HIV/AIDS community, the allocation of scarce resources is politically charged. Should more funds be directed toward prevention, or should treatment take priority? How can research funds have the greatest impact: through a return to basic science or expanded and accelerated clinical trials? What is the appropriate funding relationship between medical services and social services? Certainly no easy answers exist for these questions, and powerful interest groups can be found on every side. While debate about priorities is healthy, there is potential for conflict that does a disservice to persons with HIV/AIDS. Developing partnerships and networks to effectively organize and deliver health and social services is paramount.

## Health Policy Issues and Options

As HIV increases in communities of color and among the poor, the financial burden on public payers and health care providers will inevitably increase. Reliance on Medicaid has profound implications for persons with HIV/AIDS as public support for Medicaid has waned. In addition, new federal eligibility mandates of the 1980s and 1990s have increased the cost of Medicaid to states. As a result, many state legislatures are searching for ways to effectively control the costs of the program. Rate setting of provider payments is one way states have attempted to control their Medicaid costs. In many states, payment levels have not kept up with inflation; Medicaid generally pays providers less than their costs of care. As providers limit the number of Medicaid patients they serve, access to care may deteriorate for those dependent on this public benefit.

Medicare currently pays for a very small portion of AIDS expenditures because of the twenty-nine-month waiting period from the onset date of disability. A policy alternative proposed is to significantly reduce or entirely eliminate this waiting period.[59] The Congressional Budget Office estimated that a reduced AIDS-specific waiting period would cost the federal government $3 billion over five years, while it would generate $550 million in Medicaid savings to the states.[60] Medicare administrators may be unwilling to support another disease-specific expansion of the program, given the agency's experience with end-stage renal disease, whose costs have ballooned since the program's implementation. It is important to note that Medicare eligibility is only a partial solution for persons with AIDS because Medicare has no outpatient prescription drug benefit and most treatments for HIV disease are pharmacological.

Expansion of employer-based insurance is highly unlikely with the demise of the Clinton administration's proposed 1993 Health Security Act and its employer mandate provision. Attention should be directed toward the maintenance of private health insurance of persons with HIV. Some states have programs that pay private health insurance and Consolidated Omnibus Budget Reconciliation Act (COBRA) premiums of persons with AIDS and other high-cost illnesses; California and New York are the largest examples. These programs represent a win-win situation for persons with AIDS and public agencies. Persons with AIDS are able to remain with their current health care providers and maintain continuity of care. At the same time, public providers and payers are relieved of a substantial portion of the burden of care and treatment by shifting it to the private sector.

While Medicaid has covered much of the medical care for HIV/AIDS, funding of community-based care began to expand beyond nonprofit organizations with the passage of the Ryan White Comprehensive AIDS Resources (CARE) Act in 1990. The HIV/AIDS programs funded by the CARE Act enabled those without health insurance to access treatment. In addition, other services (such as legal, advocacy, and mental health services) were developed to support community living. Another intent of the CARE Act was to meet the needs of those with limited access to services, due to either provider availability or geography (that is, rural versus urban). The effectiveness of the act has been limited by the growing needs of persons with AIDS in all communities.

## Needs of Special Populations

Certain special populations deserve attention: HIV+ women, children, and adolescents, and certain ethnic groups who are at a higher risk of contracting HIV. These groups face additional barriers to early intervention and access to care when their vulnerability is considered.

**Women.** By the year 2000, the number of new AIDS cases reported annually in women is predicted to equal that of men.[61] AIDS is the leading cause of death for twenty- to forty-year-old women in major cities. African American and Latina women account for 75 percent of infected women.[62] The course of clinical care varies as women present to the medical care system at more advanced stages of the disease than do men and are less likely than men to receive zidovudine.[63] Most studies indicate that differences between men and women in their use of services such as the emergency room and inpatient and outpatient sites may be explained by factors such as insurance status, stage of illness, and transmission risk.[64]

Obstetric and gynecological conditions and procedures may contribute substantially to the health service use of women.[65] The availability of obstetric and gynecological services and of licensing and funding for trained health care providers, shortage of obstetricians, and the limited HIV experience of health care providers may influence health service access and utilization. Other gender-specific factors that may influence utilization include misdiagnosis or undiagnosed HIV-related conditions, sexual or domestic violence, commercial sex work, and the responsibilities of child care.

*Children.* An estimated ten to twenty thousand children in the country have HIV infection. As of June 1993, 1.5 percent ($n = 4,710$) of AIDS cases had been reported in children less than thirteen years old; 53 percent of childhood AIDS cases are African American, and 25 percent are Hispanic.[66] Most infected children acquire the disease perinatally, and most (90 percent) have mothers with known HIV infection.[67] Almost two-thirds of mothers of perinatally infected children were IDUs or had a sexual partner who injected drugs. About 25 percent of children born to HIV+ mothers are infected.[68]

The costs of pediatric AIDS are higher than the costs of adult AIDS, largely due to higher hospital costs. They are estimated at $35,000 per year on average for pediatric inpatients.[69] Medicaid is the primary payer for both hospital and community-based services for pediatric AIDS.[70] Contributing to the high costs are the complications of medical management by the absence, disability, or death of one or both parents through AIDS or drug use, urban poverty, and complex social conditions.[71]

*Adolescents.* AIDS is the sixth leading cause of death in people aged fifteen to twenty-four and contributes to premature mortality of those who are supposed to be healthy, productive, and likely to live a normal life.[72] This population is of particular concern because of the number of sexual contacts and behaviors that contribute to increased risk and likelihood of infection.[73] Although adolescents are now more aware of HIV transmission risks and AIDS, many still have misperceptions about sexual activity, drug use, and prevention measures. Despite adequate knowledge, most adolescents continue to participate in unprotected sex.[74]

*Ethnic Groups.* HIV/AIDS disproportionately affects certain ethnic groups. Hispanics and African Americans often experience institutional barriers to both access and outreach. Many may not be aware of the benefits of receiving early treatment. Geographical barriers to care also pose access concerns. Sites of care for HIV/AIDS may not be in familiar neighborhood settings. Agencies may not be prepared to deal with cultural needs.[75] These issues may exacerbate the vulnerability already experienced by people with HIV/AIDS in receiving the full range of health care services that are needed and available.

# Future Focus of HIV/AIDS Health Services Research

Ideally, policy and planning options are based on evidence of the effectiveness of treatment and acceptable levels of cost effectiveness in delivering such treatment. However, there is very little empirical evidence for the cost effectiveness of various types of AIDS care. Several studies are nearing completion that will provide relevant starting points for developing coherent HIV/AIDS health policy as well as for guiding program development, implementation, and evaluation.

Public policy related to the HIV epidemic has thus far relied solely on limited studies, that is, studies not based on a national probability sample of persons with HIV. While purposive or convenience samples may be useful during early stages of inquiry as a method of better defining new research questions, such studies cannot be used to make inferences to the broader populations of interest because of reliability and validity concerns. Generalizability of findings to new HIV populations is problematic.[76]

The AHCPR and RAND have just begun the HIV Costs and Services Utilization Study (HCSUS), a cooperative study that should vastly improve policy-relevant AIDS health services data. This study will provide data relevant to a wide range of issues pertinent to HIV policy, including costs and utilization in different delivery systems, transitions among providers, access and barriers to care, satisfaction, quality of life, social support services, mental health, dental health, and quality of care. New research efforts must include the changing clinical profile of the epidemic. In addition, research efforts must provide insights into national trends, such as regional variation in the patterns of HIV-related disease complications. Changes in treatment patterns and changes in the prices of medications over time make predictions of future costs even more difficult. The many nonmedical costs of HIV/AIDS should be examined: direct costs of transportation, nutrition, and housing as well as indirect costs of disability—such as days lost from work as a result of treatment or deteriorating health.

Supplemental studies with national probability samples of special populations will also be needed: women, children, adolescents, IDUs, persons in rural communities, and the racial/ethnic minorities who constitute a growing proportion of the HIV-infected population. Data collected on cost and utilization will enable policy makers to compare patterns of costs and utilization across the spectrum of HIV disease, across geographical areas, across the range of institutional and individual providers (including managed care settings), and for both the insured and the uninsured populations, as well as variations with different financing and provider arrangements.

Lack of insurance, poverty, and underutilization of ambulatory services often coincide for members of the groups in which the epidemic is spreading most rapidly. Disadvantaged groups (minorities, women, IDUs, and the poor) experience difficulty more often than others in obtaining access to outpatient care. In addition, they may not receive treatment, and this may account for greater mortality in those populations.[77] People with impaired access to health services often utilize costly sources of medical care (for example, emergency and acute inpatient care) and use them for longer durations. Furthermore, the variation of AIDS care by geographical region, subpopulation, and type of provider likely reflect poor quality of care for certain individuals.

In view of these concerns, the important characteristics of the changing epidemiology of AIDS and clinical treatment patterns need to be examined using better measures of access, costs, and quality. Health service delivery systems need to be developed to address the emerging needs of diverse population groups affected by HIV/AIDS. Neither the arena of formal medical services nor the continuum of care can be overlooked. The need for finance and delivery systems developed in the context of long-range planning and evaluation is paramount. Existing knowledge and critical gaps in information about HIV/AIDS have been reviewed to provide a framework for addressing the current and future challenges that HIV/AIDS presents for development of relevant health policy and health and social services planning and program implementation.

# Notes

1. F. Kirchhoff, T. C. Greenbough, D. B. Brettler, et al., "Brief Report: Absence of Intact *nef* Sequences in a Long-Term Survivor with Nonprogressive HIV-1 Infection," *New England Journal of Medicine* 332 (January 26, 1995): 228–232.

2. R. A. Kaslow, J. P. Phair, H. B. Friedman, et al., "Infection with the Human Immunodeficiency Virus: Clinical Manifestations and Their Relationship to Immune Deficiency," *Annals of Internal Medicine* 107 (October 1987): 474–480.

3. G. Pantaleo, S. Menso, M. Vaccarezza, and C. Graziosi, "Studies in Subjects with Long-Term Nonprogressive Human Immunodeficiency Virus Infection," *New England Journal of Medicine* 332 (January 26, 1995): 209–216.

4. Centers for Disease Control and Prevention HIV/AIDS Surveillance Report, 7, 1 (1995); and American Association for World Health, *AIDS and Families: Protect and Care for the Ones We Love.* (Washington, D.C.: American Association for World Health, 1994).

5. Gerald J. Stine, *AIDS: Biological, Medical, Social and Legal Issues* (Englewood Cliffs, N.J.: Prentice Hall, 1993).

6. Centers for Disease Control, "Projections of Persons Diagnosed with AIDS and the Number of Immunosuppressed HIV-Infected Persons, 1992–1994, *Morbidity and Mortality Weekly Report* 41 (1992): 1–29.

7. Stine, *AIDS: Biological, Medical, Social and Legal Issues,* pp. 238–239.

8. William V. Valenti, *Early Intervention in the Management of HIV: A Handbook for Managed Health Care Professionals* (n.p.: Burroughs-Wellcome, January 1992); and American Foundation for AIDS Research, *AIDS/HIV Treatment Directory,* vol. 7, no. 3 (New York: American Foundation for AIDS Research, June 10, 1994).

9. D. I. Abrams, "Alternative Therapies in AIDS," *AIDS* 4 (1990): 1179–1187; and G. Laifer et al., "A Frequent Use of Alternative Therapies and Higher Subjective Benefit Compared to Traditional Medicine in HIV Infected Patients," Abstract PoB 3395, International Conference on AIDS, 1992; and R. M. Greenblatt, H. Hollander, J. R. McMaster, and C. J. Henke, "Polypharmacy Among Patients Attending an AIDS Clinic: Utilization of Prescribed, Unorthodox and Investigational Treatments," *Journal of AIDS* 4 (1991): 136–143.

10. Gail Wilensky, "Financing Care for Patients With AIDS," *Journal of the American Medical Association* 266 (December 25, 1991): 3404.

11. Robert J. Buchanan and Fred G. Kircher, "Medicaid Policies for AIDS-Related Hospital Care," *Health Care Financing Review* 15 (Summer 1994): 33–41.

12. L. E. Markson, L. McKee, J. Mauskopf, et al., "Patterns of Medicaid Expenditures After AIDS Diagnosis," *Health Care Financing Review* 15 (Summer 1994): 43–59.

13. J. Green and P. S. Arno, "The 'Medicaidization' of AIDS," *JAMA* 264 (1990): 1261–1266.

14. V. Mor, J. Fleishman, M. Dresser, and J. Piette, "Variation in Health Service Use Among HIV-Infected Patients," *Medical Care* 30 (1992): 17–29.

15. H. J. Makadon, G. R. Seage, K. E. Thorpe, and H. V. Fineberg, "Paying the Medical Cost of the HIV Epidemic: A Review of Policy Options," *Journal of Acquired Immune Deficiency Syndromes* (1990): 123–133.

16. P. J. Easterbrook, J. C. Keruly, T. Kirk-Creagh, et al., "Racial and Ethnic Differences in Outcome in Zidovudine-Treated Patients with Advanced HIV Disease," *JAMA* 266 (1991): 2713–2718; R. D. Moore, J. Hidalgo, B. W. Sugland, and R. E. Chaisson, "Zidovudine and the Natural History of Acquired Immunodeficiency," *New England Journal of Medicine* 324 (1991): 1412–141; and Mor, Fleishman, Dresser, and Piette, "Variation in Health Service Use Among HIV-Infected Patients."

17. S. Gaveler and D. H. VanTheil, "The Non-Emergency in the Emergency Room," *Journal of the National Medical Association* 72 (1980): 33–35; and J. P. Geyman, "Trends and Concerns in Emergency Room Utilization," *Journal of Family Practice* 11 (1980): 23.

18. W. E. Cunningham, R. D. Hays, K. W. Williams, K. C. Beck, W. J. Dixon, and M. F. Shapiro, "Access to Medical Care and Health-Related Quality of Life for Low-Income Persons with Symptomatic Human Immunodeficiency Virus," *Medical Care* 33, 7 (July 1995): 739–754.

19. Fred J. Hellinger, "The Lifetime Cost of Treating a Person with HIV," *JAMA* 270 (1993): 474–478.

20. Fred J. Hellinger, "Forecasts of the Costs of Medical Costs with HIV Epidemic: 1992–1995," *Inquiry* 29 (1992): 356–365.

21. Bruce Japsen, "AIDS: Better Ways to Care," *Modern Healthcare* (October 3, 1994): 81–86.

22. J. J. Kelly, S. Y. Chu, and J. W. Buehler, "AIDS Deaths Shift from Hospital to Home," *American Journal of Public Health* 83 (1993): 1433–1437.

23. Seage, Landers, Lamp, and Epstein, "Effect of Changing Patterns of Care and Duration of Survival on the Cost of Treating the Acquired Immune Deficiency Syndrome"; and G. R. Seage, T. Hertz, V. E. Stone, and A. M. Epstein, "The Effects of Intravenous Drug Use and Gender on the Cost of Hospitalization for Patients with AIDS," *Journal of Acquired Immune Deficiency Syndrome* 6 (1993): 831–839.

24. A. A. Scitovsky, M. W. Cline, and D. I. Abrams, "Effects of the Use of AZT on the Medical Care Costs of Person with AIDS in the First 12 Months," *Journal of AIDS,* 3 (1990): 904–912.

25. World Health Organization, "The Alma-Alta Conference on Primary Health Care," *WHO Chronicle* 32 (1978): 182–188.

26. Ron D. Hays and Martin F. Shapiro, "An Overview of Generic Health-Related Quality of Life Measures for HIV Research," *Quality of Life Research* 1 (1992): 91–97.

27. R. M. Kaplan, J. P. Anderson, A. W. Wu, et al., "The Quality of Well-Being Scale: Applications in AIDS, Cystic Fibrosis and Arthritis," *Medical Care* 27 (1989): S27–S43; and A. W. Wu, W. C. Mathews, L. T. Brysk, et al., "Quality of Life in a Placebo-Controlled Trial of Zidovudine in Patients with AIDS and AIDS-Related Complex," *Journal of AIDS* 3 (1990): 683–690.

28. P. D. Cleary, F. J. Fowler, J. Weissman, et al., "Health-Related Quality of Life in Persons with Acquired Immune Deficiency Syndrome," *Medical Care* 31 (1993): 569–580; and T. Wachtel, J. Piette, V. Mor, M. Stein, et al., "Quality of Life in Persons with Human Immunodeficiency Infection: Measurement by Medical Outcomes Instrument," *Annals of Internal Medicine* 116 (1992): 1359–1366.

29. J. A. Hall, M. A. Milburn, and A. A. Epstein. "A Causal Model of Health Status and Satisfaction with Medical Care," *Medical Care* 31 (1993): 84–94; and C. Donald-Sherbourne, R. D. Hays, L. Ordway, et al., "Antecedents of Adherence to Medical Recommendations: Results from the Medical Outcomes Study," *Journal of Behavioral Medicine* 15 (1992): 447–468.

30. M. D. Stein, J. Fleishman, V. Mor, and M. Dresser, "Factors Associated with Patient Satisfaction Among Symptomatic HIV Persons," *Medical Care* 31 (1993): 182–188.

31. D. C. Hadorn and R. H. Brook, "The Health Care Resource Allocation Debate: Defining Our Terms," *JAMA* 266 (1991): 3328–3331.

32. R. D. Hays, W. E. Cunningham, M. K. Ettl, et al., "Health-Related Quality of Life in HIV Disease," *Assessment* 2 (1995): 363–380; A. W. Wu and H. Rubin, "Measuring Health Status and Quality of Life in HIV and AIDS," *Psychology and Health* 6 (1992): 251–264; and Ron D. Hays and Martin F. Shapiro, "An Overview of Generic Health-Related Quality of Life Measures for HIV Research."

33. D. P. Lubeck and J. F. Fries, "Changes in Quality of Life Among People with HIV Infection," *Quality of Life Research* 1 (1992): 359–366.

34. Centers for Disease Control, "Public Health Service Guidelines for Counseling and Antibody Testing to Prevent HIV Infection and AIDS," *MMWR* 36 (August 14, 1987): 509–515.

35. Eve K. Nichols, *Mobilizing Against AIDS* (Cambridge, Mass.: Harvard University Press, 1989).

36. S. W. Perry, "Organic Mental Disorders Caused by HIV: Update on Early Diagnosis and Treatment," *American Journal of Psychiatry* 147 (1990): 696–710; E. G. Bing, K. Wells, and B. Visscher, "Effect of Depression on Utilization of Mental Health and General Medical Outpatient Services by HIV-Infected Men: The Multicenter AIDS Cohort Study," in *Proceedings of the RWJ Clinical Scholars Program Annual Meeting* (Ft. Lauderdale, Fla.: Robert Wood Johnson Clinical Scholars Program, 1993); and J. Mintz, L. I. Mintz, M. J. Arruda, et al. "Treatment of Depression and the Functional Capacity to Work," *Archives of General Psychiatry* 49 (1992): 761–768.

37. C. Donald-Sherbourne, L. S. Meredith, W. Rogers, and J. E. Ware, Jr., "Social Support and Stressful Life Events: Age Differences in Their Effects on Health Related Quality of Life Among the Chronically Ill," *Quality of Life Research* 1 (1992): 235–246.

38. J. Zich and L. Temoshok, "Perceptions of Social Support in Men with AIDS and ARC: Relationships with Distress and Hardiness," *Journal of Applied Social Psychology* 17 (1987): 193–215; and R. D. Hays, S. Chauncey, and L. Toby, "The Social Support Networks of Gay Men with AIDS," *Journal of Community Psychiatry* 18 (1990): 374–385.

39. Cathy Donald-Sherbourne, "The Role of Social Support and Life Stress Events in Use of Mental Health Services," *Social Science and Medicine* 27 (1988): 1393–1400.

40. J. D. Piette, J. A. Fleishman, M. D. Stein, et al., "Perceived Needs and Unmet Needs for Formal Services Among People with HIV Disease," *Journal of Community Health* 18 (1993): 11–23; and E. I. Capiluoto, J. D. Piette, B. A. White, and J. A. Fleishman, "Perceived Need for Dental Care Among Persons Living with Acquired Immune Deficiency Syndrome," *Medical Care* 29 (1991): 745–754.

41. A. C. Verrusio et al., "The Dentist and Infectious Diseases: A National Survey of Attitudes and Behaviors," *Journal of the American Dental Association* 118 (1989): 533–562.

42. Piette, Fleishman, Stein, et al., "Perceived Needs and Unmet Needs."

43. P. Mohr, *Patterns of Health Care Use in IV-Infected Adults: Preliminary Results,* AIDS Costs and Utilization Survey, AHCPR Pub. No. 94–0105 (Rockville, Md.: U.S. Department of Health and Human Services, Public Health Service, Agency for Health Care and Policy Research, 1994).

44. C. L. Schur et al., *Measuring the Utilization and Costs of AIDS Health Care Services* (Rockville, MD.: Health Resources and Services Administration, 1992); and M. Widman, D. W. Light, and J. J. Platt, "Expert Opinion on Barriers to Hospital Discharge for AIDS Patients," *AIDS & Public Policy Journal* 5, 3 (1991): 132–136.

45. Mark S. Senak, "Legal Issues Facing AIDS Patients," in *AIDS: A Healthcare Management Response,* ed. Kevin D. Blanchet (Rockville, Md.: Aspen, 1988).

46. Office of Technology Assessment, *AIDS and Health Insurance: An OTA Survey,* staff paper (Washington, D.C.: Office of Technology Assessment, 1988).

47. J. Green, G. M. Oppenheimer, and N. Wintfield, "The $147,000 Misunderstanding: Repercussions of Overestimating the Costs of AIDS," *Journal of Health Politics, Policy, and Law* 19 (Spring 1994): 69–90.

48. Nichols, *Mobilizing Against AIDS.*

49. Makadon, Seage, Thorpe, and Fineberg, "Paying the Medical Cost of the HIV Epidemic."

50. V. Mor, J. A. Fleishman, S. A. Allen, and J. D. Piette, *Networking AIDS Services* (Ann Arbor, Mich.: Health Administration Press, 1994).

51. J. S. Hart and K. L. Redding, "A Physician's Perspective on the Advantage of Home Medical Care: The Other Side of Case Management," *Texas Medicine* 90 (February 1994): 50–54.

52. R. L. Sowell, R. L. Gueldner, M. R. Killeen, et al., "Impact of Case Management on Hospital Charges of PWAs in Georgia," *Journal of the Association of Nurses in AIDS Care* 3 (April-June 1992): 24–31.

53. R. S. Falck, H. A. Siegal, and R. G. Carlson, "Case Management to Enhance AIDS Risk Reduction for Injection Drug Users and Crack Cocaine Users: Practical and Philosophical Considerations," *National Institute of Drug Abuse Research Monograph* 127 (1992): 167–180.

54. Cathy Donald-Sherbourne et al., "Population-Based Measures of Access and Consumer Satisfaction with Health Care," in *Proceedings of Consumer Survey Information in a Reformed Health Care System* (Vienna, Va.: Agency for Health Care Policy and Research & Robert Wood Johnson Foundation, September 1994).

55. James J. Goedert and William A. Blattner, "The Epidemiology of AIDS and Related Conditions," in *AIDS: Etiology, Diagnosis, Treatment and Prevention,* eds. V. T. DeVita, S. Hellman, and S. A. Rosenberg (Philadelphia: Lippincott, 1985), pp. 1–30.

56. Markson, McKee, Mauskopf, et al., "Patterns of Medicaid Expenditures After AIDS Diagnosis."

57. L. Solomon, R. Frank, D. Vlahov, and J. Astemborski, "Utilization of Health Services in a Cohort of Intravenous Drug Users with Known HIV-1 Serostatus," *AJPH* 81 (1991): 1285–1290; and A. A. Scitovsky, M. Cline, and P. R. Lee, "Medical Care Costs of AIDS Patients in San Francisco," *JAMA* 256 (1986): 3103–3106.

58. U.S. Department of Health and Human Services, *Determining Unit Cost of Services: A Guide for Estimating the Costs of Services Funded by the Ryan White CARE Act* (Washington, D.C.: U.S. Government Printing Office, 1994).

59. Makadon, Seage, Thorpe, and Fineberg, "Paying the Medical Cost of the HIV Epidemic."

60. Congressional Budget Office, Cost Estimates, HR 276 (1987).

61. M. Gwinn, M. Pappaioanou, J. R. George, et al., "Prevalence of HIV Infection in Childbearing Women in the United States: Surveillance Using Newborn Samples," *JAMA* 265 (1991): 1704–1708.

62. E. E. Schoenbaum and M. P. Webber, "The Underrecognition of HIV Infection in Women in an Inner-City Emergency Room," *AJPH* 83 (1993): 363–368.

63. M. D. Stein, B. Leibman, T. J. Wachtel, et al., "HIV Positive Women: Reasons They Are Tested for HIV and Their Clinical Characteristics on Entry into the Health Care System," *Journal of General Internal Medicine* 6 (1991): 286–289; and Fred J. Hellinger, "The Use of Health Services by Women with HIV Infection," *Health Services Research* 28 (1991): 543–561.

64. Mor, Fleishman, Dresser, and Piette, "Variation in Health Service Use Among HIV-Infected Patients."

65. C.C.J. Carpenter, K. H. Mayer, M. D. Stein, et al., "Human Immunodeficiency Virus Infection in North American Women: Experience with 200 Women and a Review of the Literature," *Medicine* 10 (1991): 307–325.

66. Centers for Disease Control and Prevention, *HIV Surveillance, Third Quarter* (Rockville, Md.: U.S. Department of Health and Human Serivices, Public Health Service, 1993); and National Pediatric HIV Resource Center, *Getting a Head Start on HIV: A Resource Manual for Enhancing Services to HIV-Affected Children in Head Start* (n.p., N.J.: National Pediatric HIV Resource Center, 1992).

67. G. B. Scott and W. P. Parks, "Pediatric AIDS," in *Principles and Practice of Pediatrics,* eds. F. A. Oski, C. D. DeAngelis, R. D. Feigin, et al. (Philadelphia: Lippincott, 1994); and Centers for Disease Control and Prevention, *HIV Surveillance, Third Quarter.*

68. Centers for Disease Control and Prevention, *HIV Surveillance, Third Quarter.*

69. R. Conviser, C. M. Arant, and M. S. Coye, "Pediatric Acquired Immunodeficiency Syndrome Hospitalizations in New Jersey," *Pediatrics* 28 (1991): 642–653; and C. Muller et al., "Hospital Costs for Pediatric AIDS, 1988–89: A Study of Costs and Social Severity," manuscript under review, 1992.

70. J. K. Ball and S. Thaul, *Pediatric AIDS-Related Discharges in a Sample of U.S. Hospitals: Demographics, Diagnoses and Resources Use,* AHCPR Pub. No. 92–0031; Division of Provider Studies Research Note 16 (Rockville, Md.: U.S. Department of Health and Human Services, Public Health Service, Agency for Health Care Policy and Research, 1992).

71. A. E. Burn, et al., "Pediatric AIDS in the United States: Epidemiological Reality Versus Government Policy," *International Journal of Health Policy* 20 (1991): 617–630.

72. Karen Hein, "Adolescents at Risk for HIV Infection," in *Adolescents and AIDS,* ed. Ralph J. DiClemente (Newbury Park, Calif.: Sage, 1992).

73. Karen Hein, "AIDS in Adolescence: The Next Wave of the HIV Epidemic?" *Journal of Pediatrics* 114 (1989): 144–149.

74. Ralph Hingson and Lee Strunin, "Monitoring Adolescents' Response to the AIDS Epidemic: Changes in Knowledge, Attitudes, Beliefs and Behaviors," in *Adolescents and AIDS,* ed. Ralph J. DiClemente (Newbury Park, Calif.: Sage, 1992).

75. U.S. Department of Health and Human Services, *HIV/AIDS Work Group on Health Care Issues for Hispanic Americans,* Pub. No. HRSA RD–SP–93–8 (Rockville, Md.: U.S. Department of Health and Human Services, December 1991).

76. W. E. Cunningham, R. D. Hays, K. W. Williams, et al., "Comparison of Health-Related Quality of Life in Clinical Trial and Nonclinical Trial Human Immunodeficiency Virus-Infected Cohorts," *Medical Care* 33 (1995): AS15–AS25.

77. J. R. Curtis and D. L. Patrick, "Race and Survival Time: A Synthesis of the Literature," *AJPH* 83 (1993): 1425–1428.

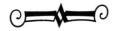

CHAPTER TEN

# HEALTH CARE REFORM FOR CHILDREN AND FAMILIES

## Refinancing and Restructuring the U.S. Child Health System

Neal Halfon, Moira Inkelas, David L. Wood, and Mark A. Schuster

Throughout the past century, expert panels and government commissions have highlighted the importance of certain basic principles for children's health care. Over the past decade, the Health Care Financing Administration and Maternal and Child Health Bureau's jointly sponsored Bright Futures Project have reiterated that health care for children should be comprehensive, continuous, coordinated, and accountable.[1] Despite great technical advances and the development of important programs that have improved the health and changed the lives of many children, the system of care for children in the United States has yet to embody the principles of Bright Futures and other expert panels. A growing number of U.S. children lack insurance and experience numerous barriers to receiving appropriate care; the infrastructure of safety-net programs and clinics available to low-income children and children with special health needs continues to erode; the medical, developmental, and environmental threats to children have changed in nature and complexity; and the system of care that has evolved to meet these changing needs is fragmented, disorganized, and difficult to navigate.

Addressing the problems of children's health services is even more complicated given the dramatic changes currently underway in the U.S. health care

*Note:* The authors would like to thank Stephen Berman, Peter Margolis, Margaret McManus, Jessica Laufer, and Jonathan Fielding for their helpful comments on earlier drafts of this manuscript.

delivery system. The reconstruction of the health care system is being spurred by government and large-employer cost control policies and by private business decisions aimed at controlling the emerging health care markets and delivery mechanisms in order to maximize profits.[2] This marketplace restructuring can be characterized by at least three important trends: the growth of managed care, with rapid development of vertically integrated delivery systems that align incentives across a wide range of providers and spread financial risk across the system; the increasing role of managed competition as a way of introducing competition in the purchase of health care products, thus enabling both large and small purchasers to aggressively bargain on the basis of price; and the replacement of community not-for-profit providers and health plans with for-profit organizations that must deliver a return to stockholders and investors. Given the failure of comprehensive health care reform at a federal level, emerging government policies designed to restructure the system now are focusing increasingly on containing costs through control of expenditures and elimination of the entitlement status of Medicaid in favor of block grants. Other government policies, like the proposed Medicare changes, are aimed at making it easier for private business to continue market consolidation efforts.

As the marketplace changes, attention should be directed toward how these transformations will affect the availability and quality of essential child health services. For example, will there be sufficient numbers of providers trained to care for children who are victims of child abuse? Can sophisticated tertiary pediatric medical care services be sustained when such centers rely on one to two million enrolled lives in order to operate? It is also unclear what role government can and should play in safeguarding local, state, and regional child health resources.

While the changing marketplace poses its own set of challenges, the massive changes that are underway provide new opportunities to fashion and construct a child health system that is more responsive to the emerging health needs of children and able to overcome deficiencies in the current system. Unfortunately, many of the design elements that should be included in a new system might not meet the narrow financial goals of a given managed care organization. How can government support the development of child health systems that provide home visitation for families at risk, early intervention services for children with potential developmental delay, preventive mental health services for children with serious medical needs, and other services that may not be profitable to the health care industry? What happens to the growing number of children who are uninsured or underinsured and the publicly supported services in community clinics and school-based health centers that constitute the health care safety net?

Whether marketplace transformations and federal and state health financing policies will improve the organization of children's health services and children's overall health status depends upon the extent to which these and other questions are addressed: How will children fare under health system restructuring driven primarily by cost control considerations? How will the unique health care needs of children be addressed as traditional medical services are reconfigured into managed care? Will current access barriers for comprehensive, coordinated health services be resolved? How can the principles outlined in *Bright Futures* guide the transformation of children's health services? By what standard should we evaluate effectiveness of the new system?

This chapter examines the key issues underlying the incongruities between the needs of children and families and the current and evolving structure of health services in the United States. We describe the unique health needs of children and the rationale for a child standard of care to ensure that emerging systems can meet these needs. Next, we examine characteristics of the U.S. health care system that influence children's access to care, including the disjointed organization of health services, and financial and structural barriers to health care. In the context of failed federal reforms, proliferating state-based initiatives, proposed downsizing of the federal health financing safety net, and sweeping market-based reforms in the health system, we present several options for accommodating the special needs of children. Finally, we describe ways in which emerging models of care can be modified to provide more effective, organized, and family-centered health services for children.

# Special Health Needs of Children

Children's health needs and risks fundamentally differ from those of adults and thus require special consideration in structuring, organizing, and delivering health services.[3] Among the unique characteristics of childhood that have important implications for health system design are a child's developmental vulnerability, dependency, and differential patterns of morbidity and mortality.

## Developmental Vulnerability

*Developmental vulnerability* refers to the rapid and cumulative physical and emotional changes that characterize childhood, and the potential impact that illness, injury, or untoward family and social circumstances can have on a child's life-course trajectory. Physical health conditions (for example, low birthweight or prematurity or asthma) as well as the child's social environment (severe poverty, unstable family, exposure to lead or other environmental hazards) can harm the developmental process.[4] Several conceptual models have been used to elucidate the dynamic relationships between factors that can promote or adversely affect children's capacity to achieve their physical, emotional, and cognitive potential.[5] Studies demonstrate two phenomena: the substantial, cumulative impact of early exposures and adverse social conditions on health status throughout the life course, and the role of critical developmental periods in which early insults cause long-term consequences.[6] Research linking the impact of various risks and insults on developmental pathways supports a broader conceptualization of health determinants and of health services.

The potential to alter the life-course trajectory is illustrated by studies that demonstrate the effectiveness of timely interventions in modifying adverse biological and social conditions that may harm a child's development. For example, cognitive development and behavioral competence at preschool age is higher for low-birthweight children who receive supportive family and educational services.[7] Such studies support the notion that timely and appropriately organized services can prevent the loss of developmental potential and highlight the mutability of various risks and their effects on the life course.

The continuity of children's development also implies that interventions must be sustained over time to appropriately address periodic, recurrent, and continuous biological and environmental threats. For example, while comprehensive early childhood intervention programs that serve socially disadvantaged children have improved young children's cognitive abilities, postintervention exposure to ongoing social disadvantage may offset earlier gains.[8] Discontinuities in health care and interruptions in eligibility for early childhood intervention programs are examples of modifiable threats to sustained developmental improvements for at-risk children.

## New and Differential Morbidities

Declining prevalence in the United States of nutritional and infectious disease and the changing patterns of childhood risk have increased the prominence of other causes of morbidity and mortality. Children increasingly are affected by a broad and complex array of conditions termed *new morbidities,* including drug and alcohol use, family and neighborhood violence, emotional disorders, and learning problems. These new morbidities originate in complex family or socioeconomic conditions rather than exclusively biological etiologies and cannot be adequately addressed by traditional medical services.[9] Instead, such conditions require a continuum of comprehensive services that includes multidisciplinary assessment, treatment, and rehabilitation as well as community-based prevention strategies in order to sustain positive outcomes.[10] Such multidisciplinary approaches often incorporate and integrate public- and private-sector services. For example, early intervention, family preservation, and violence prevention programs involve broad-based, multisector approaches that transcend agency and service-sector boundaries.[11]

Not only are the types and patterns of conditions for children changing, but patterns of morbidity and manifestations of medical conditions in children fundamentally differ in their pathophysiology and treatment as compared to adults.[12] Serious, chronic medical conditions are less prevalent in children and usually are related to birth or congenital conditions, rather than the degenerative conditions that affect adults and especially the elderly. Age-specific drug metabolism, disease expression, and health status assessments differentiate children from adults. For example, in children, cardiac conditions may result from any number of distinct congenital malformations, whereas in adults, cardiac conditions are dominated by a single degenerative disorder (atherosclerotic heart disease). Age-related differences in disease prevalence, expression, and management have important implications for issues such as ensuring appropriate access to care, developing age-specific quality assessment measures, guaranteeing availability of adequately trained providers, and assuring regional distribution of pediatric health professionals and services.[13]

## Dependency

Children also have complex and changing dependency relationships that influence their development and also affect their utilization of health services. Children are dependent on their parents or other caregivers to recognize and respond to their health needs, to organize their care and authorize treatment, and to comply with recommended treatment regimens. The importance of this dependency for children's access to health care is illustrated by studies comparing maternal utilization of health services with children's use of care. Studies find that maternal and child use of care is highly correlated irrespective of levels of health status.[14] Recent reports such as those by the National Commission on Children and the Carnegie Commission on Early Childhood further address the interdependency of family and social environments and their impacts upon children's health and development.

# Health Service Delivery for U.S. Children

While the principle that children's health services should be organized into a comprehensive, coordinated, continuous, and accessible system of health services has broad support, it is not yet clear whether changes in the health care marketplace and restructuring of the delivery system will advance this principle for all children. Children's health care encompasses health promotion and disease prevention strategies that are necessarily broad and that increasingly specify multisector approaches integrating medical, public health, educational, and social services. Consequently, consolidating personal medical care services and other services heretofore delivered by the community health sector into privately managed, vertically integrated delivery systems may not provide the scope and horizontal integration of health and related services needed to rationalize the delivery system for many children. Managed care arrangements may effectively organize primary and specialty medical services for relatively healthy populations. However, the increasingly prevalent new morbidities and the complex socioeconomic and environmental conditions faced by many families often require intense, sustained, and coordinated health services that neither the current system nor the emerging managed care arrangement is structured to provide.

## Child Health Service Sectors in the United States

The U.S. child health system has been characterized as a patchwork of disconnected programs, each with distinct eligibility, administrative, and funding criteria.[15] The three distinct yet interdependent sectors that comprise the child health services have unique histories, mandates, organizational characteristics and constraints, and funding streams.[16] These sectors include the personal medical and preventive services sector, the population-based community health services sector, and the health-related support services sector.

## Personal Medical and Preventive Services

Personal medical and preventive health services include primary and specialty medical services, which are generally delivered in private and public medical offices, hospitals, and laboratories. Restructuring the organization of the personal health service care sector, where the majority of health care dollars are spent, is the major focus of current health system change. Personal medical services are principally funded by private insurance and health plans, by the federal Medicaid and Medicare programs, and by out-of-pocket payments by families.[17]

## Population-Based Community Health Services

The second sector of child health services includes population-based health promotion and disease prevention services, such as immunization delivery and monitoring programs, lead screening and abatement programs, and child abuse prevention. Other community health services include special child abuse treatment programs and rehabilitative services for children with complex congenital conditions or other chronic and debilitating diseases. Community-based programs provide assurance and coordination functions for children's health services, such as case management and referral programs for children with chronic diseases and early interventions and monitoring programs for infants at risk for developmental disabilities. Funding for this sector comes from federal programs such as Medicaid's Early Periodic Screening, Diagnosis, and Treatment program (EPSDT), Title V (Maternal and Child Health) of the Social Security Act, and many other categorical programs.[18]

## Health-Related Support Services

The third sector of the child health system includes health-related support services, such as nutrition education, early intervention, rehabilitation, and family support programs. Services in this sector include parent education and skill building in families with infants at risk for developmental delay due to physiological or social conditions (such as low birthweight or very low income), and special education and psychotherapy for children with HIV. Funding for these services comes from diverse agencies such as the U.S. Department of Agriculture, which funds the Supplemental Food Program for Women, Infants, and Children (WIC), and the Department of Education, which funds the Individuals with Disabilities Education Act (IDEA).

## Disjointed Nature of Child Health Service Sectors

These three child health sectors have evolved separately, and the patchwork of programs that each sector comprises poses real challenges to providing integrated services.[19] Incremental federal and state funding for children's health programs has produced this array of categorical, condition-specific, means-tested programs that are not well integrated within or between the child health service sectors. Many of these programs were developed to fill gaps or to address an emerging need such as child abuse, HIV, mental health problems, or lead toxicity, and there is often little coordination within the federal, state, or local governing authorities; nor are there any attempts to link with private-sector efforts. Program administrative mandates and categorical or block grant criteria often determine the numbers of children that can be served.

Some states have moved to establish omnibus coordinating agencies or administrative councils for children and family services. In contrast, the Bureau of Maternal and Child Health is the single federal agency charged with improving the health status and organization of service systems for children, but it has little authority or funding to achieve its mission.

## Integration of Child Health Service Sectors

Achieving better health outcomes for the growing number of children afflicted with multiple and complex problems requires coordinated health and health-related services that may include primary and specialty medical care, case management, early intervention, and special education. Recent efforts to rationalize the organization and allocation of child health services is exemplified by the infant and toddler portion of the IDEA legislation. The 1986 amendments to this legislation mandate interagency collaboration and regional service integration as part of a state planning process for early childhood intervention services. In many states, this has resulted in organized comprehensive and coordinated assessment and treatment services for infants and young children at risk for development disabilities due to a variety of adverse perinatal outcomes or environmental factors.

Other examples of integrated delivery models developed for children at risk demonstrate efficiencies in providing coordinated, multisector services for children. The Child and Adolescent Service System Program (CASSP) is the National Institutes of Mental Health initiative to increase states' capacity to create coordinated systems of care in mental health for children and youth.[20] An example of such a mental health service integration model was developed in Ventura County, California, and has involved the collaboration of health, juvenile justice, mental health, and education agencies for the purpose of coordinating service delivery to children and reducing out-of-home placements for children with severe mental health conditions. Evaluations of the Ventura model demonstrate improved mental health outcomes in children and lower frequency of out-of-home placements.[21]

Innovative models, designed to facilitate service coordination by decategorizing funding streams and creating flexible funding pools, include a series of ongoing demonstration projects funded by the Robert Wood Johnson Foundation in ten small and medium-sized U.S. cities.[22] These projects illustrate that strategies to integrate services and cut across all three sectors can increase children's access to appropriate services and rationalize the provision of publicly funded health services.

Part of the difficulty in integrating health services comes from the sheer volume of categorical programs as well as the scope of eligibility and financial constraints that inhibit greater coordination.[23] Table 10.1 illustrates part of this problem. This figure demonstrates that a comprehensive approach to the provision of preventive, diagnostic, treatment, and rehabilitative services across the

### TABLE 10.1. PUBLIC PROGRAMS IN CHILD HEALTH SERVICE AND HEALTH NEED DOMAINS.

| *Health Service* | *Health Need* | | | | |
|---|---|---|---|---|---|
| | *Physical* | *Emotional* | *Cognitive* | *Family* | *Social* |
| Prevention | Title XIX<br>Title V<br>Title X<br>WIC<br>MCH Block<br>Grant | Title X<br>PL 99–457 | Title XIX<br>Title X<br>PL 99–457<br>Head Start | Title X<br>SSI<br>Head Start<br>AFDC<br>PL 99–457 | Title IV<br>HUD<br>AFDC |
| Early<br>Identification | Title XIX<br>Title V<br>Title X<br>WIC<br>MCH Block<br>Grant | Title XIX<br>PL 99–457 | Title XIX<br>PL 99–457 | Title XX<br>Title IV | Title IV |
| Diagnosis | Title XIX<br>Title V<br>PL 99–457 | Title XIX<br>PL 99–457 | Title XIX<br>PL 99–457 | Title XX<br>Title IV<br>PL 99–457 | Title IV |
| Treatment | Title XIX<br>Title V<br>PL 99–457 | Title XIX<br>PL 99–457 | Title XIX<br>PL 99–457 | Title XX<br>PL 99–457 | Title IV |
| Rehabilitation | Title XIX<br>Title V | Title XIX<br>PL 99–457 | Title XIX<br>PL 99–457 | PL 99–457 | |

*Source:* Halfon and Berkowitz, "Health Care Entitlements for Children: Providing Health Services as If Children Really Mattered," in *Visions of Entitlement: The Care and Education of America's Children,* eds. M. A. Jensen and S. G. Goffin (Albany: State University of New York Press, 1993), p. 195. Reprinted by permission.

physical, emotional, cognitive, and social domains would require integration of many different programs and funding sources.

## Financing of Children's Health Care

Financial barriers to health care primarily result from lack of insurance or the lack of coverage for primary care services such as well-child care or immunizations or for specialty care such as mental health services or rehabilitative therapy.

### Uninsured Children

The proportion of uninsured children in the United States has increased over the last twenty years. From 1977 to 1987, the proportion of children uninsured increased by 40 percent;[24] by 1989, 13.3 percent of children were uninsured.[25] While insurance rates for children have been relatively stable over the past five years, the percentage of children covered by employer-based insurance has dropped steadily for over a decade. The decline in private insurance coverage for children has resulted from the elimination of dependent coverage by some employers and from economic shifts toward service jobs without generous health benefits. By 1992, the percentage of children with employer-based coverage had declined to 56.2 percent (from 60.7 percent in 1987), accounting for nearly three million children losing coverage.[26] The number of uninsured children would have been even greater if expansions of the Medicaid program had not partially compensated for this erosion in employer-based insurance.[27] Between 1989 and 1993, the number of children covered by Medicaid increased by 54 percent, from 13.6 percent of U.S. children in 1989 (8.9 million children) to 19.9 percent in 1993 (13.7 million children).[28]

There is also a continuing gap in health insurance coverage for children from near-poor families. Definitions of *near-poor* differ but generally describe families earning at or above the federal poverty level but not more than 150 percent to 199 percent of that level.[29] Children from near-poor families are particularly vulnerable to declining employer-based coverage. Public health safety-net services originally were designed for poor or chronically disabled children and lack the capacity to meet the needs of near-poor families. Two-thirds of uninsured children live in families with incomes above the poverty level.[30] In 1992, 21 percent of children with family incomes of 100 percent to 199 percent of the federal poverty level were uninsured, and 74 percent of uninsured children lived in families with one or more working parents.[31] Recently authorized Medicaid expansions extended coverage to 11 percent of these near-poor children.[32]

Children without health insurance are less likely to have routine doctor visits or to receive care for injuries, and are more likely to delay seeking care.[33] Delay in care for common childhood conditions that have potentially disabling effects (for example, ear infections leading to hearing loss) has been attributed to families' lack of health coverage for the child.[34] Uninsured preschoolers have lower immunization coverage rates and lower compliance with well-child visit schedules.[35] Uninsured families are also more likely to rely on emergency rooms for their regular sources of care and to inappropriately use costly emergency rooms and hospital outpatient departments for the child's primary care needs.[36]

## Medicaid

While increasing numbers of children are insured by Medicaid due to eligibility expansions initiated in the late 1980s, programmatic obstacles have inhibited access to care for low-income children due to low reimbursement levels, bureaucratic and regulatory complexities, and frequent discontinuities of eligibility.[37] Complex Medicaid eligibility criteria and bureaucratic regulations result in significant turnover in enrollees each year. It is estimated that 40 percent of Medicaid AFDC enrollees lose Medicaid coverage each year.[38] Historically, many Medicaid-insured children have received medical care in safety-net public health facilities, where provider continuity and comprehensive health care may not be available.[39] Rapid expansion of Medicaid managed care is beginning to alter some of these utilization patterns, but with unclear results.[40]

## Private Insurance

Children with employment-based health coverage also are at risk for loss of insurance and disruption of care. Health insurance for children covered under a parent's employment is jeopardized when job loss or job changes occur as the economy shifts from high-paying benefit-rich manufacturing jobs to lower-paying benefit-poor service jobs with less-assured dependent coverage. For example, 25 percent of children from thirteen to eighteen months old in a large health maintenance organization had experienced some disruption of coverage during the previous five-month period.[41] For families with children who have preexisting conditions, obtaining health insurance or maintaining health insurance after a job change can be a real challenge.

Even those children and families with health insurance frequently have been underinsured for essential primary medical care, including well-child care, immunizations, and specialty care. In 1992, 50 percent of indemnity insurance health plans covered well-child care, and 65 percent of preferred provider organizations covered immunizations.[42] In 1992, 70 percent of health plans contracting with medium and large businesses offered no coverage for immunizations.[43] Special health care needs due to congenital conditions, chronic illness, or injury are also more likely to lack adequate private medical coverage—especially for services such as speech therapy, behavioral therapy, physical therapy, and other essential services.[44] Moreover, despite the proven efficacy of nonmedical social support benefits on health and developmental outcomes, services such as home visitation, transportation, and health-related social service consultations are rarely provided under most plans. In contrast, Medicaid coverage for children with chronic and disabling conditions routinely covers these so-called wraparound services as well as providing for home visitation and other kinds of health-related support services.

## Cost Sharing

Nearly all health plans apply cost-sharing mechanisms that are designed to minimize unnecessary use of medical services and thus limit expenditures. The RAND Health Insurance Study found that placing cost-sharing requirements on families for primary and preventive care services reduced children's use of these services.[45] Although adverse outcomes from reduced use of medical care were not detected in the RAND study, the sensitivity of children's basic ambulatory medical services to cost sharing was demonstrated.[46] With the expansion of managed care, more preventive services such as immunizations and well-child care are routinely covered, and administration fees, deductibles, co-payments, and other cost-sharing mechanisms are less often applied for preventive and primary care visits. In contrast, greater cost sharing has been applied to acute and chronic care services including hospital services, in an attempt to discourage their use. For many poor, near-poor, and even middle-income families, even nominal cost sharing poses a significant barrier to care.

## Nonfinancial Barriers to Care

Children's access to medical care traditionally has been measured by analyzing utilization patterns for specific provider services (such as number of annual physician visits), designated populations (such as adolescents or children in foster care), groups with specific conditions (such as children with asthma), or specific services (such as immunization or prenatal care).[47] These analyses have identified many factors that impede use of care and that appear to account for differential usage rates (for example, ethnicity, income, and residence) when controlling for health need (as measured by health status indicators and number and type of conditions).[48] Nonfinancial barriers to care include structural, environmental, and personal barriers such as bureaucratic complexities in the organization of child health services, cultural barriers based on ethnicity or language, and provider distribution or shortages, among others.[49] The reader is referred to other sources for a more exhaustive review of this subject.[50]

*Race.* In addition to income, differential access has been consistently documented on the basis of race. Differential access and utilization based on race and ethnicity can be the result of different modes of utilization as well as discriminating practices. Nonwhite children and adolescents have fewer physician visits and experience reduced continuity of care as compared to Caucasian children.[51] Inadequate utilization of care and poorer health outcomes for African American children can be minimized by targeted interventions designed to overcome organizational barriers.[52] A study of African American women receiving prenatal care in an environment with equal access to care (a U.S. Army base) detected lower infant mortality rates than the average rates for African American women, underscoring the important role that special barriers have on poor health outcomes in children.[53]

***Provider Training.*** Emerging patterns of morbidity in children, including complex risks, health conditions, and social problems pose new challenges to health care providers and delivery systems.[54] Surveys and anecdotal reports document inadequacies in the clinical training of health professionals and their inability to identify, treat, or refer children suffering from complex medical conditions, mental disorders, developmental problems, complex psychosocial problems, and abuse and neglect.[55] In one study, physicians' assessments identified less than 50 percent of emotional problems of the children who were screened.[56] These inadequacies are a function of provider training and knowledge, systemic undervaluing of assessment for new morbidities, and the shortage of community-based treatment resources for these problems.[57]

***Distribution of Providers.*** Geographical access barriers pose problems for both insured and uninsured poor families. Travel time for families in underserved urban areas or rural locations may be substantial[58] and result in reduced utilization of care.[59] For example, for poor children, lower local physician supply is associated with reduced access to preventive care services and routine emergency room use for nonemergent sick care.[60] The shortage of local primary care providers for poor children has been further compromised in recent years; the number of office-based physicians delivering primary care services in low-income areas declined by 45.1 percent between 1963 and 1980.[61]

Children who receive care in an office-based setting are more likely to receive continuity of care and coordination of services. One effect of the shortage in available office-based primary care providers has been the high, and often inappropriate, rate of emergency department utilization. Persons who identify their regular provider of care as a hospital outpatient department rather than a medical office are significantly less likely to see the same provider on a subsequent visit,[62] and young children receive less preventive care, including immunizations, in these settings.[63] In recent years, outpatient departments of hospitals increasingly replaced offices of private physicians as the site of the regular source of care for poor children.[64]

## Considerations for a New Child Health System

Current efforts to reform the health system by expanding insurance coverage and market penetration of managed care arrangements may improve children's access to primary medical care services. However, health insurance reforms and managed care arrangements may not be sufficient for children who have special health care needs or multiple conditions, and for children whose care requires integrated services from different sectors. The task of integrating personal medical services with complementary community-based health, social, and educational services will demand substantial coordination as well as financial incentives.

## Health Insurance and the Removal of Financial Barriers

In 1994, it seemed that national health care reform might provide the means to provide universal coverage and usher in a more rationally organized system. By 1995, state-initiated efforts to expand health insurance had taken center stage. Several states have obtained Section 1115 Medicaid demonstration waivers that provide the flexibility to transform Medicaid programs into managed care systems and expand coverage to previously uninsured groups.[65] As of February 1995, thirty-four states had expanded the federal mandate for eligibility for pregnant women and infants, and eighteen states had expanded income eligibility requirements for additional groups of children. Other states have embarked on health insurance expansions for children using state funding (such as Pennsylvania's Child Health Insurance Program) or have developed programs that combine public and private revenues (such as Colorado's Child Health Plan). Another form of insurance expansion has grown out of the Blue Cross and Blue Shield Caring Program for Children that was initiated by two ministers in 1984. The ministers approached Western Pennsylvania Blue Cross and Blue Shield on behalf of steelworkers who had lost their jobs as a result of steel industry collapse in the early 1980s. As of 1995, Caring Programs for Children are currently operating in twenty states and are serving more that 170,000 children.[66] Because these programs primarily provide well-child care, acute care, chronic care, and nonacute trauma care but do not cover hospitalizations, their costs are relatively modest. A 1994 analysis of 808 children enrolled in the Colorado Child Health Plan resulted in an average monthly cost of $24; an analysis of the Alabama Blue Cross Caring Program for Children demonstrated a similar cost at $20 per month.[67]

Current federal proposals to eliminate Medicaid entitlements and to substitute block grant funding to the states will provide additional impetus for reforms designed and driven by states. The Urban Institute estimates that the proposed Medicaid cut could result in 4.4 million children losing publicly supported health care coverage over the next seven years. While Medicaid program transitions to managed care may introduce some efficiencies, it is not evident that resultant cost savings will be sufficient to finance expanded eligibility under a fixed cap or to maintain or improve current levels of access and quality. Even if states choose to expand coverage to children for a modest primary care benefit package, there is growing concern that many of the most needy children will have some of their benefits curtailed.

## Health System Integration and the Removal of Nonfinancial Barriers

Expansion of health insurance coverage and system reorganization based on managed care cannot guarantee children's access to a system of health care that is comprehensive and coordinated. Structural and organizational characteristics of the current health system that are independent of insurance-related factors must be addressed to improve the allocation and quality of health services for children and families.

The principles of comprehensive, continuous, and coordinated care originally embodied in Medicaid's EPSDT program and reinforced in 1989 amendments to Title XIX recognize that access to basic ambulatory medical care will not suffice to meet the needs of children with complex health conditions and environmental risks. For such children, screening, diagnostic, and treatment services must be supplemented with a constellation of support services, including outreach, comprehensive case management, home visiting, and family counseling services.[68] Several authors have suggested that an appropriately responsive package of services would address both existing health conditions and potential risks to the health of the child and family and that such services would be sensitive to the functional and developmental capacities of the child as well as to the family's needs and the specific community environment.[69]

In an increasingly cost-conscious era, initiatives to broaden the scope of services and develop linkages across sectors should demonstrate both effectiveness (improved health outcomes) and efficiency (cost impact).[70] Home visiting and other early intervention programs targeted to at-risk families have proven cost effective in improving children's health status, cognitive functioning, and academic performance, while decreasing dependence on public assistance.[71] However, few of these successful demonstration and local community projects have been implemented on a large statewide scale, with the exception of Hawaii's Healthy Start Program.

The fate of integrated service programs, such as early intervention or school-linked health services, is even more uncertain given the current political environment. First, these programs are not likely to meet the narrow, short-term economic interests of managed care organizations by reducing hospitalizations and other high-cost medical expenditures. Instead, the savings from these programs are realized in lower special education rates, better family function, and lower welfare payments, and these savings are likely to accrue to the education, mental health, juvenile justice, and other business sectors. States may bear increased responsibility for building appropriate continuums of care if financial and programmatic building blocks are transferred from the federal government through proposed block grants. State and local policy makers will need to negotiate productive public-private partnerships if they are to meet this challenge.

The fate of our current public health care system—including community clinics, county health department services, school-based clinics, disease prevention and monitoring services, and even public hospitals—is also being reconsidered in many states and communities around the country. These services are important for all children, especially for the growing number of poor children and those who are uninsured or underinsured. Even children who have private insurance coverage through managed care plans may be referred to community health centers for basic services like immunizations.[72] The current collapse of the publicly financed and publicly delivered health services in Los Angeles, the move to turn the District of Columbia's general hospital over to private management, and the ongoing challenges to the fiscal solvency of the New York Hospital Corporation are all part of this disturbing trend.

It might also be more difficult for states to continue to support integrated cross-sector delivery efforts like early intervention programs, school-based clinics, or many public health safety-net programs regardless of their importance. Over the past decade, many of these services have been paid for (in the case of early intervention and school-based clinics) or heavily subsidized (in the case of FQHCs and public hospitals) with Medicaid funds. In fact, the disproportionate share of Medicaid dollars allocated to states has accounted for the fastest-growing component of federal medical expenditures. As Medicaid funds are increasingly diverted into commercial managed care contracts, the ability of state or local communities to use these funds for community health programs and health-related support services will be reduced, and continued development of integrated continuums will pose a fundamental challenge to states and localities.

## Public Accountability and Monitoring Systems

Mechanisms of public accountability to ensure that all children have access to comprehensive health care are largely absent in the United States. In European nations that maintain population-based service delivery models and utilize public health nurses and other providers to track and monitor infants through the preschool years, compliance with immunization schedules and age-appropriate preventive care visits is substantially higher than in the United States.[73] A combination of universal access to preventive care and integrated health information systems permits such population-based assurance.

Despite recent advances in health information systems, current U.S. data systems are frequently adult oriented (containing relatively little data on children), not population-based, and provide little information on quality of care or health outcomes. Data systems currently are not structured or capable of providing child-focused information on encounters with the broader child health system, including the public health, nutrition, and school-based health sectors.

Efforts are underway across the United States to introduce model systems that can be used to assure delivery of the most basic of medical services for children. Programs such as the All Kids Count immunization information and monitoring systems and the Robert Wood Johnson Foundation Child Health Initiative are implementing population-based report cards and monitoring systems.[74] These initiatives may serve as initial steps toward the population-based accountability that has been lacking for children and families.

## Child-Specific Standards and Guidelines

Normative definitions of comprehensive primary care have been developed by government agencies, medical professional organizations, and multidisciplinary expert working groups.[75] For example, standards have been issued by the federal Maternal and Child Health Bureau (MCHB) and by the American Academy of Pediatrics for children's medical care, and by the Child Welfare League of America for the health needs of children in foster care. The recent Bright Futures recommendations, funded by the MCHB and the Health Care Financing Administration (HCFA), set forth a comprehensive set of standards for the content of well-child services.[76] The principles embodied in *Bright Futures* reaffirm the need for an integrated health care system that is comprehensive, continuous, accessible, coordinated, and accountable. In addition to these broad public and professional standard-setting exercises, many professional organizations and managed care organizations are developing practice guidelines, focused on a particular service or medical condition.[77]

To assess the extent to which children's health needs are met in the current and evolving health system, performance measures and standards of care for children and families will require further development.[78] In order to capture the potential contribution to children's health from the different sectors responsible for their care, performance should be measured at three different levels: the individual patient-provider level, the health plan level, and the community level. Such measures are necessary not only to ensure quality of care within a particular relationship, organization, or sector but also to provide information critical to determining the direction indicated for health system reform. For policy and planning purposes, this three-level strategy is essential.[79]

Evaluating the quality of each child sector's performance will require further technical developments and support for the development of necessary infrastructure. Current methodologies for measuring quality of care for individual children and families also are quite limited.[80] Given the current shortcomings of assessing quality of care and of measuring performance of the health system on a larger scale, several public- and private-sector initiatives are under development to pursue these research areas. The central role that quality assurance will play in making sure that children's health needs are met is reflected in the Agency for Health Care and Policy Research (AHCPR) effort to develop more appropriate indicators.

In the private sector, the National Commission for Quality Assurance (NCQA) is adapting indicators from the Health Employer Data Information Set (HEDIS), used by commercial managed care plans to measure quality, for use in the Medicaid managed care setting.[81] The Medicaid HEDIS set of indicators will use administrative data to more adequately reflect health risks and services to low-income mothers and children. However, it is important to recognize that HEDIS and other quality assurance systems based on administrative data are limited in their ability to capture all domains of quality measurement for prudent and necessary care. Family satisfaction information collected from patients can supplement utilization and administrative data. Measures of service and system integration will also require development in order to evaluate performance within and among the three child health service sectors. Each of these tasks should become part of a national health service research agenda to measure our progress toward implementing effective family-centered models of care.

## Managed Care for Children

In early studies, health maintenance organizations (HMOs) demonstrated marginally higher preventive care utilization rates for maternal and child health services.[82] In a recent study of families randomized to managed care or fee-for-service arrangements, managed care plans successfully reduced emergency room use and diminished ambulatory visits for nonsevere conditions, but did not appear to reduce medical services for children with acute needs. Thus, the authors conclude that managed care can rationalize care without inappropriate rationing of care.[83]

While managed care models construct incentives to maintain enrollees' health status and to reduce demand for expensive health services such as inpatient care, this potential has not yet been realized in serving children with special health care needs.[84] Managed care arrangements are largely untested in terms of their ability to cost-effectively manage the care of vulnerable children. Many children with special health needs (including serious medical conditions) or with special circumstances (for example, foster children or homeless children) have either been excluded from previous studies of health outcomes, utilization, or costs or are such a small proportion of study populations that evaluation of the impact of managed care on their health outcomes has not taken place.

In fact, current managed care models may be inadequate for serving the needs of children with chronic illness, due to organizational priorities, lack of experience with comprehensive delivery systems of care for children, and tendency to control rather than coordinate service utilization.[85] Pediatricians participating in managed care plans reported high rates of denied referrals to specialists and inpatient services for children.[86] Analyses of HMOs' management of children with special health care needs reveal that HMOs often provide specialty services only when the child's health is expected to immediately improve. They also tend to limit mental health and related services, and to limit access to specialists.[87] A survey of administrators from twenty-two managed care plans found that few plans make special efforts to assure the appropriate participation of pediatric providers.[88] Although long-term management of children with special health care needs involves educational components, plans have tended to limit services that are perceived as educational rather than medical.[89]

The Medicaid Competition Demonstrations contrasted capitated and fee-for-service arrangements for children and pregnant women and found similar rates of prenatal care utilization and immunization.[90] However, HMOs currently serving inner-city Medicaid children may not provide children with greater access to immunizations than fee-for-service arrangements.[91] A health department survey following the 1989–1990 measles epidemic in Milwaukee revealed that of the confirmed measles cases among preschoolers, 83 percent were enrolled in Medicaid HMOs; more than two-thirds were inadequately immunized; and 30 percent were using emergency departments for primary care.[92]

As managed care expands in the U.S. marketplace, research on the outcomes and effectiveness in such systems is increasingly important. However, variation in managed care structures, benefits, and implementation across regions makes generalization difficult. For example, Fox and McManus identify four alternative arrangements used by managed care organizations that deliver services to Medicaid children with special health care needs. These include contracting with a child health network to provide all health and related services, contracting with specialty managed care programs for certain special needs children, contracting with in-plan providers or fee-for-service providers for certain services, and contracting only for a limited package of services under capitated arrangements while reimbursing specialty services on a fee-for-service basis.[93] It will become increasingly important to evaluate how these different contracting arrangements and the financial incentives engendered affect the diagnosis and treatment of new morbidities, the provision of timely access to care and allocation of resources for the management of children with special health needs, and the provision of integrated health and support services for children at risk for developmental delay and other conditions due to environmental risks.[94]

***Impact of Medicaid Managed Care on Systems Integration.*** Until recently, the categorical nature of publicly funded child health services (WIC, school nutrition programs, lead screening and treatment, and so forth) has prohibited managed care providers from providing and coordinating these services. The speed at which states are adopting managed care arrangements to serve their Medicaid populations reflects a dramatic change in the delivery of personal medical services and has ramifications for the administration of community health and health-related services. While managed care has the potential to improve children's access to primary care services, such models must be examined in the context of children's unique needs and of the need for integrated systems of personal medical services, community health, and supportive services. As the diversion of Medicaid funds into managed care health plans eliminates the flexibility that certain states and localities have employed to develop more coordinated delivery models, alternative resources and mechanisms for integration will have to be developed.

***Social HMOs.*** Some obstacles to comprehensive and coordinated management of health services for high-risk children and families could be overcome through the development of Social HMOs (SHMOs) that augment vertically integrated medical services with additional health promotion, social, and educational services and with enhanced coordination mechanisms to provide more appropriate horizontal integration.[95] SHMOs tailored for the frail elderly population have offered multifaceted risk assessment, an inclusive set of services and resources, and case management and coordination. Evaluation of the SHMO experience for the elderly has resulted in mixed outcomes.[96] Nonetheless, the design and delivery concepts embodied in the SHMO have enormous potential to maximize the fit between the true health needs of children and appropriately constructed integrated delivery system. Capitated models have been developed for pregnant women to provide a mix of medical and social services within one site of care, and several states currently are exploring the possibility of using this approach in the managed care setting.

An example of delivery systems that have adopted the SHMO model is the Los Angeles County Protective Service Child Health System for children at risk due to abuse and neglect. This system will use regional multidisciplinary assessment sites to evaluate and monitor children entering the foster care system and to coordinate the care received by these children from a range of providers of health and related services. The system utilizes and blends funds from Title XIX (Medicaid) and Title IV-E (Foster Care) to integrate health and social service functions into a coherent system. Such HMO hybrids could provide the mechanism to develop the horizontal integration of health care services (including medical and health-related care) that is so important for high-risk children and families. However, most organized continuums of health care for children remain as demonstration projects and have not yet been implemented systematically across the United States.

## Summary

Population-based, integrated service delivery systems have been developed in European nations and in localized demonstration projects in the United States. Most European countries provide universal health, developmental, and social services to children beginning at conception, including nationally insured health care, maternity leave and support, and child care and development programs.[97] The U.S. health care system continues to produce many important innovations in addressing the special medical and developmental needs of children. The use of managed care to rationalize the delivery of personal medical services may substantially improve children's access to basic medical care. Nonetheless, many health needs, especially for children with complex medical or socially based health problems, may not be adequately addressed.

The evolution of the U.S. health care system into distinct sectors, with fragmented services and categorical funding mechanisms, poses significant barriers to improved organization of care. Reforming the health care delivery system for children must integrate the activities of largely publicly funded community-based health services with privately delivered managed care models. Whether or not the emerging health system will more adequately meet the health needs of children and successfully address the newer morbidities will depend not only on insurance coverage but also upon the integration of the disparate sectors of the child health system.

Opportunities exist during this time of great structural change to fashion delivery systems that provide all children with access to a continuum of services. However, in the public policy area, insufficient attention has been paid to the unique needs of children and to the design of a system that will meet children's needs. The move to managed care may facilitate some of the changes necessary to improve services delivered to children, if essential components and safeguards are included. One mechanism to facilitate this focus is to operate under a child standard of coverage.[98] Policy makers, health care providers, and the public at large will have to consider how to ensure that children's unique needs are met under the evolving health system if health outcomes are to be improved.

## Notes

1. M. Green (ed.), *Bright Futures: National Guidelines for Health Supervision of Infants, Children, and Adolescents* (Arlington, Va.: National Center for Education in Maternal and Child Health, 1994).

2. The structure of this analysis was suggested by Stephen Berman, Professor of Pediatrics, University of Colorado.

3. E. J. Jameson and E. Wehr, "Drafting National Health Care Reform Legislation to Protect the Health Interests of Children," *Stanford Law and Policy Review* 5, 1 (1994): 152–176; and N. Halfon, M. Inkelas, and D. Wood, "Nonfinancial Barriers to Care for Children and Youth," *Annual Review of Public Health* 16 (1995): 447–472.

4. J. P. Shonkoff and S. J. Meisels, "Early Childhood Intervention: The Evolution of a Concept," in *Handbook of Early Childhood Intervention*, eds. S. J. Meisels and J. P. Shonkoff (Cambridge, England: Cambridge University Press, 1990), pp. 119–149.

5. C. Hertzman, "The Lifelong Impact of Childhood Experiences: A Population Health Perspective," Proceedings of the American Academy of Arts and Sciences, *Daedalus: Health and Wealth*, 123, 4 (1994): 167–180.

6. Hertzman, "The Lifelong Impact of Childhood Experiences"; R. G. Evans, "Introduction," in *Why Are Some People Healthy and Others Not? The Determinants of Health of Populations*, eds. R. G. Evans, M. L. Barer, and T. R. Marmor (Hawthorne, N.Y.: Aldine de Gruyter, 1994); D. J. Barker, C. Osmond, S. J. Simmonds, et al. "The Relation of Small Head Circumference and Thinness at Birth to Death from Cardiovascular Disease in Adult Life," *British Medical Journal* 306 (1993): 422–426; L. S. Bakketeig, G. Jacobsen, L. J. Hoffman, et al. "Pre-Pregnancy Risk Factors of Small-for-Gestational-Age Births Among Parous Women in Scandinavia," *Acta Obstetrica et Gynecologica Scandinavica* 72 (1993): 273–279; E. E. Werner, "High Risk Children in Young Adulthood: A Longitudinal Study from Birth to Age 32 Years," *American Journal of Orthopsychiatry* 59, 1 (1989):72–81; J. Freeman, *Prenatal and Perinatal Factors Associated with Brain Disorders*, NIH Pub. No. 85–1149. (Washington, D.C.: U.S. Department of Health and Human Services, 1985).

7. J. Brooks-Gunn, C. M. McCarton, P. H. Casey, M. C. McCormick, C. R. Bauer, et al., "Early Intervention in Low Birthweight Premature Infants: Results Through Age 5 Years from the Infant Health and Development Program," *Journal of the American Medical Association* 272, 16 (1994): 1257–1262; and The Infant Health and Development Program, "Enhancing the Outcomes of Low-Birthweight, Premature Infants: A Multisite Randomized Trial," *JAMA* 263, 22 (1990): 3035–3042.

8. Brooks-Gunn, McCarton, Casey, McCormick, Bauer, et al. "Early Intervention in Low Birthweight Premature Infants"; and E. F. Zigler, "Early Childhood Intervention: A Promising Preventative for Juvenile Delinquency," *American Psychologist* 47 (1992): 997–1006.

9. R. J. Haggerty, K. J. Roghmann, and I. B. Pless, *Child Health and the Community* (New York: Wiley, 1975); and B. Starfield, "Child and Adolescent Health Measures," *Future of Children* 2, 2 (Winter 1992): 25–39.

10. N. Halfon and G. Berkowitz, "Health Care Entitlements for Children: Providing Health Services as If Children Really Mattered," in *Visions of Entitlement: The Care and Education of America's Children*, eds. M. A. Jensen and S. G. Goffin (Albany: State University of New York Press, 1993).

11. J. E. Fielding and N. Halfon, "Where Is the Health in Health Reform?" *JAMA* 272 (1994): 1292–1296.

12. Jameson and Wehr, "Drafting National Health Care Reform Legislation to Protect the Health Interests of Children."

13. E. McGlynn, N. Halfon, and A. Leibowitz, "Assessing the Quality of Care for Children: Prospects Under Health Care Reform," *Archives of Pediatric and Adolescent Medicine* 149 (1995): 359–368.

14. P. W. Newacheck and N. Halfon, "The Association Between Mothers' and Children's Use of Physician Services," *Medical Care* 24, 1 (1986): 30–38.

15. Select Panel for the Promotion of Child Health, *Better Health for Our Children: A National Strategy* (Washington, D.C.: U.S. Department of Health and Human Services, 1981); B. Harvey, "Why We Need a National Child Health Policy," *Pediatrics* 87, 1 (1991): 1–6; M. Schlesinger and L. Eisenberg, "Little People in a Big Policy World: Lasting Questions and New Directions in Health Policy for Children," in *Children in a Changing Health System: Assessments and Proposals for Reform*, eds. M. Schlesinger and L. Eisenberg (Baltimore, Md.: Johns Hopkins University Press, 1990), pp. 325–359.

16. N. Halfon, P. Newacheck, D. Wood, and R. St. Peter, "Routine Emergency Room Use for Sick Care by U.S. Children," *Pediatrics* in press.

17. E. Lewitt and A. Monheit, "Expenditure on Health Care for Children and Pregnant Women," *Future of Children* 2, 2 (1992): 95–114.

18. Harvey, "Why We Need a National Child Health Policy."

19. Schlesinger and Eisenberg, "Little People in a Big Policy World."

20. A. J. Kahn and S. B. Kamerman, *Integrating Services Integration: An Overview of Initiatives, Issues, and Possibilities* (New York: Columbia University School of Public Health, National Center for Children in Poverty, 1992).

21. A. Rosenblatt and C. C. Attkisson, "Integrating Systems of Care in California for Youth with Severe Emotional Disturbance; I: A Descriptive Overview of the California AB377 Evaluation Project," *Journal of Child and Family Studies* 1, 1 (1992): 93–113; and A. Rosenblatt, C. C. Attkisson, and A. J. Fernandez, "Integrating Systems of Care in California for Youth with Severe Emotional Disturbance; II: Initial Group Home Expenditure and Utilization Findings from the California AB377 Evaluation Project," *Journal of Child and Family Studies* 1, 3 (1992): 263–286.

22. P. W. Newacheck, D. C. Hughes, C. Brindis, and N. Halfon, "Decategorizing Health Services: Interim Findings from the Robert Wood Johnson Foundation's Child Health Initiative," *Health Affairs* 14, 3 (1995): 232–242.

23. Halfon and Berkowitz, "Health Care Entitlements for Children."

24. Employee Benefit Research Institute, *Sources of Health Insurance and Characteristics of the Uninsured: Analysis of the March 1992 Current Population Survey*, No. 133 (Washington, D.C.: Employee Benefit Research Institute, 1993).

25. U.S. General Accounting Office, *Preventive Care for Children in Selected Countries*, GAO/HRD–93–62. (Washington, D.C.: U.S. Government Printing Office, 1993).

26. P. W. Newacheck, D. C. Hughes, and M. Cisternas, "Children and Health Insurance: An Overview of Recent Trends," *Health Affairs* 14, 1 (Spring 1995): 224–254.

27. Newacheck, Hughes, and Cisternas, "Children and Health Insurance"; and M. Teitelbaum, *The Health Insurance Crisis for America's Children* (Washington, D.C.: Children's Defense Fund, 1994).

28. U.S. General Accounting Office, *Preventive Care for Children in Selected Countries.*

29. U.S. General Accounting Office, *Preventive Care for Children in Selected Countries;* Newacheck, Hughes, and Cisternas, "Children and Health Insurance"; and Teitelbaum, *The Health Insurance Crisis for America's Children.*

30. Teitelbaum, *The Health Insurance Crisis for America's Children.*

31. Newacheck, Hughes, and Cisternas, "Children and Health Insurance"; and Teitelbaum, *The Health Insurance Crisis for America's Children.*

32. U.S. General Accounting Office, *Preventive Care for Children in Selected Countries.*

33. J. Stoddard, R. St. Peter, and P. Newacheck, "Health Insurance Status and Ambulatory Care for Children," *New England Journal of Medicine* 330, 20 (1994): 1421–1425.

34. Stoddard, St. Peter, and Newacheck, "Health Insurance Status and Ambulatory Care for Children."

35. D. L. Wood, R. A. Hayward, C. R. Corey, H. E. Freeman, and M. F. Shapiro, "Access to Medical Care for Children and Adolescents in the United States," *Pediatrics* 86, 5 (1990): 666–673; and P. F. Short and D. C. Lefkowitz, "Encouraging Preventive Services for Low-Income Children: The Effect of Expanding Medicaid," *Medical Care* 30, 9 (1992): 766–780.

36. Wood, Hayward, Corey, Freeman, and Shapiro, "Access to Medical Care for Children and Adolescents in the United States"; and P. Newacheck, D. Hughes, and J. Stoddard, "Children's Access to Primary Care: Differences by Race, Income, and Insurance Status" *Pediatrics* 97, 1 (1996): 26–32.

37. J. Perloff, P. Kletke, and K. Neckerman, "Recent Trends in Pediatrician Participation in Medicaid," *Medical Care* 24, 8 (1986): 749–760; and S. Davidson, J. Perloff, P. Kletke, D. Schiff, and J. Connelly, "Full and Limited Medicaid Participation Among Pediatricians," *Pediatrics* 72, 4 (1983): 552–559.

38. U.S. General Accounting Office, *Preventive Care for Children in Selected Countries.*

39. D. Dutton, "Children's Health Care: The Myth of Equal Access," in *Better Health for Our Children;* vol. 4: *Select Panel for the Promotion of Child Health,* DHHS Pub. No. (PHS) 79–55071 (Washington, D.C. U.S. Government Printing Office, 1981), pp. 357–440; J. Lion and S. Altman, "Case-Mix Differences Between Hospital Outpatient Departments and Private Practice," *Health Care Financing Reviews* 4, 1 (September 1982): 89–98; N. Halfon and P. W. Newacheck, "Childhood Asthma and Poverty: Differential Impacts and Utilization of Health Services," *Pediatrics* 91 (1993): 56–61; and R. St. Peter, P. Newacheck, and N. Halfon, "Access to Care for Poor Children: Separate and Unequal?" *JAMA* 267, 20 (1992): 2760–2764.

40. U.S. General Accounting Office, *Medicaid: States Turn to Managed Care to Improve Access and Control Costs* GAO/HRD–93–46 (Washington, D.C.: U.S. Government Printing Office, 1993).

41. T. A. Lieu, S. B. Black, P. Ray, M. Chellino, H. R. Shinefield, and N. E. Adler, "Risk Factors for Delayed Immunization Among Children in an HMO," *American Journal of Public Health* 84, 10 (1994): 1621–1625.

42. U.S. Department of Labor, *Employee Benefits in Medium and Large Establishments,* Bulletin 2422 (Washington, D.C.: Bureau of Labor Statistics, 1993).

43. R. Curtis, *Policy Bulletin: Report on the Employer-Sponsored Health Benefit Plan Survey* (Washington, D.C.: Health Insurance Association of America, 1991).

44. H. B. Fox and P. W. Newacheck, "Private Health Insurance Coverage of Chronically Ill Children," *Pediatrics* 85 (1990): 50–57.

45. R. Valdez, *The Effects of Cost Sharing on the Health of Children,* RAND Pub. No. R–3720–HHS (Santa Monica, Calif.: RAND Corporation, 1986).

46. R. Valdez, J. Ware, W. Manning, R. Brook, W. Rogers, G. Goldberg, and J. Newhouse, "Prepaid Group Practice Effects on the Utilization of Medical Services and Health Outcomes for Children: Results from a Controlled Trial," *Pediatrics* 83, 2 (1989): 168–180.

47. Halfon, Inkelas, and Wood, "Nonfinancial Barriers to Care for Children and Youth."

48. Newacheck and Halfon, "The Association Between Mothers' and Children's Use of Physician Services"; P. W. Newacheck, "Characteristics of Children with High and Low Usage of Physician Services," *Medical Care* 30, 1 (1992): 30–42; D. L. Wood, C. Corey, H. E. Freeman, and M. Shapiro, "Are Poor Families Satisfied with the Medical Care Their Children Receive?" *Pediatrics* 90 (1992): 66–70; S. Guendelman and J. Schwalbe, "Medical Care Utilization by Hispanic Children: How Does It Differ from Black and White Peers? *Medical Care* 24, 10 (1986): 925–940; B. L. Wolfe, "Children's Utilization of Medical Care," *Medical Care* 18, 12 (1980): 1196–1207; D. B. Dutton, "Explaining the Low Use of Health Services by the Poor: Costs, Attitudes, or Delivery Systems?" *American Sociological Review* 43 (1978): 348–368; and L. A. Aday and R. M. Andersen, "A Framework for the Study of Access to Medical Care," *Health Services Research* 9 (1974): 208–220.

49. Halfon, Inkelas, and Wood, "Nonfinancial Barriers to Care for Children and Youth"; Newacheck, "Characteristics of Children with High and Low Usage of Physician Services"; Wood, Corey, Freeman, and Shapiro, "Are Poor Families Satisfied with the Medical Care Their Children Receive?"; and Dutton, "Explaining the Low Use of Health Services by the Poor."

50. Halfon, Inkelas, and Wood, "Nonfinancial Barriers to Care for Children and Youth."

51. Wood, Hayward, Corey, Freeman, and Shapiro, "Access to Medical Care for Children and Adolescents in the United States"; A. W. Riley, J. W. Finney, E. D. Mellits, B. Starfield, S. Kidwell, et al., "Determinants of Health Care Use: An Investigation of Psychosocial Factors," *Medical Care* 31 (1993): 767–783; and T. A. Lieu, P. W. Newacheck, and M. A. Mc-Manus, "Race, Ethnicity, and Access to Ambulatory Care Among U.S. Adolescents," *AJPH* 83 (1993): 960–965.

52. S. T. Orr, E. Charney, and J. Straus, "Use of Health Services by Black Children According to Payment Mechanism," *Medical Care* 26, 10 (1988): 939–947; and S. T. Orr, E. Charney, J. Straus, and B. Bloom, "Emergency Room Use by Low Income Children with a Regular Source of Health Care," *Medical Care* 29 (1991): 283–286.

53. J. S. Rawlings and M. R. Weir, "Race- and Rank-Specific Mortality in a U.S. Military Population," *American Journal of Diseases in Children* 146 (1992): 313–316; and P. A. Margolis, T. Carey, C. M. Lannon, J. L. Earp, and L. Leininger, "The Rest of the Access-to-Care Puzzle," *Archives of Pediatric and Adolescent Medicine* 149 (1995): 541–545.

54. B. Starfield and P. Newacheck, "Children's Health Status, Health Risks, and Use of Health Services," in *Children in a Changing Health System*, eds. M. Schlesinger and L. Eisenberg (Baltimore: Johns Hopkins University Press, 1990), 3–26; L. H. Bearinger, L. Wildey, J. Gephart, and R. W. Blum, "Nursing Competence in Adolescent Health: Anticipating the Future Needs of Youth," *Journal of Professional Nursing* 8, 2 (1992): 80–86; and R. W. Blum and L. H. Bearinger, "Knowledge and Attitudes of Health Professionals Toward Adolescent Health Care," *Journal of Adolescent Health Care* 11 (1990): 289–294.

55. L. S. Friedman, B. Johnson, and A. S. Brett, "Evaluation of Substance-Abusing Adolescents by Primary Care Physicians," *Journal of Adolescent Health Care* 11 (1990): 227–230; M. I. Singer, M. K. Petchers, and J. M. Anglin, "Detection of Adolescent Substance Abuse in a Pediatric Outpatient Department: A Double-Blind Study," *Journal of Pediatrics* 111, 6 (1987): 938–941; and I. D. Goldberg, K. J. Roghmann, T. K. McInerny, and J. D. Burke, "Mental Health Problems Among Children Seen in Pediatric Practice: Prevalence and Management," *Pediatrics* 73 (1984): 278–293.

56. E. J. Costello, "Primary Care Pediatrics and Child Psychopathology: A Review of Diagnostic, Treatment, and Referral Practices," *Pediatrics* 78 (1986): 1044–1051.

57. Singer, Petchers, and Anglin, "Detection of Adolescent Substance Abuse in a Pediatric Outpatient Department"; Office of Technology Assessment, *Adolescent Health;* vol. 3: *Cross-Cutting Issues in the Delivery of Health and Health-Related Services,* OTA–H–469 (Washington, D.C.: U.S. Government Printing Office, 1991); and D. Kamerow, H. Pincus, and D. Macdonald, "Alcohol Abuse, Other Drug Abuse, and Mental Disorders in Medical Practice," *JAMA* 255, 15 (1986): 2054–2057.

58. D. Hughes and S. Rosenbaum, "An Overview of Maternal and Child Health Services in Rural America," *Journal of Rural Health* 5 (1989): 299–319.

59. Dutton, "Children's Health Care."

60. Halfon, Newacheck, Wood, and St. Peter, "Routine Emergency Room Use for Sick Care by U.S. Children"; and Short and Lefkowitz, "Encouraging Preventive Services for Low-Income Children."

61. D. Kindig, H. Movassaghi, N. Dunham, D. Zwick, and C. Taylor, "Trends in Physician Availability in 10 Urban Areas from 1963 to 1980," *Inquiry* 24 (1987): 136–146.

62. J. A. Butler, W. D. Winter, J. D. Singer, and M. Wenger, "Medical Care Use and Expenditures among Children and Youth in the United States: An Analysis of a National Probability Sample," *Pediatrics* 76 (1985): 495–507.

63. J. D. Kasper, "The Importance of Type of Usual Source of Care for Children's Physician Access and Expenditures," *Medical Care* 25, 5 (1987): 386–398.

64. M. Schlesinger, "On the Limits of Expanding Health Care Reform: Chronic Care in Prepaid Settings," *Milbank Quarterly* 64 (1990): 189–215.

65. S. Rosenbaum and J. Darnell, *Medicaid Section 1115 Demonstration Waivers: Approved and Proposed Activities as of November 1994* (Washington, D.C.: Center for Health Policy Research, George Washington University, 1994).

66. D. Perry, "Children's Health Insurance: Beyond Medicaid Coverage," *Health Policy and Child Health,* 2, 3 Special Supplement (1995): 1–4.

67. Perry, "Children's Health Insurance."

68. W. S. Barnett and C. M. Escobar, "Economic Costs and Benefits of Early Intervention," in *Handbook of Early Childhood Intervention,* eds. S. J. Meisels and J. P. Shonkoff (New York: Cambridge University Press, 1990), pp. 560–582; and D. Olds, "Home Visitation for Pregnant Women and Parents of Young Children," *American Journal of the Diseases of Children* 146 (1992): 704–708.

69. Starfield, "Child and Adolescent Health Measures"; and Starfield and Newacheck, "Children's Health Status, Health Risks, and Use of Health Services."

70. J. L. Wagner, R. C. Herdman, and D. W. Alberts, "Well-Child Care: How Much Is Enough?" *Health Affairs* (September 1989): 147–157.

71. Barnett and Escobar, "Economic Costs and Benefits of Early Intervention"; D. Olds, C. Henderson, C. Phelps, H. Kitzman, and C. Hanks, "Effect of Prenatal and Infancy Nurse Home Visitation on Government Spending," *Medical Care* 31, 2 (1993): 155–174; D. Olds and H. Kitzman, "Can Home Visitation Improve the Health of Women and Children at Environmental Risk?" *Pediatrics* 86, 1 (1990): 108–116; and J. R. Berrueta-Clement, L. J. Schweinhart, W. S. Barnett, A. S. Epstein, and D. P. Weikart, *Changed Lives: The Effects of the Perry Preschool Program on Youths Through Age 19* (Ypsilanti, Mich.: High/Scope, 1984).

72. D. L. Wood, N. Halfon, C. Sherbourne, and M. Grabowsky, "Access to Infant Immunization for Poor Inner-City Families: What Is the Impact of Managed Care?" *Journal of Health Care for the Poor and Underserved* 5, 2 (1994): 112–123.

73. U.S. General Accounting Office, *Medicaid: States Turn to Managed Care.*

74. Newacheck, Hughes, Brindis, and Halfon, "Decategorizing Health Services."

75. Starfield, "Child and Adolescent Health Measures."

76. Green, *Bright Futures.*

77. Physician Payment Review Commission, *Annual Report to Congress* (Washington, D.C.: Physician Payment Review Commission, 1995).

78. McGlynn, Halfon, and Leibowitz, "Assessing the Quality of Care for Children"; and J. Durch (ed.), *Protecting and Improving Quality of Care for Children Under Health Care Reform: Workshop Highlights* (Washington, D.C.: Institute of Medicine, 1994).

79. H. Grayson and B. Guyer, *MCH Quality Systems Functions Framework* (Baltimore, Md.: Johns Hopkins School of Hygiene and Public Health, 1995).

80. McGlynn, Halfon, and Leibowitz, "Assessing the Quality of Care for Children."

81. Physician Payment Review Commission, *Annual Report to Congress.*

82. D. A. Freund, L. F. Rossiter, P. D. Fox, J. A. Meyer, R. E. Hurley, et al., "Evaluation of the Medicaid Competition Demonstrations," *Health Care Financing Review* 11, 2 (1989): 81–97.

83. J. Mauldon, A. Leibowitz, J. L. Buchanan, et al., "Rationing or Rationalizing Children's Medical Care: Comparison of a Medicaid HMO with Fee-for-Service Care," *AJPH* 84 (1994): 899–904.

84. P. Newacheck, D. Hughes, J. Stoddard, and N. Halfon, "Children with Chronic Illness and Medicaid Managed Care," *Pediatrics* 93 (1994): 497–500.

85. S. M. Horwitz and R.E.K. Stein, "Health Maintenance Organizations vs. Indemnity Insurance for Children with Chronic Illness: Trading Gaps in Coverage," *American Journal of Diseases of Children* 144, 5 (1990): 581–586.

86. J.D.C. Cartland and B. K. Yudkowsky, "Barriers to Pediatric Referral in Managed Care Systems," *Pediatrics* 89 (1992): 183–192.

87. H. B. Fox, L. B. Wicks, and P. W. Newacheck, "Health Maintenance Organizations and Children with Special Health Needs: A Suitable Match?" *American Journal of Diseases in Children* 147 (1993): 546–552; and U.S. General Accounting Office, *Preventive Care for Children in Selected Countries.*

88. H. B. Fox and M. A. McManus, *Strategies to Enhance Preventive and Primary Care Services for High-Risk Children in Health Maintenance Organizations* (Washington, D.C.: Child and Adolescent Health Policy Center, 1995).

89. H. B. Fox, L. B. Wicks, M. McManus, and P. W. Newacheck, "Private and Public Insurance for Early Intervention Services," *Journal of Early Intervention* 16 (1992): 109–122.

90. Freund, Rossiter, Fox, Meyer, Hurley, et al., "Evaluation of the Medicaid Competition Demonstrations."

91. Wood, Halfon, Sherbourne, and Grabowsky, "Access to Infant Immunization for Poor Inner-City Families."

92. P. Nannis, *Strengthening Urban MCH Capacity: Highlights of the 1992 Urban MCH Leadership Conference,* ed. Magda Peck (Washington, D.C.: U.S. Department of Health and Human Services, 1993).

93. Fox and McManus, *Strategies to Enhance Preventive and Primary Care Services for High-Risk Children in Health Maintenance Organizations.*

94. H. Ireys, "Children with Special Health Care Needs: Evaluating Their Needs and Relevant Service Structures," background paper for the Institute of Medicine, Johns Hopkins University, 1994.

95. Halfon and Berkowitz, "Health Care Entitlements for Children."

96. W. N. Leutz, M. R. Greenlick, and J. A. Capitman, "Integrating Acute and Long-Term Care," *Health Affairs* 13, 4 (1994): 58–74.

97. Kahn and Kamerman, *Integrating Services Integration;* U.S. General Accounting Office, *Preventive Care for Children in Selected Countries;* B. C. Williams and C. A. Miller, "Preventive Health Care for Children: Findings from a 10-Country Study and Directions for United States Policy," *Pediatrics* 89, 5 Supplement (1992): 983–998.

98. Jameson and Wehr, "Drafting National Health Care Reform Legislation to Protect the Health Interests of Children."

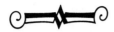

CHAPTER ELEVEN

# WOMEN'S HEALTH

## Key Issues in Access to Insurance Coverage and to Services Among Non-Elderly Women

Roberta Wyn and E. Richard Brown

Analysis of the current health care system and debates on alternative solutions to increasing coverage, improving access, and controlling costs have often proceeded without regard to the specific implications of the effects on women of alternative approaches. Although women and men share the same need for affordable, accessible, and quality care, there are specific health concerns and patterns of use unique to women that are often overlooked. Many health conditions are particular to women, occur with greater frequency among women, or have different consequences for women than for men. These differences affect the amount and kind of health care services needed and suggest different priorities regarding which services should be funded and different conclusions about what are appropriate funding mechanisms.

Women have a large stake in how health care services are financed and delivered. They are primary users of the health care system both for themselves and as the coordinators of care for their families. They have higher physician use rates than do men at all ages and higher hospital use rates among the non-elderly.[1] Furthermore, women's less advantaged and less stable economic status places them at particular financial risk for the costs of medical care.

This chapter examines some of the key policy factors related to the financing and delivery of services for women under sixty-five years of age. First, we examine the adequacy of women's access to health insurance coverage and the ability of that coverage to protect against the costs of health services. This includes an analysis of the advantages and disadvantages of the current insurance system for women, gaps in coverage and benefits, and the economic importance of coverage. Second, we examine how health insurance coverage and other financial barriers affect women's access to care and health status. Lastly, we look beyond financial barriers to other aspects of the health care system that influence access. The population is limited to the non-elderly because much of the chapter focuses on health insurance coverage. Although women over sixty-five years of age also face health insurance access problems, most older women have insurance coverage through Medicare; therefore, their insurance coverage issues are different.

## Women's Access to Insurance Coverage

The mechanisms for obtaining health insurance coverage are embedded in complex social and economic situations that differ between women and men and among subgroups of women. The current health insurance structure in the United States is a voluntary system that relies primarily on health insurance obtained from one's own employment or the employment of a spouse or parent, augmented by individually purchased private insurance and by public systems for eligible low-income individuals and families (Medicaid) and for the elderly (Medicare). This patchwork of coverage options leaves many women dependent on coverage through a spouse; reliant on an isolated, precarious public system; or uninsured. Even though women have lower uninsured rates than men, as shown in Table 11.1, they must rely on complicated arrangements to obtain coverage.[2]

The main source of coverage for both women and men is through employment. This dependence of health insurance coverage on employment is unique in the United States. Pairing coverage with employment connects two distributive systems: work and insurance. Thus, the factors that determine the distribution of jobs in the society also determine access to employment-based health insurance coverage.[3] This places women at a distinct disadvantage as they have less attachment to the labor market than do men. Women are more likely than men to work part-time, to receive lower wages, and to have interruptions in their work histories[4]—all factors that reduce the likelihood of receiving employment-based coverage through one's own work and increase the risk of being uninsured.[5]

Although nearly equal proportions of non-elderly women and men have employment-based coverage, Table 11.1 shows some interesting distinctions. Women are more likely than men to be covered as a dependent (that is, covered through a spouse or parent) and less likely than men to have coverage directly through their own employer. Another distinction is women's greater reliance on Medicaid.

## TABLE 11.1. HEALTH INSURANCE COVERAGE BY GENDER, AGES 18–64, UNITED STATES, 1993.

| Health Insurance Coverage | Women ( percent) | Men ( percent) |
|---|---|---|
| Employment-based, primary | 38 | 53 |
| Employment-based, dependent | 24 | 10 |
| Privately purchased | 10 | 10 |
| Medicaid | 9 | 4 |
| Medicare | >1 | 1 |
| CHAMPUS | 2 | 1 |
| Uninsured | 16 | 21 |
| Total[a] | 100 | 100 |

[a]Due to rounding may not equal 100 percent.

Source: Authors' analysis of the *March 1994 Current Population Survey.*

Women are twice as likely as men to receive this benefit because of its link to Aid to Families with Dependent Children (AFDC). Despite women's greater access to Medicaid, this program fails to reach many poor women. The national average cutoff level for Medicaid eligibility in 1992 for the non-elderly was 44 percent of poverty and more than half of all states set eligibility at below 50 percent of poverty.[6] Not surprisingly, approximately one-third of poor women between the ages of eighteen and sixty-five are uninsured.[7]

The patterns of coverage vary considerably among women by ethnicity. Ethnic minority women are less likely than Anglo women to receive employment-based coverage, with striking differences seen in access to coverage as a dependent. Table 11.2 explores these patterns. Differences in family structure[8] (both Latinas and African American women are more likely to live in families headed by a woman) and differences in coverage rates of minority men (who are less likely to be employed and when employed have lower wages than Anglo men[9]) account for these lower rates. Medicaid coverage is also higher among African American women and Latinas compared with Anglo women.

Given women's less advantaged economic position and employment status, one would assume that they would have less access than men to insurance coverage. Women are, however, less likely to be uninsured than are men (16 percent versus 21 percent, respectively) because of women's greater access to Medicaid and dependent coverage (as shown in Table 11.1). This apparent paradox is due to compensating mechanisms in the system that reduce the effects of women's less advantaged position but in many ways help to shape and reinforce the notion of

## TABLE 11.2. HEALTH INSURANCE COVERAGE BY ETHNICITY, WOMEN AGES 18–64, UNITED STATES, 1993

| Health Insurance Coverage | Latina | African American | Anglo | Asian |
|---|---|---|---|---|
| Employment-based, primary | 25 | 37 | 40 | 35 |
| Employment-based, dependent | 16 | 12 | 28 | 22 |
| Privately purchased | 6 | 7 | 11 | 12 |
| Medicaid | 18 | 22 | 6 | 6 |
| Medicare | <1 | <1 | <1 | <1 |
| CHAMPUS | 1 | 1 | 1 | 3 |
| Uninsured | 32 | 20 | 13 | 21 |
| Total[a] | 100 | 100 | 100 | 100 |

[a]Due to rounding may not equal 100 percent.

*Source:* Authors' analysis of the *March 1994 Current Population Survey.*

women's dependency. Both Medicaid and dependent coverage are insurance sources that pertain to the gendered roles of women.

Among women, rates of lack of coverage vary by ethnicity. Anglo women have the lowest uninsured rate (13 percent lack coverage), increasing to 20 percent of African American women, 21 percent of Asian women, and 32 percent of Latinas. Other groups of women with high uninsured rates include younger women, those with low incomes, and those who are not married.[10]

## Concerns with Women's Current Coverage Options

Both employment-based dependent coverage and Medicaid compensate for the disadvantages to women of an insuring system that is structured around employment. However, both may well be more vulnerable to economic constraints and to political changes than is employment-based primary coverage.

In the absence of effective cost controls, it is likely that dependent coverage benefits will become increasingly more difficult to obtain as employers attempt to reduce health insurance costs. Employers with a high proportion of workers with family coverage face higher health care costs. Employers who offer dependent coverage are subsidizing the health costs of businesses that do not provide coverage for their workers or for the dependents of workers. This concern with cost shifting has led some employers to increasingly limit dependent coverage, offering it only to those dependents without other coverage options.[11] The percentage of employees required to contribute to family coverage has steadily increased, rising from 46 percent to 69 percent of full-time employees in medium and large private firms between 1980 and 1991.[12] This same study showed these employees are more likely to be required to contribute toward family coverage than toward self-coverage (51 percent were required to contribute to the latter in 1991).

Medicaid is also vulnerable to economic constraints as well as policy changes. Because Medicaid is among the largest and fastest-growing costs for state governments,[13] it has increasingly become the target of many state efforts to control costs. Low-income women and children account for nearly three-quarters of Medicaid beneficiaries, although they generated only 27 percent of total program spending in 1993.[14] Efforts have focused on controlling both the demand for and the supply of services by limiting the types of services covered, moving to managed care delivery systems, tightening eligibility requirements, and reducing the reimbursements to health care providers and hospitals.[15]

One of the most dramatic changes in Medicaid is the shift from fee-for-service to managed care. Many states have developed or are developing Medicaid managed care systems, using waivers under section 1115 of the Social Security Act. The populations enrolled in these managed care plans have been mainly AFDC recipients (who are primarily low-income women and children) and eligible pregnant women and their children.[16] Many features of managed care, such as its focus on coordinated care and emphasis on primary care, have the potential to improve access. Studies comparing Medicaid fee-for-service with Medicaid managed care enrollees generally show that access to care and quality of care are fairly equal between the two groups.[17] Medicaid managed care is being implemented primarily to save costs, and concerns over access and quality have been raised as a result. The incentives in managed care, with the fixed payment reimbursement, could lead to underservice.[18] Furthermore, the limited experience of many managed care plans in working with low-income populations may create barriers to care or insufficient understanding of the range of services low-income populations may need. The Medicaid population is fluid, with considerable turnover in eligibility. This could limit the development of stable relationships with managed care providers and diminish the incentives to provide preventive care. Nonetheless, managed care does have the potential to improve access to care and in particular to primary and preventive care.

Another overarching issue with Medicaid is eligibility determination. Because Medicaid eligibility remains closely associated with federal public assistance programs for many women, women's access to Medicaid is threatened by AFDC policies that tighten eligibility requirements, lessen the duration of coverage, or eliminate altogether the entitlement to public assistance.

Medicaid has played a pivotal role in improving the access of poor women to medical care, and in the absence of alternative options for poor women, it remains a primary reason why the uninsured rate among women is not even higher. However, there are several limitations to the program. The federal government establishes minimum eligibility and coverage mandates that states must adhere to, but some major decisions are left to the states. The downside of this state flexibility and autonomy is the geographical inequity among women in eligibility level, benefit scope and duration (beyond those services that are mandatory), and provider reimbursement amount (which affects provider participation).[19] Furthermore, eligibility and benefit level determinations are subject to yearly fluctuations based on each state's current economic and political priorities, making this an unstable source of coverage for many women. In addition, the stigma attached to receiving Medicaid, administrative paperwork, and insufficient reimbursement often result in low provider participation rates and beneficiary difficulty with finding a provider.[20]

Recent federal legislation has tried to reverse some of the erosion in access to Medicaid for pregnant women and their children by extending coverage to those whose incomes are above the eligibility level for AFDC and also by raising physician fees for prenatal care and delivery.[21] This incremental expansion has improved financial access to care for the poor and demonstrates the importance of policy solutions to improve access, although difficulties in finding providers still persist for women on Medicaid.[22]

## Coverage Gaps of Particular Importance to Women

Even among women with health insurance, gaps in benefit coverage discourage women from seeking medical and preventive services. Contraceptive services are not well funded, and are among the most poorly covered reproductive health care services. Women of childbearing age paid 56 percent of the cost of contraceptives in 1993, with the majority of the expenditures for prescribed contraceptives.[23] Many nonsurgical contraceptors (such as the diaphragm, Norplant implants, the IUD, and oral contraceptives) are either not covered by insurance or are inadequately covered. One-half of health plans provide no coverage for these reversible contraceptors.[24] Oral contraceptives, the most widely used form of reversible contraception, are covered by only 33 percent of large employer group fee-for-service plans. Health maintenance organizations (HMOs) provide better coverage, but still 15 percent do not cover this basic contraceptive method.[25]

Overall, HMOs are more likely than fee-for-service plans to offer contraceptive services, with almost all HMOs providing some contraceptive option and contraceptive counseling.[26] Even among HMO plans that do provide some coverage, however, the scope of the coverage is restrained; most do not offer women a full range of choice of reversible contraception options. Less than half of HMOs provide women with a full range of nonsurgical medical family planning options. In contrast, coverage for surgical procedures is higher; 90 percent of plans cover sterilization and two-thirds cover abortion,[27] suggesting a bias toward funding of surgical procedures, as is seen in other aspects of medicine.

Also inadequately funded are certain clinical preventive services. Historically, the delivery of care and its financing have been structured around acute curative care, with a bias toward better financing for inpatient care and procedures. This bias is reflected by the insufficient coverage of clinical preventive services in private-sector financing and, to a lesser extent, in the public sector. Clinical preventive services attempt to identify a disease at its early stages. The use of screening tests for early detection of disease is credited with major reductions in morbidity and mortality.[28] Coverage of mammography screening for breast cancer and the Pap test for cervical cancer illustrate some of the deficiencies in preventive care coverage.

HMOs are more likely to cover preventive services than are conventional (fee-for-service) plans. According to a 1990 study, nearly all HMOs provide coverage for the Pap test and mammogram; in comparison, slightly under 60 percent of conventional fee-for-service plans and 70 percent of preferred provider organizations cover these services.[29] In the late 1980s, there was a flurry of state-mandated benefit laws requiring third-party payers to cover screening mammography, and by 1990, two-thirds of states had such laws.[30] Legislation requiring third-party payers to cover the Pap test is not as widespread. As of 1990, only eight states mandated this benefit.

In the public sector, coverage for the Pap test and mammogram are state optional under Medicaid. Although optional, as of 1991, almost all state Medicaid programs covered the Pap test, and thirty-nine provided some coverage for screening mammography.[31] However, many states have age and frequency restrictions that often conflict with recommended guidelines.[32] Medicare recently enacted legislation mandating coverage of the Pap test and screening mammography after years of policy debate.[33]

Many women report that they do not have coverage for basic clinical preventive services or are not sure if these services are covered by their policies. Among non-elderly women, four out of ten women do not have coverage for the Pap test or are unclear about their coverage: 15 percent of women are completely uninsured; 17 percent are insured, but their coverage does not cover cervical cancer screening; and 7 percent are insured, but are uncertain if their coverage pays for the Pap test.[34] A very similar pattern is seen for mammography coverage for women fifty to sixty-four years of age. Fourteen percent are completely uninsured; 16 percent are insured but not covered for mammography; and another 11 percent do not know whether their policy covers this benefit.

# Economic Importance of Coverage: Women and Economic Disadvantage

The financing of health care and the distribution of health care costs are particularly important for women. Across all ages, women are more likely than men to use physician services. Some of the largest gaps in use rates between men and women are seen during the reproductive years. Per capita expenditures for women ages fifteen to forty-four are $2,123 compared with $1,272 for men, a differential attributable in part to the expenses associated with reproductive services for women.[35]

Financial barriers are often cited by women as a reason for not receiving care. Among women who did not receive clinical preventive services during a yearlong period, the most frequently cited barrier was the cost of care, reported by four out of ten non-elderly women and almost two out of ten elderly women.[36] Not surprisingly, uninsured women were the most likely to experience cost barriers, with seven out of ten uninsured women reporting cost as a reason for not receiving a clinical preventive service.

Having insurance coverage does not guarantee that medical or preventive services will be affordable. Nearly one-third of non-elderly women with insurance coverage reported that costs were a barrier to use.[37] Lack of coverage for specific health services and out-of-pocket expenses even when insured (to meet deductibles, co-payments, or coinsurance obligations) increase the financial risk for insured women. Studies have shown that use of services is highest when there is no cost sharing and that cost sharing reduces the amount of both effective and less effective medical care.[38] Furthermore, coinsurance appears to have a greater effect on low-income persons, reducing their use of effective services relative to use rates for higher income persons. Not all effects of cost sharing are viewed as detrimental, however. Cost sharing reduces the demand for services and therefore health care expenditures, and cost-sharing obligations can also reduce the use of health care services with little or no value.[39] However, cost sharing does impose a disproportionate burden on low-income persons and can inhibit the use of important medical and preventive services.

It is difficult for women to shoulder the expenses of health care without adequate subsidies or affordable cost-sharing arrangements. Thirty-two percent of women ages eighteen to sixty-four had family incomes below 200 percent of poverty in 1993, with the highest rates of low income among racial and ethnic minority subgroups of women.[40] Over fifty percent of Latinas and African American women report incomes below 200 percent of poverty, placing them at very high risk of financial liability for health care costs in the absence of affordable coverage. Services essential to women's health that are not covered or inadequately covered may simply not be available to women. Approximately 13 percent of women report that they did not receive necessary health care within a yearlong period.[41] Of these women, one-half report that costs were the reason for the lack of needed care.

As we highlighted in the section on covered benefits, there are several services that are either specific to women or used more by women that are not covered or are inadequately covered. Women ages fifteen to forty-four spend a larger proportion of their income on out-of-pocket medical costs than men the same ages, in part because of the inadequacy of coverage for preventive and reproductive services.[42] Twice as many women as men (7.4 million versus 3.4 million, respectively) had out-of-pocket expenditures for health care services in 1993 that exceeded 10 percent of their incomes. Even among those with health insurance coverage, women had higher out-of-pocket expenses than did men.

Furthermore, among women, those who are poor assume a disproportionate share of the burden. One out of four poor women have out-of-pocket expenditures exceeding 10 percent of their incomes, compared with 5 percent of higher-income women.[43]

# Health Insurance Coverage: Effects on Women's Access to Health Care Services

Several studies have documented the relationship between insurance coverage and access to care, building upon the conceptual framework developed by Aday and Andersen[44] and measuring such access indicators as utilization of physician and hospital visits, delayed care, and receipt of preventive care. Most of these studies, except for those specifically designed to assess gender-specific preventive screenings or services, do not distinguish differences for women and men. Even without this distinction, however, they do provide important information about the role of insurance coverage on use and show the disadvantage that the uninsured have in an insurance-based health care system.

### Physician Visits and Hospital Use Rates

The uninsured are less likely than insured persons to receive services, including preventive care. The uninsured have fewer inpatient hospital days and, in most studies, fewer physician visits than those with coverage.[45] This differential remains even after controlling for differences in demographic factors and, to the extent possible, differences in need for services.

## Clinical Preventive Service Use

A more specific measure of access than physician and hospital visits is the use of clinical preventive services. There is considerable agreement about the efficacy of these services and, in most cases, the frequency at which services should be received. This consensus provides an independent criterion of use that can be applied across subgroups of women.

Several studies have shown that after controlling for demographic factors, women who lack coverage are less likely than women with coverage to receive such screenings as blood pressure testing, glaucoma testing, clinical breast examinations, mammograms, and Pap tests.[46] For example, 70 percent of uninsured women ages fifty to sixty-four had not had a mammogram within the past two years, compared with 36 percent of women with coverage.[47] Among women ages eighteen to sixty-four, 52 percent of those without coverage have not had a Pap test within the past year, compared with one-third of those with coverage.[48] Many uninsured women also have low incomes, a factor associated with elevated risk for many of the conditions that these screenings are intended to discover. Thus, the burden of paying for preventive services often falls on those women who are the least able to afford such costs and most in need of them. Lack of insurance coverage may well force women and medical providers to prioritize urgent health care problems, compromising access to preventive screenings. This creates an ineffective health care system, one in which advances in prevention and early diagnosis are not fully and adequately used. Diagnosis of disease at an early stage is particularly important for cervical and breast cancer; both morbidity and mortality are reduced if these cancers are detected early.[49]

## Prenatal Service Use

A further indicator of access for women is use of prenatal services. Several studies have documented that uninsured women do not receive adequate prenatal services, as measured by the point during pregnancy when care was initiated and the number of physician visits throughout the pregnancy.[50] In 1987, it was estimated that over fourteen million women of childbearing age had inadequate or no coverage for prenatal services.[51] The 1978 Pregnancy Discrimination Act, which requires all employee group health policies to cover pregnancy and related services, guards against an even higher proportion of women being uninsured for these services.[52] However, this act excludes from its provisions individually purchased health insurance policies and health insurance policies not covered by state mandates.

## Delayed or Forgone Care

Delay in care or forgone care is another indicator often used as a measure of access. Studies have consistently found that the uninsured are likely to delay care or not to receive needed care. In 1993, 71 percent of the uninsured (both women and men) postponed getting needed care, compared with 21 percent of those with private coverage and 28 percent of those covered by Medicaid.[53] Additionally, one-third of these uninsured respondents did not receive needed care, compared with 8 percent of the privately insured and 10 percent of those on Medicaid. Among the uninsured, women are more likely to delay needed care than are men (35 percent versus 24 percent, respectively) and less likely to receive needed care (36 percent versus 23 percent).[54]

## Health Outcomes

Lack of health insurance coverage not only reduces access to health care but appears to affect health outcomes. Women without health insurance coverage have a more advanced stage of breast cancer at diagnosis, and among those with local and regional disease, poorer survival than women with private coverage.[55] Lack of coverage also affects birth outcomes among women[56] and increases the risk of in-hospital mortality (for both women and men).[57] As access measures increasingly include health status as an outcome, rather than focusing mainly on health care use, more will be known about the connection between access and health status.

## Differences in Access by Insurance Type

The influence of health insurance coverage is more complex, however, than whether or not a person is insured. Some of the indicators of poor access seen for uninsured women are also seen for women on Medicaid, such as delayed initiation of prenatal care.[58] However, the factors associated with poorer access may differ between these two groups of women. For example, among women on Medicaid, low provider reimbursement fees, administrative delays, and complications in the Medicaid application and eligibility process may affect timely care. Overall, Medicaid has improved access to care for its enrollees, although full integration into mainstream care has not occurred and serious access barriers remain.

Among those with private coverage, the benefits covered (the comprehensiveness of coverage) and the extent of cost sharing influence use. Among the insured, lack of coverage for a specific benefit or cost-sharing features that inhibit use of services can pose formidable access barriers for women. Clinical preventive service use is related not only to coverage but to whether or not a particular benefit or procedure is covered.[59] Cost sharing reduces the use of both medical and preventive services, and has a stronger effect on the poor.[60]

Given that women are higher users of the health care system, that they spend more out-of-pocket than men, and that costs appear to inhibit use more for women than for men (potentially affecting the use of needed services) the effects of health care financing on the costs of care for women warrant primary consideration in any policy, programmatic, or management decision.

## Beyond Health Insurance and Cost: Health Care System Factors Affecting Use

There are several other access barriers that women report in addition to the costs of services. In this next section, we highlight some of the access barriers that are potentially amenable to change through policy, administrative, and management decisions.

The availability of primary care providers for Medicaid recipients and other poor women is often hampered by an inadequate geographical distribution of providers and by low reimbursement fees.[61] For both economic and noneconomic reasons, providers prefer to practice in urban, wealthier areas. A recent study found that primary care providers were less likely than other physicians to accept new Medicaid patients.[62] Surveyed physicians cited low fees as the most serious problem with the Medicaid program, and a substantial proportion also identified paperwork and billing difficulties as problematic. These distributional issues affect women's access to primary care services, including prenatal care, and particularly affect poor women and women living in rural areas.[63]

Studies indicate the importance of having a regular connection to the health care system. Having a usual source of care is associated with women's increased use of clinical preventive services and general medical checkups.[64] Even among insured women, those with a usual source of care are up to twice as likely to receive a cervical or breast cancer screening than those without a regular place where they receive care.[65]

Access to a regular provider of care is also an important component of women's health. Women's health care has been characterized as fragmented; many women typically see more than one provider for primary care needs—in part because women's health is often split into reproductive needs and all other needs.[66] Because of this fragmentation, women may not receive needed services or may receive repeated services. Studies have shown that the type of provider seen influences the receipt of certain services for women. Women who see an obstetrician/gynecologist are more likely to be screened for breast and cervical cancer than are those whose primary physician is an internist or family practitioner.[67] Physician specialty also affects access to health promotion advice. Internists and family practitioners are more likely to counsel their patients in such areas as exercise, nutrition and diet, and mental health issues, whereas obstetricians/gynecologists are more likely to ask about sexual practices and sexually transmitted diseases.[68] Practice and referral patterns of physicians are important determinants of the use of clinical preventive services for women; nearly three-quarters of women who have mammograms reported physician recommendation as the reason for the screening.[69]

Enhancing the accessibility of services for women is also crucial. Factors such as geographical location of services, availability of child care, and cultural sensitivity of services all influence access to the health care system.[70] Time constraints also impede women's access to care. Multiple roles and responsibilities (paid employment, care of children and parents, household work, and so on) all compete for women's time. Women often make trade-offs to allocate the time and resources available. In one study, over one-quarter of women who did not receive a recommended clinical preventive service reported time constraints as a factor.[71]

## Policy Implications and Future Research

The current insurance system leaves many women uninsured or with coverage as a dependent or through Medicaid. Women's coverage options differ from those of men. Women without insurance coverage are at serious risk of delaying or not receiving needed care and of not being screened for early detection of disease. Costs remain a barrier even for insured women, suggesting that any coverage that imposes large deductibles and coinsurance obligations would hinder the use of necessary services, especially for economically disadvantaged women. Lack of coverage for specific services also reduces the use of necessary care, such as preventive screenings. Limited coverage of important services, such as reproductive care, restricts the choices that women have available to them. These problems with benefit coverage emphasize the importance of comprehensive coverage. Particular consideration of low-income women is required in the formulation of new health policy regarding the financing of services. They have the lowest rates of screening for certain clinical preventive services, the poorest health status, and are the most vulnerable to the effects of costs.

Providing only financial access to health services will not sufficiently improve women's use of services, however. Services need to be organized to facilitate access to a regular source and provider of care to increase the continuity of care women receive. Appropriate incentives need to be in place in the health care system to encourage physician promotion of primary and preventive care. Women may benefit from having a women's health specialist as a primary care provider,[72] an area that requires additional consideration and research. The trend toward defining gynecologists as primary care providers would increase access to certain types of preventive screenings for women, but it is not clear what effect this designation would have on women's overall access to non-reproductive-related primary care services.

Managed care plans are well positioned to promote a more cohesive delivery approach and to educate their practitioners about the value of primary and preventive care. The literature suggests that women enrolled in health maintenance organizations (HMOs) have cancer screening rates equal to or higher than women in indemnity plans,[73] but the studies do not differentiate among HMO type, therefore limiting our understanding of the organizational structures and processes that promote better primary care. A meta-analysis shows that compared with indemnity plans, managed care plans generally had lower hospital admission rates and used fewer tests, procedures, or treatments that were expensive in absolute terms or had cheaper alternatives.[74] Such financial incentives in managed care could lead to underservice.[75]

We need further research on special measures needed to reach women who historically have been underserved by the health care system, such as ethnic minority women, low-income women, and women with less formal education. These population groups often experience the worst health status, are typically less likely to have access to primary care and preventive care services, and once in the system, may also experience disparities in medical treatment.

In addition to the financial and structural barriers that women face, many women experience competing social roles and responsibilities that interfere with their own needs for appropriate health care. Many women report time constraints as a deterrent to use of services. Some of these barriers can be addressed by the health care system—extending hours, bringing services into the communities where women live and work, and providing child-care access could remove some of these barriers.

Facilitating access to the health care system is only part of the process of improving the health of women. Additional research is needed on the coordination and process of care once a women has been screened and identified as needing further diagnostic work and treatment. Disparities in access to services, treatment approaches, and clinical outcomes between women and men and among subgroups of women need continuing investigation to allow us to understand and eliminate the causes of inequities in the health care system.[76]

## Notes

1. Karen Scott Collins, Diane Rowland, Alina Salganicoff, and Elizabeth Chait, *Assessing and Improving Women's Health* (Washington, D.C.: Women's Research and Education Institute, 1994); and P. Adams and V. Benson, "Current Estimates from the National Health Interview Survey, 1989," *Vital and Health Statistics* 10 (1990), 115.

2. Roberta Wyn, "Women's Access to Health Insurance Coverage," unpublished Ph.D. dissertation, University of California, Los Angeles, 1995.

3. Nancy Jecker, "Can an Employer-Based Health Insurance System Be Just?" *Journal of Health, Politics, Policy, and Law* 18 (1993): 657–673.

4. U.S. Bureau of the Census, *Statistical Abstract of the United States: 1990* (Washington, D.C.: U.S. Government Printing Office, 1990); U.S. Bureau of the Census, *Current Population Reports, Health Insurance Coverage: 1986–88,* Series P–70, No. 17, (Washington, D.C.: U.S. Government Printing Office, 1990).

5. U.S. Bureau of the Census, *Statistical Abstract of the United States: 1990.*

6. Diane Rowland, Judith Feder, Barbara Lyons, and Alina Salganicoff, *Medicaid at the Crossroads: A Report of the Kaiser Commission on the Future of Medicaid, 1992* (Washington, D.C.: Kaiser Commission on the Future of Medicaid.

7. Collins, Rowland, Salganicoff, and Chait, *Assessing and Improving Women's Health,* p. 38

8. U.S. Bureau of the Census, Current Population Reports, *How We're Changing: Demographic State of the Nation: 1990,* Series P–23, No. 170 (Washington, D.C.: U.S. Government Printing Office, 1990).

9. U.S. Bureau of the Census, *Statistical Abstract of the United States: 1990.*

10. Wyn, "Women's Access to Health Insurance Coverage."

11. F. Ham, "The Future of Dependent Health Benefits," *Business and Health* 7 (1989): 19–26; and D. Holzman, "Are You Paying Other Companies' Health Bills?" *Business and Health* 9 (1991): 19–25.

12. Laura Scofea, "The Development and Growth of Employer-Provided Health Insurance," *Monthly Labor Review* (March 1994): 3–10.

13. U.S. General Accounting Office, *Medicaid: States Turn to Managed Care to Improve Access and Control Costs,* GAO/HRD–93–46 (Washington, D.C.: U.S. General Accounting Office, March 1993).

14. Kaiser Commission on the Future of Medicaid, *Medicaid and Managed Care Policy Brief* (Washington, D.C.: Kaiser Commission on the Future of Medicaid, April, 1995).

15. U.S. General Accounting Office, *Medicaid: States Turn to Managed Care to Improve Access and Control Costs.*

16. Kaiser Commission on the Future of Medicaid, *Medicaid and Managed Care Policy Brief.*

17. Diane Rowland, Sara Rosenbaum, Lois Simon, and Elizabeth Chait, *Medicaid Managed Care: Lessons from the Literature,* (Washington, D.C.: Kaiser Commission on the Future of Medicaid, March 1995).

18. Rowland, Rosenbaum, Simon, and Chait, *Medicaid Managed Care: Lessons form the Literature.*

19. Physician Payment Review Commission, *Physician Payment Under Medicaid* (Washington, D.C.: Physician Payment Review Commission, 1991); and Diane Rowland, Judy Feder, and J. Ed-

wards, "Health Care for the Poor in the Reagan Era," *Annual Review of Public Health* 9 (1988): 427–450.

20. Physician Payment Review Commission, *Physician Payment Under Medicaid;* and Rowland, Feder, and Edwards, "Health Care for the Poor."

21. Embry Howell and Marilyn Rymer Ellwood, "Medicaid and Pregnancy: Issues in Expanding Eligibility," *Family Planning Perspectives* 23 (1991): 123–128.

22. Joyce Piper, Wayne Ray, and Marie Griffin, "Effects of Medicaid Eligibility Expansion on Prenatal Care and Pregnancy Outcome in Tennessee," *Journal of the American Medical Association* 264 (1990): 2219–2223.

23. Women's Research and Education Institute, *Women's Health Insurance Costs and Experiences* (Washington, D.C.: Women's Research and Education Institute, 1994).

24. Alan Guttmacher Institute, *Uneven and Unequal: Insurance Coverage and Reproductive Health Services* (Washington, D.C.: Alan Guttmacher Institute, 1994).

25. Alan Guttmacher Institute, *Uneven and Unequal,* pp. 16–17.

26. Alan Guttmacher Institute, *Uneven and Unequal,* pp. 17–19.

27. Alan Guttmacher Institute, *Uneven and Unequal,* pp. 17–19.

28. National Cancer Institute, *Cancer Screening Summary—Cervical Cancer Screening* (Washington, D.C.: National Cancer Institute, October 31, 1993); and National Cancer Institute, *Cancer Facts: Updating the Guidelines for Breast Cancer Screening* (Washington, D.C.: National Cancer Institute, October 21, 1993).

29. Health Insurance Association of America, *Source Book of Health Insurance Data,* (Washington, D.C.: Health Insurance Association of America, 1991).

30. Leslie P. Boss and Frederick Guckes, "Medicaid Coverage of Screening Tests for Breast and Cervical Cancer," *American Journal of Public Health* 82 (1992): 252–253; and Kathryn Glovier Moore, "States Enact Mammography Coverage Laws," *Women's Health Issues* 2 (1991): 102–108.

31. Boss and Guckes, "Medicaid Coverage of Screening Tests."

32. Kathryn Glovier Moore, "Survey of State Medicaid Policies for Coverage of Screening Mammography and Pap Smear Services," *Women's Health Issues* 2 (1992): 40–49; and Boss and Guckes, "Medicaid Coverage of Screening Tests."

33. Helen Schauffler, "Disease Prevention Policy Under Medicare: A Historical and Political Analysis," *American Journal of Public Health* 9, 2 (1993): 71–77.

34. Roberta Wyn, E. Richard Brown, and Hongjian Yu, "Women's Use of Clinical Preventive Services," in *Women's Health and Care Seeking Behavior,* eds. Karen Scott Collins and Marilyn Falik (Baltimore, Md.: Johns Hopkins University Press, in press).

35. Women's Research and Education Institute, *Women's Health Insurance Costs,* p. 11.

36. Wyn, Brown, and Yu, "Women's Use of Clinical Preventive Services."

37. Wyn, Brown, and Yu, "Women's Use of Clinical Preventive Services."

38. Kathleen Lohr, Robert Brook, Caren Kamberg, George Goldberg, Arleen Leibowitz, Joan Keesey, David Reboussin, and Joseph Newhouse, "Effect of Cost-Sharing on Use of Medically Effective and Less Effective Care," *Medical Care* 24, 9 Supplement (1986): S31–S38.

39. Thomas Rice and Kathleen Morrison, "Patient Cost Sharing for Medical Services: A Review of the Literature and Implications for Health Care Reform," *Medical Care Review* 51, 3 (1994): 235–287.

40. Authors' analysis of the *March 1994 Current Population Survey.*

41. Joan Leiman, Anne Reisinger, Karen Scott Collins, Karen Davis, Mary Duncan, Mary Johnson, and Jane Meyer, *Health Care Reform: What Is at Stake for Women?* Policy Report of the Commonwealth Fund Commission on Women's Health (New York: Commonwealth Fund Commission on Women's Health, 1994).

42. Women's Research and Education Institute, *Women's Health Insurance Costs,* pp. 6–10.

43. Women's Research and Education Institute, *Women's Health Insurance Costs,* p. 10.

44. Lu Ann Aday and Ronald Andersen, "A Framework for the Study of Access to Medical Care," *Health Services Research* 9 (1974): 208–220.

45. Howard Freeman, Linda Aiken, Robert Blendon, and Christopher Corey, "Uninsured Working-Age Adults: Characteristics and Consequences," *Health Services Research* 24 (1990): 811–23; and Llewellyn Cornelius, "Access to Medical Care for Black Americans with an Episode of Illness," *Journal of the National Medical Association* 83 (1991): 617–26.

46. E. Richard Brown, Roberta Wyn, W. G. Cumberland, Hongjian Yu, Emily Abel, Lillian Gelberg, and Lyra Ng, *Women's Health-Related Behaviors and Use of Preventive Services: Report to the Commonwealth Fund* (New York: Commonwealth Fund, Commission on Women's Health, 1995); Wyn, Brown, and Yu, "Women's Use of Clinical Preventive Services," pp. 16–18; Women's Research and Education Institute, *Women's Health Care Costs and Experiences,* pp. 13–15; and Steffie Woolhandler and David Himmelstein, "Reverse Targeting of Preventive Care Due to Lack of Health Insurance," *JAMA* 259, 29 (1988): 2872–2874.

47. Brown, Wyn, Cumberland, Yu, Abel, Gelberg, and Ng, *Women's Health-Related Behaviors,* pp. 70–78

48. Brown, Wyn, Cumberland, Yu, Abel, Gelberg, and Ng, *Women's Health-Related Behaviors,* pp. 64–69.

49. National Cancer Institute, *Cancer Screening Summary;* and National Cancer Institute, *Cancer Facts.*

50. U.S. General Accounting Office, *Prenatal Care: Medicaid Recipients and Uninsured Women Obtain Insufficient Care,* Pub. No. GAO/HRD–87–137 (Washington, D.C.: U.S. General Accounting Office, 1987); and Howard Freeman, Robert Blendon, and Linda Aiken, "Americans Report on Their Access to Health Care," *Health Affairs* (1987): 6–18.

51. Alan Guttmacher Institute, *Blessed Events and the Bottom Line: Financing Maternity Care in the United States.* (New York: Alan Guttmacher Institute, 1987).

52. Alan Guttmacher Institute, *Uneven and Unequal,* p. 12.

53. Henry J. Kaiser Family Foundation and Commonwealth Fund, *Survey of Americans and Their Health Insurance* (New York: Louis Harris and Associates, 1993).

54. Commonwealth Fund, *The Health of American Women* (New York: Louis Harris and Associates, 1993).

55. John Ayanian, Betsy Kohler, Toshi Abe, and Arnold Epstein, "The Relation Between Health Insurance Coverage and Clinical Outcomes Among Women with Breast Cancer," *New England Journal of Medicine* 329 (1993): 326–331.

56. Paula Braverman, Geraldine Oliva, and Marie Graham Miller, "Adverse Outcomes and Lack of Health Insurance Among Newborns in an Eight-County Area of California, 1982–1986," *New England Journal of Medicine* 321 (1989): 508–513.

57. Jack Hadley, Earl P. Steinberg, and Judith Feder, "Comparisons of Uninsured and Privately Insured Hospital Patients: Condition on Admissions, Resource Use, and Outcome," *JAMA* 265 (1991): 374–379.

58. Paula Braverman, Trude Bennett, Charlotte Lewis, Susan Egerter, and Jonathan Showstack, "Access to Prenatal Care Following Major Medical Eligibility Expansions," *JAMA* 269 (1993): 1285–1289.

59. Wyn, Brown, and Yu, "Women's Use of Clinical Preventive Services," pp. 19–21.

60. K. Lohr, R. Brook, C. J. Kamberg, G. Goldberg, A. Leibowitz, J. Keesey, D. Reboussin, and J. Newhouse, "Use of Medical Care in the RAND Health Insurance Experiment: Diag-

nosis and Service-Specific Analyses in a Randomized Controlled Trial," *Medical Care* 24, Supplement (1986): S1–S86.

61. Physician Payment Review Commission, *Report to Congress* (Washington, D.C.: Physician Payment Review Commission, 1994); and Janet Mitchell, "Physician Participation in Medicaid Revisited," *Medical Care* 29 (1991): 645–653.

62. Louis Harris and Associates, *Physicians and the Medicare Fee Schedule: A Look at the Medicare Program and Other Payers in a Changing Practice Environment* (New York: Louis Harris and Associates, 1993). This report was prepared under contract to the Physician Payment Review Commission.

63. Jacob's Institute of Women's Health, *The Women's Health Data Book* (Washington, D.C.: Jacob's Institute of Women's Health, 1992).

64. Wyn, Brown, and Yu, "Women's Use of Clinical Preventive Services"; Brown, Wyn, Cumberland, Yu, Abel, Gelberg, and Ng, *Women's Health-Related Behaviors;* and Ronald Hayward, Howard Feeman, and C. Corey, "Who Gets Screened for Cervical and Breast Cancer? Results from a New National Study," *Archives of Internal Medicine* 148 (1988): 1177–1181.

65. Brown, Wyn, Cumberland, Yu, Abel, Gelberg, and Ng, "Women's Health-Related Behaviors."

66. Carolyn Clancy and Charlea Massion, "American Women's Health Care: A Patchwork Quilt with Gaps," *JAMA* (1992) 268: 1918–1920.

67. Wyn, Brown, and Yu, "Women's Use of Clinical Preventive Services"; and Nicole Lurie, Jonathan Slater, Paul McGovern, Jacqueline Ekstrum, Lois Quam, and Karen Margolis, "Preventive Care for Women: Does the Sex of the Physician Matter?" *New England Journal of Medicine* (1993): 478–482.

68. American College of Obstetricians and Gynecologists, ACOG News Release, "Issues in Women's Health," October 29, 1993.

69. M. C. Romans, D. J. Marchant, W. H. Pearse, J. F. Gravenstine, and S. M. Sutton, "Utilization of Screening Mammography 1990," *Women's Health Issues* 1 (1991): 68–73.

70. Wyn, Brown, and Yu, "Women's Use of Clinical Preventive Services"; Leiman, Reisinger, Collins, Davis, Duncan, Johnson, and Meyer, *Health Care Reform;* Steven Woloshin, Nina Bickell, Lisa Schwartz, Francesca Gany, and Gilbert Welch, "Language Barriers in Medicine in the United States," *JAMA* 273 (1995): 724–728; and Julia Solis, Gary Marks, Melinda Garcia, and David Shelton, "Acculturation, Access to Care, and Use of Preventive Services by Hispanics: Findings from HHANES 1982–84," *American Journal of Public Health* 80 (1990): 11–19.

71. Wyn, Brown, and Yu, "Women's Use of Clinical Preventive Services."

72. Clancy and Massion, "American Women's Health Care"; and Karen Johnson and Eileen Hoffman, "Women's Health: Designing and Implementing an Interdisciplinary Specialty," *Women's Health Issues* 3 (1993): 115–119.

73. Karen Davis, Karen Scott Collins, Cathy Schoen, and Catherine Morris, "Choice Matters: Enrollees' Views of Their Health Plans," *Health Affairs* 14 (1995): 99–112.

74. Robert Miller and Hal Luft, "Managed Care Plan Performance Since 1980: A Literature Analysis," *JAMA* 271 (1994): 1512–1519.

75. Miller and Luft, "Managed Care Plan Performance."

76. Council on Ethical and Judicial Affairs, American Medical Association, "Gender Disparities in Clinical Decision Making," *JAMA* 266 (1991): 559–562; and Council on Ethical and Judicial Affairs, American Medical Association, "Black-White Disparities in Health Care," *JAMA* 263 (1990): 2344–2346.

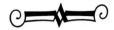

CHAPTER TWELVE

# HOMELESS PERSONS

Lillian Gelberg

H omelessness has reached crisis proportions in the United States today. It is
estimated that 600,000[1] to 3 million[2] people are currently without a home.
However, the crisis is much worse than this; nationally, 14 percent of the U.S. population (26 million people) have been homeless at some time in their lives, and 5
percent (8.5 million people) have been homeless within the past five years.[3] Los
Angeles is known as the homeless capital although some would argue that New
York holds this infamous record. While a majority of homeless persons live in our
major urban areas, 19 percent live in rural areas.[4]

The picture of the homeless population of the United States has changed
over the years.[5] "Skid rows" developed as a result of industry's need for a mobile semiskilled labor class. The term derived from the *skid roads*, or *skidways*, used
by Seattle's lumberjacks employed as seasonal labor to slide logs to the mills.[6]
These skid roads (later, skid rows), with their flophouses, taverns, brothels, labor
agencies, inexpensive eating places, and location near transportation stations,
served as centers for unattached seasonal laborers. Skid rows were populated by
middle-aged white men, predominately Northern European immigrants, employed in seasonal and temporary work.[7] During the nineteenth and twentieth
centuries, skid row populations grew during depressions and at the ends of wars
in proportion to increases in the unemployment rate. The Great Depression, with
25 percent unemployment, brought a large cross section of the general population to skid row in search of work and housing.[8] With the economic boom years

after World War II and welfare reform, skid rows decreased in size. With less need for an unskilled labor pool, skid rows became havens for mainly white, middle-aged alcoholic men.[9] However, skid rows did not disappear. In the 1950s, with the civil rights movement, development of psychotropic drugs, loss of funding for state mental institutions, and inadequate funding of community-based mental health services, we began to see increasing numbers of alcoholic and mentally ill men and women living on the streets.[10] In the 1970s, 1980s, and 1990s, with urban development, loss of low-income housing, reduction in welfare benefits relative to inflation, and high unemployment rates, increasing numbers of homeless persons were members of minority groups and families with children. Not since the Great Depression have we seen such large numbers of homeless persons and such a broad cross section of society represented.[11]

As we face homeless individuals lining the streets of our major cities (and in rural areas as well), casual observation reveals that they are burdened with unattended mental and physical health problems. Because of high rates of infectious diseases, they have the potential to spread diseases such as tuberculosis to other homeless persons and the general population. Planning for appropriate and effective health services for homeless persons requires attention to the unique characteristics of the homeless population, both as individuals and as patients, in terms of health status, barriers to obtaining and adhering to prescribed medical care, and integration of housing and health services.

## Who Are the Homeless?

While in prior generations the homeless population primarily consisted of middle-aged alcoholic white men, the homeless population of today includes single men (70 percent) and single women (7 percent), adolescents (2 percent), and children (13 percent). Eight percent are parents with children.[12] The fastest-growing segment of this population is composed of families (23 percent) and ethnic minority groups (60 percent).[13] Homeless persons are young: most children are under the age of six[14] and most adults are in their mid thirties,[15] but only 3 percent of the homeless are older than sixty-five years.[16] About one-third of homeless men are veterans.[17]

The economic picture of homeless persons is dismal, as would be expected, and suggests that they are severely lacking in the financial and educational resources necessary to access health care. In 1987, their average monthly income was $137—28 percent of the federal poverty level for a one-person household. Further, almost half have not graduated from high school and on average they have been unemployed for four years. Despite these figures, only 20 percent receive income maintenance.[18] Only 26 percent have health insurance.[19]

Homelessness represents a continuum. On average, homeless persons have been without a home for three years. However, half of the homeless population may be considered to be the newly homeless (homeless one year or less) and one-fifth comprise the very long-term homeless (homeless for more than four years.[20] Further, the distinction between homeless and nonhomeless impoverished persons is not a clear one, since persons cycle in and out of homelessness during their lifetimes.[21]

The shortage of adequate low-income housing is the major precipitating factor for homelessness. Unemployment, personal or family life crises, increases in rent out of proportion to inflation, and reduction in public benefits can also directly result in the loss of a home. Illness, on the other hand, tends to result in the loss of a home in a more indirect manner, via these more direct precipitating factors. Other indirect precipitants of homelessness include deinstitutionalization from public mental hospitals, substance abuse, and overcrowded prisons and jails.[22]

## Health Status

The homeless, adults and children, have a very high prevalence of untreated acute and chronic medical, mental health, and substance abuse problems. Their increased risk for illness as compared to the general population may be due to a variety of factors. Persons may become homeless because of a physical or mental illness, and homelessness itself may lead to the development of physical and mental disability.

Homeless persons are subject to the same risk factors for physical illness as the general population, but they may be exposed to excessive levels of such risk, and they also experience risk factors more unique to homelessness. Risk factors include the excessive use of alcohol, illegal drugs, and cigarettes; sleeping in an upright position (resulting in venous stasis and its consequences); extensive walking in poorly fitting shoes; and inadequate nutrition.[23]

Further, homelessness itself is physically dangerous, as homeless persons are at risk of assault and victimization, as well as exposure to the elements. Homeless people are at great risk of being victimized due to lack of personal security, whether they live in a shelter or in the outdoors. And they are exposed to illness due to overcrowding in shelters and exposure to heat and cold.[24] This relationship between lack of housing and health is important and suggests why we must view the entire ecology of homelessness, including lack of housing, rather than focus narrowly on the health and mental health problems of the homeless.

## Physical Illness

The homeless have much higher rates of physical illness than the general population. Whereas 39 percent of homeless men rate their health as poor, only 21 percent of housed men in the same community rate their health as poor.[25] Studies have found that one-third to one-half of homeless adults have some form of physical illness.[26] This illness appears to be taking its toll, preventing some of the homeless from escaping their predicament. For example, one-quarter of homeless adults report that their poor health prevented them from working or going to school.[27] Even more seriously, rates of mortality are three to four times higher in the homeless population than they are in the general population.[28] As for the physical health of homeless children, at least half have a physical illness,[29] and they are twice as likely as housed children to have such illnesses.[30]

The most common physical illnesses among homeless persons include upper respiratory tract infections, trauma, female genitourinary problems, hypertension, skin and ear disorders, gastrointestinal diseases, peripheral vascular disease, musculoskeletal problems, dental problems, and vision problems.[31] Inadequate immunization, while not a physical illness, reflects the lack of preventive health care in this population.[32]

## Communicable Disease

The data suggest that the prevention, diagnosis, and treatment of infectious diseases among homeless populations will need to be addressed by health care, housing, and social service providers. Contagious diseases such as tuberculosis[33] and HIV infection[34] are more common among the homeless than the general population.

The prevalence of tuberculosis infection among homeless adults ranges from 32 percent in San Francisco[35] to 43 percent in New York.[36] The rate of active tuberculosis among men in a New York shelter clinic is 6 percent.[37] The rate of positive tuberculosis skin tests has been found to be related to duration of homelessness,[38] living in crowded shelters or single-room occupancy hotels,[39] and injection drug use.[40] And the homeless can spread communicable diseases such as tuberculosis to others. A homeless person with undiagnosed pulmonary tuberculosis who frequented a neighborhood bar infected 42 percent of the regular customers of that bar.[41] Tuberculosis may be more difficult to treat among the homeless because of the difficulty of screening, following, and maintaining tuberculosis treatment for this population, and because many have multidrug-resistant organisms.[42]

The prevalence of HIV infection among the homeless population is higher than in the housed population. Studies reveal an HIV infection rate of 9 percent among San Francisco's homeless adults,[43] 1.3 percent among African American homeless women in Los Angeles,[44] 19 percent among homeless psychiatric patients in a New York City men's shelter,[45] 62 percent among homeless men who visited a New York City shelter clinic,[46] and 5 percent among homeless youth in a New York City shelter clinic.[47]

Further evidence of contagious disease among homeless persons are the outbreaks of infection that have occurred in this population. This includes meningococcal disease in the skid rows of the Northwest,[48] pneumococcal pneumonia in a Boston shelter,[49] tuberculosis in shelters in Boston,[50] Cincinnati,[51] and Columbus;[52] and diphtheria in an Omaha mission[53] and in Seattle's skid row.[54]

## Women's Health

Homeless women are severely lacking in women's health services,[55] and yet pregnancy and recent births are risk factors for becoming homeless.[56] Ninety-five percent of homeless women are sexually active,[57] and yet 72 percent do not use birth control.[58] Less than 10 percent use condoms, despite life-styles that place them at great risk for AIDS and other sexually transmitted diseases;[59] 60 percent of homeless family planning clinic users had a history of a sexually transmitted disease and 28 percent had a history of pelvic inflammatory disease.[60] In addition, more than one-fifth have not had a Pap smear in the past five years,[61] compared to less than 9 percent of women in the general population.[62] This is alarming given that 23 percent of homeless family planning clinic users had an abnormal Pap smear.[63]

Regarding homeless women's obstetrical history, 74 percent have had children, and 54 percent are currently at risk for unintended pregnancy; however, nearly three-quarters do not have their children living with them.[64] Homeless women are more likely to be pregnant (11 percent of homeless adults, 24 percent of sixteen- to nineteen-year-old homeless youth) than their poor but housed peers (5 percent).[65] In addition, they are more likely to receive inadequate prenatal care than poor but housed women (56 percent versus 15 percent).[66] It follows that homeless women are more likely than impoverished housed women to have poor birth outcomes[67] (16 percent versus 7 percent low-birthweight newborns).[68] In New York City, infant mortality was highest among the homeless (24.9 per 1,000 live births) as compared to poor housed women (16.6 per 1,000 live births), and nonpoor housed women (12.0 per 1,000 live births).[69] In Great Britain, homeless women had higher rates of premature births (11 percent versus 7 percent of the general population), while their rates of infant mortality were the same as those of housed women.[70]

## Dental Health

One of the more overt identifiers of poverty in the United States is poor dental health. It is one of the major health problems reported by homeless individuals.[71] Ten percent of homeless clinic patients have been found to have poor dental health, a rate thirty-one times that found in the general population.[72] Homeless persons living in the community are one-third as likely as domiciled adults to have obtained dental care in the past year, and consequently are twice as likely to have gross dental decay (57 percent versus 23 percent).[73] Given this high rate of dental disease, dental care should be an integral part of any health care services package developed for the homeless population.

## Mental Illness and Substance Abuse

The media has made the public aware of the high prevalence of mental illness among the homeless and their desperate need for effective mental health treatment. One-third of homeless adults suffer from current major mental illness, including schizophrenic disorders, affective disorders, personality or character disorder, and cognitive impairment.[74] Further, one-third have a substance abuse disorder.[75] About 12 percent have dual diagnoses of chronic mental illness and chronic substance use. These latter individuals pose a challenge to developing services that will successfully address both aspects of their illness.[76] In addition to intrinsic illness processes, environmental stresses and homeless appearance must be considered in order to avoid inaccurate diagnosis of mental illness among homeless individuals. These individuals may experience chronic isolation, geographical mobility, disturbed sleep, and fear of victimization and may exhibit disheveled appearance and signs of lack of self-care.[77]

A similarly high prevalence of mental problems has been found among homeless children. It has been reported that 47 percent of homeless children aged five or younger are developmentally delayed, and 31 percent of those older than age five are clinically depressed.[78]

## Access to Health Care

Homeless persons' patterns of health services use suggest inappropriate health care delivery. The high rates of hospitalization in this young population represent the substitution of inpatient care for outpatient care that results from poor access to ambulatory services. This poor access is due to individual factors (competing needs, substance dependence, and mental illness) as well as to system factors (availability, cost, convenience, and appropriateness of care).

## Use of Physical Health Services

Homeless people are at least twice as likely as the general population to report having had a medical hospitalization during the preceding year.[79] A Hawaiian study found that homeless persons' age- and sex-adjusted acute care hospitalization rate was 542/1,000 person-years as compared with the general population rate of 96/1,000 person-years. Homeless persons were admitted to acute care hospitals for 4,766 days compared with a predicted 640 days, resulting in costs of $2.8 million for excess hospitalization.[80] Another study found that homeless adults' hospital lengths of stay exceeded the mean general admission by 12 percent to 23 percent. Following hospital discharge, 40 percent of these homeless individuals were readmitted to the hospital within fourteen months, usually with the same diagnosis as on the initial hospitalization. These high hospitalization and readmission rates resulted in costs at a major urban hospital of more than $1.8 million during the three-month study.[81] The finding that most of the homeless inpatients were admitted for problems that could have been treated less expensively in an outpatient setting suggests difficulty in sustaining treatment intensity for homeless persons outside the hospital. These data imply an ineffective local service delivery system for the homeless population.

Despite higher rates of medical hospitalization and higher rates of disease, the homeless are in fact less likely to use medical outpatient services than the general population. One study found that whereas only 24 percent of the homeless had used outpatient medical services during the preceding year, 43 percent of the general population had made such a visit during the same time period.[82] This suggests that the homeless may delay seeking medical attention at a time when more severe stages of illness could be prevented.

Once homeless persons do get needed medical services, they may find it difficult to comply with treatment. For example, only 50 percent of homeless patients in New York City who were referred from a satellite clinic to a hospital clinic kept their appointments,[83] and only 25 percent with cardiovascular disease remained in long-term therapy.[84] Further, in a New York City shelter, only six out of fifty homeless individuals requiring isoniazid prophylaxis for tuberculosis were found to be taking their medications, and not one completed the full year of treatment.[85] And only four of thirty acutely psychotic homeless patients were taking the psychotropic medications that had been prescribed to them.[86]

Success of interventions and compliance with medical regimens is affected by the social situation of the homeless.[87] Their social conditions, competing needs, and unique life-styles all combine to make more traditional approaches to health care delivery less effective for homeless patients even when compared to poor domiciled patients. Homeless persons obtain their health care primarily from the public health system and not from private doctors' offices (the main source of care for the general population). This is explained by their lack of health insurance and inability to pay for health care, as well as lack of availability of facilities and providers willing to treat them. They receive most of their outpatient care from emergency rooms,[88] but also seek care from public hospital clinics and community clinics that are free of charge.[89] When hospitalized, homeless persons are most likely to be admitted to general county hospitals.[90]

## Use of Mental Health Services

As noted above, mental illness is more prevalent among homeless people than in the general population. Consequently, a large proportion (15 percent to 44 percent) of homeless adults report having had a previous psychiatric hospitalization.[91] The age- and sex-adjusted rate of admission of homeless persons to Hawaiian state psychiatric hospitals was 105/1,000 person-years, compared with the general population rate of 0.8/1,000 person-years.[92]

Despite their high prevalence of current mental illness and prior psychiatric hospitalization, most homeless persons do not use the existing outpatient mental health system for care. Only 18 percent of homeless people in Baltimore's shelters had used outpatient mental health services during the six months preceding a study,[93] and the majority of persons with a previous mental hospitalization had not made an outpatient mental health visit in the past five years,[94] Further, possibly in combination with their homeless plight, there is a high prevalence of inadequately treated mental illness within the homeless population: 25 percent of homeless adults considered committing suicide, and 7 percent attempted suicide during a yearlong period.[95]

## Barriers to Health Care

Compounding their increased risk for disease, there is evidence that homeless people encounter major obstacles to obtaining needed medical and psychiatric services. The majority of homeless adults state that they did not obtain needed medical care in the previous year.[96] Even among those with a chronic medical condition, half had not seen a doctor within the previous year.[97] While some homeless persons do seek care for their health problems, certain segments of the population are less likely to obtain care even if they are sick. The only empirical examination of this situation found that homeless adults with little education and without health insurance were less likely to seek care even if they were sick.[98] Such delay in seeking care may result in health care practitioners having to manage conditions that would have been easier to treat had the individual sought help earlier.

Homeless individuals face numerous problems in obtaining appropriate health care. These include cost, transportation, competing needs, mental illness, the homeless life-style, personal barriers, lack of availability of health services, medical provider bias, insufficient discharge planning from hospitals, and lack of recuperative care.

*First,* there are the financial barriers and problems in satisfying eligibility requirements for health insurance. One-fifth of homeless adults who had not obtained needed medical care stated that this was due to inability to pay for medical services.[99] Only one-sixth[100] to one-third[101] of the homeless in the community have any form of health insurance (Medicaid, Medicare, Veterans Services, or private insurance), and most have no cash resources at all.[102]

*Second,* accessible transportation to medical facilities is often unavailable to this population.[103]

*Third,* the homeless have competing needs, and it is understandable that they may place a greater priority on fulfilling their basic needs for food, shelter, and income than on obtaining needed health services or following through with a prescribed treatment plan.[104] Although we typically think of homeless people as having an inordinate amount of time on their hands, often they must deal with the varied schedules and locations of several service facilities to ensure that all their needs are met.[105] For instance, it is not uncommon for a homeless person to begin the day early in the morning by lining up at a soupline for breakfast, then walking to the next soupline to join the long line for lunch, and then walking back to the shelter to wait in line once again in hope of securing a bed for the night. Even medical care for an active disease may seem less important than other needs, and preventive health care often loses out completely. Only 20 percent of homeless children were reported to have up-to-date immunizations,[106] and half of the homeless adults who said they had not obtained needed medical care stated that this was because their medical problem was not sufficiently serious to warrant their attention.[107]

*Fourth,* those homeless individuals who experience psychological distress as well as disabling mental illness may be in the greatest need of health services[108] and yet may be the least able to obtain them.[109] This may be attributable to such individual characteristics of mental illness as paranoia, disorientation, unconventional health beliefs, lack of social supports, lack of organizational skills to gain access to needed services,[110] or fear of authority figures and institutions as a result of previous institutionalization.[111] Further, mentally ill homeless adults often require services, largely unavailable today, able to handle multifaceted problems including mental illness, substance abuse, physical illness, criminality, and such social-service-related problems as housing and employment.[112] What is needed is nontraditional services that would fulfill basic needs before addressing psychodynamic issues.[113] Comprehensive case management is needed that would address such homeless mentally ill persons' housing, social support, employment, vocational rehabilitation, mental health, and physical health needs. Such services would be best provided by a multidisciplinary team and health service center.

*Fifth,* the social conditions of street life itself may affect compliance with medical care. There is usually a lack of proper sanitation;[114] lack of a stable place to keep medications safe, intact, and refrigerated;[115] and an inability to obtain the proper food for a medically indicated diet required for conditions such as diabetes mellitus or hypertension.[116] Lacking social support, homeless persons often do not have anyone who can transport them to a clinic or care for them if needed after giving birth or experiencing a major illness.[117] While most homeless persons are long-term residents of their community, many are quite mobile within a city in their search for subsistence resources. This mobility makes continuity of care difficult.[118] Keeping follow-up appointments—necessary for continuous, comprehensive care—is difficult for homeless people due to their competing needs and different time orientation.[119]

*Sixth,* homeless people at times present barriers to their own care. Because an exhibition of toughness is necessary in order to survive on the streets, homeless persons may at times deny that they have health problems in an attempt to maintain a sense of their own endurance. However, while attempting to present a tough facade, they actually may be afraid to venture out of the immediate geographical area to which they have become somewhat acclimated, which presents a barrier to seeking medical services in another area. They may be too embarrassed to have medical professionals see them in a condition of poor personal hygiene. They may fear that their meager financial resources will be taken away to pay for the medical care they receive. Fear of authority figures and need for control of situations concerning themselves are additional factors that keep homeless people from seeking medical care.[120] Fear of persons in positions of authority is prevalent throughout a wide spectrum of the homeless population and can result in failure to seek medical care. For example, homeless undocumented immigrants have reason to fear that medical providers will call in Immigration and Naturalization authorities, runaway teenagers and homeless women with children may fear child protective service workers, and drug abusers or ex-convicts may fear the police.[121]

*Seventh,* there is a lack of facilities that can adequately treat homeless people. The offices of most middle-class physicians will not welcome an unwashed, ungroomed individual.[122] As a result, national health care reform and universal coverage may not solve the access problems of homeless people, as is evident in the barriers to their care in Great Britain today. Availability and accessibility of primary care for many homeless persons in Great Britain is quite limited despite the elimination of hospital and medication charges.[123]

Further, health care facilities designed for the poor, or for emergency treatment, are not set up to provide the basic care that the homeless population requires, and may not be set up to take into consideration the culture of homelessness. Homeless people often cannot keep the scheduled appointments that are required in most primary care operations, thus creating barriers to first contact as well as follow-up care. However, the purpose of emergency rooms is to provide urgent or emergent care to people who arrive without prior scheduling. This is often why homeless individuals use emergency rooms as their source of medical care, but emergency rooms cannot provide the continuous comprehensive medical care that the complex problems of the homeless require.[124]

Many primary care settings that were designed for the housed poor are not set up to treat homeless patients. Public health systems for the poor tend to be based on clinics designed for specific, targeted programs such as family planning, prenatal care, tuberculosis testing and treatment, or immunization, yet the multiple medical and social problems of homeless persons do not neatly fit into such types of services. Thus, many homeless persons end up seeking medical care late in the course of their diseases or for traumatic or life-threatening conditions.

*Eighth*, homeless people may sense from the medical profession itself a barrier to obtaining needed medical care. Medical providers may consider homeless persons to be undesirable patients because of their poor hygiene or their mental illness, or because of assumptions that they come to hospitals for shelter and not for a medical problem.[125] Being treated with a lack of respect does not encourage follow-up care or compliance with care.

Health care practitioners, usually middle class, may view various aspects of health care quite differently than do their homeless patients. The attitudes of homeless patients in regard to establishing priorities, adhering to schedules, and keeping appointments can differ from those of their providers, setting up the possibility of conflict and failure.[126] Treatment plans are often automatically based on the assumption that the patient has a home. However, most homeless persons lack reliable access to places where they can recuperate (in bed, if indicated) and properly store medication. Ordinary uncomplicated postclinic care such as the cleansing of wounds with soap and hot water may be extremely difficult to implement. Prescribed dietary regimens, which may involve taking medications with meals, are impractical when patients are without a reliable place to store groceries. Because shelters, souplines, and garbage cans provide an unreliable source of nutritious food, homeless people have little control over what they eat. Needles and medications with recreational use are highly valued on the street and can make homeless patients a target for victimization.[127]

*Ninth*, for homeless inpatients there is a lack of adequate discharge planning. Homeless inpatients are discharged directly from the hospital to the streets; even homeless mothers are discharged to the streets with their newborn infants soon after childbirth. Readmission of homeless patients to hospitals is not uncommon.[128]

*Tenth*, there is a lack of recuperative services for homeless patients. When homeless persons are inappropriately discharged from hospitals, they are often unable to manage the necessary recuperation. Recuperation cannot be adequately managed on the streets or accommodated in shelters. Few health centers that care for the homeless offer recuperative care services because of the cost as well as restrictive licensing in many cities.

# Health Programs for Homeless People

A variety of programs have been developed to address the health care needs of the homeless, but there is no effort to integrate these systems or to ensure permanent funding. Without adequate and permanent funding, their support is in jeopardy every year.[129] Within the federal government, most of the services fall under the umbrella of the 1987 Stewart B. McKinney Homeless Assistance Act (Public Law 100–77), the first comprehensive federal legislation to address the health, education, and social welfare needs of homeless persons. In this section, I will focus on several programs that have addressed the health of homeless persons.

## The Health Care for the Homeless Program

Federal efforts to provide medical services to the homeless population are primarily conducted by the Health Care for the Homeless Program. Community health centers supported by the 1985 Robert Wood Johnson Foundation/Pew Memorial Trust Health Care for the Homeless Program (HCH programs), subsequently covered by the 1987 McKinney Homeless Assistance Act, have addressed many of the access and quality of care issues raised in this chapter.[130]

A critical aspect of the program is outreach: teams of health care professionals bring a wide range of services to homeless persons in shelters, hotels, souplines, beaches and parks, train and bus stations, religious facilities, and other places where homeless people are found. This reduces barriers to care such as lack of transportation, lack of information about available facilities, and psychological problems. Outreach teams are typically based in health care centers, to which clinicians can refer homeless patients who need additional medical attention. A walk-in appointment system reduces access barriers at these medical facilities. Medical care, routine laboratory tests, substance abuse counseling, and some medications are provided free of charge to reduce the cost barrier.

HCH programs try to employ staff (physicians, nurses, case mangers, dentists, and so on) who are nonjudgmental and sympathetic to the social problems of homeless people. Physicians and nurse practitioners build trusting relationships with homeless patients. They know that this requires patience. HCH providers try to treat homeless patients with as much respect as affluent patients are customarily treated in private doctors' offices. This encourages effective interventions, better compliance, and higher quality and continuity of care. Providers learn to look beyond the presenting problem and are prepared to intervene on many fronts, some of which do not lie within the traditional boundaries of medicine. At the same time, they realize that some homeless patients will not want to address anything other than the problems for which they are seeking care, at least at first.

Medical providers are usually in the primary care disciplines, and therefore are capable of treating the common problems faced by homeless people. They can recognize and treat, or refer for treatment, most common primary care problems that are medical, mental, or social in nature, including inadequate vaccination, routine health maintenance and prevention, developmental delay, depression and anxiety, substance abuse, physical and emotional abuse, trauma, skin infestations, peripheral vascular disease, malnutrition and failure to thrive, anemia, dental decay, podiatry problems, and vision impairment.

Providers often work in teams made up of case managers, nurses, nurse practitioners, social workers, and physicians. The case manager coordinates treatment and referrals for homeless patients. Referral networks of community groups and public agencies are called upon for problems the health center does not have the capability to treat, such as basic needs for shelter, food, and clothing; subspecialty health problems, including serious mental illness and substance abuse; social problems, including lack of income, public benefits, health insurance, and employment as well as legal problems; emergency care; and hospital care. Transportation vouchers (for public transportation, taxis, or ambulances) are often provided to transport homeless patients to this network of referral facilities. In addition, some facilities provide showers, food, and clothing as well as health education and preventive care programs. Respite care is provided by a few of these facilities,[131] where the average length of stay is two weeks.[132]

National evaluations of the HCH programs have been conducted.[133] Results reveal that availability and accessibility of services was accomplished to a certain degree—the program treated 23 percent of homeless persons in smaller cities but only 8 percent of homeless persons in larger cities. The HCH programs were successful at the difficult task of maintaining continuity of care for homeless patients. Half of their clients were seen on more than one occasion. Contacts with clients with a chronic medical condition averaged 4.5, with two-thirds being seen more than once, whereas contacts with the remaining clients averaged 2.3. Compared to patients without targeted conditions, whose average stay in the system was about one month, patients with the targeted chronic medical conditions of tuberculosis, hypertension, peripheral vascular disease, diabetes, and seizure disorders were seen about every two weeks for a period of two to three months. However, these visits may represent provision of more than one type of encounter per patient, so firm conclusions about treatment frequency cannot be drawn from the available data.

There is evidence that the HCH Program also provided comprehensive care. While 47 percent of patient encounters were for primary care services, 25 percent were for case management and social services, and 28 percent were for substance abuse, mental health, and dental services or referrals to hospitals or specialists. A large-scale national evaluation of McKinney-funded HCH programs is nearing completion. No data exist on health status outcomes of the HCH program.

## Mental Health Programs

There are several federal McKinney-funded programs that provide mental health services to the homeless, most of which are located in the Center for Mental Health Services of the Substance Abuse and Mental Health Services Administration. The Mental Health Services for the Homeless Block Grant set aside funds to implement services for homeless persons with mental illness, including outreach services, community mental health services and rehabilitation, referrals to inpatient treatment and primary care and substance abuse services, case management services, and supportive services in residential settings.[134] An evaluation of one such program for homeless persons with dual diagnoses of mental illness and substance abuse revealed greater housing stability, a 66 percent decrease in contact with the criminal justice system, a 50 percent decrease in crisis contacts, a 60 percent reduction in hospital admissions, and a 75 percent reduction in use of detoxification services.[135] Projects for Assistance in Transition from Homelessness supplants this program and provides funds for outreach services for homeless persons with mental illnesses who may also have substance abuse disorders. The Access to Community Care and Effective Services and Supports Program is a demonstration program in nine states focusing on coordination of services for homeless persons with severe mental illness as well as those with dual diagnoses of mental illness and substance abuse.[136]

The McKinney Act also funded the Demonstration Program for Homeless Adults with Serious Mental Illness.[137] The funded programs provided comprehensive mental health treatment, housing, and support services (via case management) to seriously mentally ill homeless adults. Accessible, relevant community mental health treatment services resulted in increased outpatient care of the homeless, reduced mental health symptoms, improved quality of life, and a reduction in inpatient days. With appropriate levels of support that this program provided, homeless mentally ill persons were maintained in community-based housing. Substance abuse treatment was required to prevent dual diagnosed mentally ill persons from returning to the streets. Another McKinney-funded program was the National Institute on Alcohol Abuse and Alcoholism Community Demonstration Grant Projects for Alcohol and Drug Abuse Treatment of Homeless Individuals.[138]

Many local programs do not fall directly under the McKinney Act. For the homeless with mental health problems, examples include the New York City Mayor's Project Help, which funded mobile unit staff and mandated them to hospitalize homeless persons in danger to themselves because of their mental illness. At the end of two years, 28 percent were housed in the community, 27 percent were in hospital settings, 34 percent were on the streets.[139] Project Outreach in New York City has volunteer psychiatrists in community agencies that provide mental health care to the homeless.[140] The Los Angeles Skid Row Project has a three-phase approach to treating the homeless mentally ill: emergency mental health services; shelters for stabilization where clients are evaluated for their medical, mental health, and social needs; and case management with the long-term goals of securing appropriate housing, public benefits, and mental health treatment.[141] Connecticut's Homeless Outreach Team (HOT)[142] and Santa Monica's St. John's Mental Health Outreach Project[143] identify homeless mentally ill persons in facilities that serve the homeless, and provide assessment and case management services. Data for the HOT program reveal that 37 percent of the clients were successfully placed in housing.[144]

## Veterans' Programs

Services for homeless veterans are provided through the U.S. Department of Veterans Affairs. The Homeless Chronically Mentally Ill Veterans Program provides outreach, case management services, and psychiatric residential treatment for homeless mentally ill veterans in community-based facilities in forty-five U.S cities. The Domiciliary Care for Homeless Veterans Program operates in thirty-one states, addressing the health needs of veterans who have psychiatric illnesses or alcohol or drug abuse problems. Veterans with such health problems are provided with room and board in the domiciliary. Services provided include screening for health problems, medical and psychiatric examinations, treatment and rehabilitation, and postdischarge community support.[145] An evaluation of these programs reveals that one-third of homeless veterans complete residential treatment, and of those, one-third are in stable community housing and one-third are employed at the time of discharge.[146] The evaluators suggest that to be more successful, health care programs for homeless veterans should be combined with sustained vocational rehabilitation services, housing, and public benefits.

## Other Health Services

The Salvation Army provides a variety of social, rehabilitation, and support services for homeless persons. Their centers include adult rehabilitation programs, food programs, and permanent and transitional housing facilities. Travelers Aid International, a network of social agencies, provides homeless adults and youth with short-term counseling, shelter, food, and clothing.[147] The Los Angeles Homeless Outreach Project employs formerly homeless persons to go out to the homeless on the streets to provide condoms and AIDS prevention education.

The Better Homes Fund was started by *Better Homes and Gardens* magazine in 1988. The fund provides assistance to homeless families to enable them to escape from homelessness. Local service providers are funded, evaluated, and provided with training materials to help homeless families attain the social services, support, and skills they need to become and remain housed.[148]

The Homeless Families Program, a national demonstration program in nine cities, co-sponsored by the Robert Wood Johnson Foundation and the U.S. Department of Housing and Urban Development, awarded its first grants in 1990. This program provides housing combined with appropriately designed health and support services for homeless families.[149]

## Homeless Health Care: Future Work

The Health Care for the Homeless Program has provided accessible, continuous, comprehensive, appropriate, and sensitive care to homeless people. However, only 157 clinics are funded by the Health Care for the Homeless Program, and these facilities provide for only 50 percent of homeless persons in their communities.[150] Currently there are 121 HCH grantees nationally.[151] Thus, one basic starting point in addressing the health care needs of homeless people is to stabilize and increase the amount and stability of funding for this excellent program.

Access to dental care is seriously needed by homeless individuals as well as other impoverished groups in our country,[152] and yet poor oral health may prevent homeless individuals from obtaining employment and escaping from the streets.

There is also a lack of vision care for homeless persons. While they can get their vision tested by their primary care providers, such providers often do not provide eyeglasses.[153] Further, great efforts must be made to address the family planning and prenatal needs of homeless women. Without attention to health care for these women, we will be creating a second generation at risk of poverty and homelessness.

In addition, mental health professionals are seriously needed in health care facilities treating homeless persons. Their training should include placement in primary care community health centers so that they can learn to work hand in hand with generalist physicians in treating the intertwined physical and mental health problems of the homeless. Research is needed on how to integrate substance abuse support groups such as Alcoholics Anonymous and other substance abuse treatment programs into primary care health centers that treat homeless patients.

Respite care is severely lacking for the homeless, even in the majority of facilities funded by the Health Care for the Homeless Program. Currently, shelters and streets are often the sites to which homeless patients are discharged;[154] these are inappropriate environments for the sick. Since shelters are, for the most part, open only at night, where do ill homeless persons go for rest, nutrition, and simple basic care? Convalescent facilities are needed so that homeless persons, after being provided medical, surgical, or obstetrical care, are not discharged from outpatient settings or hospitals to the streets when their recuperation requires running water, a bed, refrigeration of medication, or proper nutrition.[155] Respite care would ensure that homeless persons receive care that most others with homes and families receive routinely.[156] The homeless need a protected environment in shelters or Health Care for the Homeless Program facilities for respite, convalescence, and treatment. Given their high rates of excessive hospitalization, such respite care would help homeless individuals to stay out of hospitals and reduce hospital stays.

The chronically mentally and physically ill or disabled would rapidly fill up respite care facilities. Therefore, long-term public housing is needed for the chronically ill, including housing to treat homeless persons with tuberculosis, severe mental illness, and substance abuse, as well as hospice facilities for those with terminal illnesses such as AIDS. Community-based screening must be performed to ensure early identification of persons with these illnesses.[157] Burt and Cohen[158] suggest that "at the very least, the extent of serious health disabilities suggests that housing solutions must include not simply financial assistance or public housing, but also supportive services that can help the disabled deal with the life crises that can destabilize them and ultimately result in a return to the streets." Such services must be able to treat homeless persons with the dual diagnosis of substance abuse and mental illness.[159]

The reform in medical education toward a more humanistic primary care model will, it is to be hoped, have an impact on the creation of a cadre of medical providers who are trained to care for vulnerable populations such as the homeless. Fifty percent of McKinney-funded Health Care for the Homeless clinics report that they have difficulty recruiting physicians. Perhaps medical education reform in combination with health care reform will ameliorate some of the major physician recruitment barriers experienced by these clinics: poor working conditions, inadequate salaries, physician bias against working with homeless patients, and the lack of respect this work now receives from the medical profession.[160] Since most of the care provided to homeless people is provided in emergency rooms rather than in special clinics for the homeless, all medical and surgical trainees in medical school, residency, and fellowship programs must be trained to develop an appreciation for their patients' housing and poverty status. "It is thus essential that those delivering health care to homeless persons carefully consider how their usual procedures and advice will be heard and experienced by those who do not have a home."[161] Appropriate models of care must be developed, taught to clinicians, and replicated in the community.

Currently in the United States, there is much discussion and planning of health care reform proposals. Much of the debate has focused on various managed care models. Such health care reform proposals have attempted to address the health care needs of underserved populations. As noted earlier, to be effective, health services for the diverse homeless population must address their unique health and social service needs, access to medical care, and quality of care. Typical managed care models of health care delivery have resulted in barriers to care for homeless persons and created unnecessary administrative burdens for Health Care for the Homeless programs.[162] Because homeless people are often mobile, locking them into one local managed care system reduces their access to health care providers who can treat them. Co-payments would also create serious barriers to care for homeless persons.[163] Unless such managed care plans include an HCH program, homeless patients will not have access to clinicians who are sensitive to their needs. Managed care models may do nothing to increase access to care and quality of care for homeless people, unless they address the unique needs of underserved vulnerable populations.[164] The unique characteristics of individuals who are homeless demand systems of care that are tailored to meet their unique needs.[165]

Single-payer national health care delivery is the best option for homeless people and is endorsed by the National Health Care for the Homeless Council and National Coalition for the Homeless.[166] A single-payer plan allows homeless persons to have health care regardless of whether or not they are welfare recipients. Such a plan should guarantee the right to choose one's health care provider. This would allow homeless persons to obtain medical care regardless of where they move. Further, free choice provides homeless people the opportunity to select care from programs such as HCH programs with providers who have experience in managing the intertwined health and social problems of homeless persons, and allows these programs to be reimbursed for their efforts. It would make permanent the funding of such programs, which now are funded on a year-to-year basis. A single-payer plan should also be designed to augment the reimbursements to providers for services they give to homeless and other vulnerable populations to acknowledge the more intensive effort required to assess and treat such patients' complex and intertwined medical, mental health, and social problems. It is essential that this plan be universal as well as comprehensive, and cover mental health, substance abuse, dental care, vision care, medications, case management, ancillary services, and long-term care. Such a plan would offer comprehensive coverage regardless of income or employment status; no cash contributions should be required of the homeless, given their extreme impoverishment.

## Homeless Health Care: Needed Research

Jahiel[167] carefully summarizes the serious need for health services research to evaluate the health care provided to the homeless population, including the access, cost, organization, and quality (structure, process, and outcomes) of this care. There is no way of knowing how the homeless population will fit into a managed care delivery system. Evaluation of existing programs is very limited, and lacking are cost-effectiveness studies that compare different programs. Research on how to improve the physical and social environments of the homeless people is essential. Shelters are dangerous; architecture and urban planning research could resolve this problem. Streets are dangerous, too, requiring the joint efforts of social policy experts, social workers, police, and emergency medical services personnel working together to understand how to prevent crime and its attendant psychological distress.

## Conclusion

Perhaps of greatest concern is that our nation seems to have come to accept homelessness as just another negative aspect of modern life, similar in this way to violent crime. It is difficult for health policy makers to address the problems of the homeless population when public support for homeless people is weak at best. Perhaps advocates for the homeless have done a disservice by focusing on homeless persons' medical, mental health, and substance abuse problems and needs rather than on the core issues of lack of low-income housing and the breakdown of social cohesiveness and community relations in this country.

Gary Blasi suggests that

> Mass homelessness is now seen as an acceptable feature of American life. . . . Institutional forces have been aggravated by . . . conservative political forces, aimed at demonstrating either that homelessness is not much of a problem after all or that such problems as there are flow from the personal and moral failures of those who are homeless. . . . Advocates for homeless people, as some of them now recognize, bear considerable responsibility for reinforcing some distortions and introducing others. Indeed it is possible (although by no means certain) that by redefining extreme poverty in terms of homelessness, by advocating for "the homeless" rather than for the extremely poor (including those with disabilities), and by paying inadequate attention to questions of race, advocates unwittingly harmed the ultimate cause they believed they were serving: alleviating the human suffering that attends extreme deprivation.[168]

As a nation, we should not limit our treatment of homelessness to addressing only the physical health, mental health, and substance abuse problems of homeless persons. To end homelessness, we must address our nation's attitudes toward and treatment of the poor as well as its welfare and housing policies. We need to focus our attention not only on ameliorating or managing homelessness, but on an effort to end mass homelessness.

## Notes

1. M. R. Burt and B. E. Cohen, "America's Homeless: Numbers, Characteristics, and Programs that Serve Them," (Washington, D.C.: Urban Institute Report 89–3, The Urban Institute Press, 1989): 1–22.

2. M. E. Hombs and M. Snyder, *Homelessness in America: A Forced March to Nowhere* (Washington, D.C.: Community for Creative Nonviolence, 1982).

3. B. G. Link, E. Susser, A. Stueve, et al., "Lifetime and Five-Year Prevalence of Homelessness in the United States," *American Journal of Public Health* 84, 12 (1994): 1907–1912.

4. D. Roth, J. Bean, N. Lust, and T. Saveanu, *Homelessness in Ohio: A Study of People in Need* (Columbus, Ohio: Ohio Department of Mental Health, Office of Program Evaluation and Research, 1985).

5. E. Bassuk and D. Franklin, "Homelessness Past and Present: The Case of the United States, 1890–1925," *New England Journal of Public Policy* 8 (1992): 67–86.

6. G. R. Garrett, "Homelessness, Alcohol, and Other Drug Abuse: Research, Traditions, and Policy Responses" *New England Journal of Public Policy* 8 (1992): 353–370.

7. M. Leepson, "The Homeless: Growing National Problem," *Editorial Research Reports* 11 (1982): 795–812; and R. Vanderkooi, "The Main Stem: Skid Row Revisited," in *Sociological Realities II,* eds. I. L. Horowitz and C. Nanry, (New York: HarperCollins, 1971), 305–312.

8. Hombs and Snyder, *Homelessness in America;* and Leepson, "The Homeless."

9. B. A. Lee, "The Disappearance of Skid Row: Some Ecological Evidence," *Urban Affairs Quarterly* 16 (1980): 81–107; and M. Leepson, "The Homeless: Growing National Problem," *Editorial Research Reports* 11 (1982): 795–812.

10. P. Dreier and R. Appelbaum, "The Housing Crisis Enters the 1990s," *New England Journal of Public Policy* 8 (1992): 155–167; and Hombs and Snyder, *Homelessness in America.*

11. E. Baxter and K. Hopper, *Private Lives/Public Spaces: Homeless Adults on the Streets of New York City* (New York: Community Service Society, Institute for Social Welfare and Research, 1981); and K. Hopper, E. Baxter, S. Cox, and L. Klein, *One Year Later: The Homeless Poor in New York City, 1982* (New York: Community Service Society, Institute for Social Welfare Research, 1982).

12. Burt and Cohen, "America's Homeless."; and U.S. Conference of Mayors, *A Status Report on Hunger and Homelessness in America's Cities: 1992* (Washington, D.C.: U.S. Conference of Mayors, 1992).

13. Burt and Cohen, "America's Homeless."; U.S. Conference of Mayors, *A Status Report on Hunger and Homelessness;* and Institute of Medicine, Committee on Health Care for Homeless People, *Homelessness, Health, and Human Needs* (Washington, D.C.: National Academy Press, 1988).

14. E. L. Bassuk, L. Rubin, and A. S. Lauriat, "Characteristics of Sheltered Homeless Families," *AJPH* 76 (1986): 1097–1101.

15. Institute of Medicine, Committee on Health Care for Homeless People, *Homelessness, Health, and Human Needs.*

16. Burt and Cohen, "America's Homeless."

17. Institute of Medicine, Committee on Health Care for Homeless People, *Homelessness, Health, and Human Needs.*

18. Burt and Cohen, "America's Homeless."

19. L. Gelberg, L. S. Linn, and S. A. Mayer-Oakes, "Differences in Health Status Between Older and Younger Homeless Adults," *Journal of the American Geriatrics Society* 38 (1990): 1220–1229.

20. Burt and Cohen, "America's Homeless."

21. P. Koegel, "Through a Different Lens: An Anthropological Perspective on the Homeless Mentally Ill," *Culture, Medicine and Psychiatry* 16 (1992): 1–22.

22. P. W. Brickner, L. K. Scharer, B. Conanan, et al., *Health Care of Homeless People* (New York: Springer, 1985).

23. Brickner, Scharer, Conanan, et al., *Health Care of Homeless People.*

24. Brickner, Scharer, Conanan, et al., *Health Care of Homeless People.*

25. P. J. Fischer, S. Shapiro, W. R. Breakey, et al., "Mental Health and Social Characteristics of the Homeless: A Survey of Mission Users," *American Journal of Public Health* 76 (1986): 519–524.

26. Burt and Cohen, "America's Homeless": L. Gelberg and L. S. Linn, "Assessing the Physical Health of Homeless Adults," *Journal of the American Medical Association* 262 (1989): 1973–1979; D. Roth and J. Bean, "New Perspectives on Homelessness: Findings from a Statewide Epidemiological Study," *Hospital and Community Psychiatry* 37 (1986): 712–719: E. L. Bassuk and L. Rosenberg, "Why Does Family Homelessness Occur? A Case-Control Study," *AJPH* 78 (1988): 783–788; and G. Morse and R. J. Calsyn, "Mentally Disturbed Homeless People in St. Louis: Needy, Willing, but Underserved," *International Journal of Mental Health* 14 (1986): 74–94.

27. M. J. Robertson and M. R. Cousineau, "Health Status and Access to Health Services Among the Urban Homeless," *AJPH* 76 (1986): 561–563.

28. J. D. Wright and E. Weber, *Homelessness and Health* (Washington D.C.: McGraw Hill, 1987); C. H. Alstrom, R. Lindelius, and I. Salum, "Mortality Among Homeless Men," *British Journal of Addiction* 70 (1975): 245–252; J. R. Hibbs, L. Benner, L. Klugman, et al., "Mortality in a Cohort of Homeless Adults in Philadelphia," *New England Journal of Medicine* 331, 5 (1994): 304–309; Morbidity and Mortality Weekly Report, "Deaths Among Homeless Persons—San Francisco, 1985–1990," *Morbidity and Mortality Weekly Report* 40 (1991): 877–880; R. Hanzlick and R. G. Parrish, "Deaths Among the Homeless in Fulton County, GA, 1988–90," *Public Health Reports* 108 (1993): 488–491; and Morbidity and Mortality Weekly Report, "Deaths Among Homeless Persons—San Francisco," *JAMA* 267 (1992): 484–485.

29. D. L. Wood, R. B. Valdez, T. Hayashi, and A. Shen, "Health of Homeless Children and Housed, Poor Children," *Pediatrics* 86 (1990): 858–866.

30. Wright and Weber, *Homelessness and Health*.

31. Wright and Weber, *Homelessness and Health*; J. B. Reuler, M. J. Bax, and J. H. Sampson, "Physician House Call Services for Medically Needy, Inner-City Residents," *AJPH* 76 (1986): 1131–1134; D. S. Miller and E. H. Lin, "Children in Sheltered Homeless Families: Reported Health Status and Use of Health Services," *Pediatrics* 81 (1988): 668–673; and Wood, Valdez, Hayashi, and Shen, "Health of Homeless Children and Housed, Poor Children."

32. G. Alperstein, C. Rappaport, and J. M. Flanigan, "Health Problems of Homeless Children in New York City," *AJPH* 78 (1988): 1232–1233; Wood, Valdez, Hayashi, and Shen, "Health of Homeless Children and Housed, Poor Children"; and Miller and Lin, "Children in Sheltered Homeless Families."

33. Brickner, Scharer, Conanan, et al., *Health Care of Homeless People*; Wright and Weber, *Homelessness and Health*; and A. R. Zolopa, J. A. Hahn, R. Gorter, et al., "HIV and Tuberculosis Infection in San Francisco's Homeless Adults," *JAMA* 272, 6 (1994): 455–461.

34. R. A. Torres, S. Mani, J. Altholz, and P. W. Brickner, "Human Immunodeficiency Virus Infection Among Homeless Men in a New York City Shelter," *Archives of Internal Medicine* 150 (1990): 2030–2036; and Zolopa, Hahn, Gorter, et al., "HIV and Tuberculosis Infection in San Francisco's Homeless Adults."

35. Zolopa, Hahn, Gorter, et al., "HIV and Tuberculosis Infection in San Francisco's Homeless Adults."

36. J. M. McAdam, P. W. Brickner, L. L. Scharer, et al., "The Spectrum of Tuberculosis in a New York City Men's Shelter Clinic" (1982–1988)," *Chest* 97 (1990): 798–805.

37. McAdam, Brickner, Scharer, et al., "The Spectrum of Tuberculosis in a New York City Men's Shelter Clinic."

38. Zolopa, Hahn, Gorter, et al., "HIV and Tuberculosis Infection in San Francisco's Homeless Adults."

39. McAdam, Brickner, Scharer, et al., "The Spectrum of Tuberculosis in a New York City Men's Shelter Clinic"; and Zolopa, Hahn, Gorter, et al., "HIV and Tuberculosis Infection in San Francisco's Homeless Adults."

40. Zolopa, Hahn, Gorter, et al., "HIV and Tuberculosis Infection in San Francisco's Homeless Adults."

41. S. E. Kline, L. L. Hedemark, and S. F. Davis, "Outbreak of Tuberculosis Among Regular Patrons of a Neighborhood Bar," *New England Journal of Medicine* 333 (1995): 222–227.

42. J. Bernardo, "Drug-Resistant Tuberculosis Among the Homeless: Boston," *MMWR* 34 (1985): 429–431; K. Brudney and J. Dobkin, "Resurgent Tuberculosis in New York City," *American Review of Respiratory Disease* 144 (1991): 745–749.

43. Zolopa, Hahn, Gorter, et al., "HIV and Tuberculosis Infection in San Francisco's Homeless Adults."

44. A. Nyamathi, "Comparative Study of Factors Related to HIV Risk Level of Black Homeless Women," *Journal of Acquired Immune Deficiency Syndromes* 5 (1992): 222–228.

45. E. Susser, E. Valencia, and S. Conover, "Prevalence of HIV Infection Among Psychiatric Patients in a New York City Men's Shelter," *American Journal of Public Health* 83 (1993): 568–570.

46. Torres, Mani, Altholz, and Brickner, "Human Immunodeficiency Virus Infection Among Homeless Men in a New York City Shelter."

47. R. L. Stricof, J. T. Kennedy, T. C. Nattell, et al., "HIV Seroprevalence in a Facility for Runaway and Homeless Adolescents," *Am J Public Health* 81, Supplement (1991): 50–53.

48. G. A. Filice, S. J. Englender, J. A. Jacobson, et al., "Group A Meningococcal Disease in Skid Rows: Epidemiology and Implications for Control," *AJPH* 74, 3 (1984): 253–254; and G. W. Counts, D. F. Gregory, J. G. Spearman, et al., "Group A Meningococcal Disease in the U.S. Pacific Northwest: Epidemiology, Clinical Features, and Effect of a Vaccination Control Program," *Reviews of Infectious Diseases* 6, 5 (1984): 640–648.

49. A. DeMaria, K. Browne, S. Berk, et al., "An Outbreak of Type 1 Pneumococcal Pneumonia in a Men's Shelter," *JAMA* 244, 13 (1980): 1446–1449.

50. E. Nardell, B. McInnis, B. Thomas, and S. Weidhaas, "Exogenous Reinfection with Tuberculosis in a Shelter for the Homeless," *New England Journal of Medicine* 315, 25 (1986): 1570–1575; and Bernardo, "Drug-Resistant Tuberculosis Among the Homeless."

51. Morbidity and Mortality Weekly Report, "Tuberculosis Among Residents of Shelters for the Homeless—Ohio, 1990," *MMWR* 40 (1991): 869–877.

52. Morbidity and Mortality Weekly Report, "Tuberculosis Among Residents of Shelters for the Homeless—Ohio, 1990."

53. C. W. Heath and J. Zusman, "An Outbreak of Diphtheria Among Skid-Row Men," *New England Journal of Medicine* 267, 16 (1962): 809–812.

54. A.H.B. Pedersen, J. Spearman, E. Tronca, et al., "Diphtheria on Skid Road, Seattle, Wash., 1972–75," *Public Health Reports* 92, 4 (1977): 336–342.

55. Institute of Medicine, Committee on Health Care for Homeless People, *Homelessness, Health, and Human Needs.*

56. B. C. Weitzman, "Pregnancy and Childbirth: Risk Factors for Homelessness?" *Family Planning Perspectives* 21 (1989): 175–178.

57. A. M. Nyamathi, "Sense of Coherence in Minority Women at Risk for HIV Infection," *Public Health Nursing* 10, 3 (1993): 151–158.

58. Gelberg and Linn, "Health of Homeless Adults," unpublished work, 1985.

59. Gelberg and Linn, "Health of Homeless Adults"; P. Shuler, L. Gelberg, and J. E. Davis, "Characteristics Associated with Unintended Pregnancy Among Urban Homeless Women: Use of the Shuler Nurse Practitioner Practice Model in Research," *Journal of the American Academy of Nurse Practitioners* 7 (1995): 13–22; and P. Brickner, L. K. Scharer, B. A. Conanan, et al., *Under the Safety Net: The Health and Social Welfare of the Homeless in the United States* (New York: Norton, 1990).

60. Shuler, Gelberg, and Davis, "Characteristics Associated with Unintended Pregnancy Among Urban Homeless Women."

61. Gelberg and Linn, "Health of Homeless Adults."

62. R. Hayward, M. Shapiro, H. Freeman, and C. Corey, "Who Gets Screened for Cervical and Breast Cancer? Results from a New National Survey," *Archives of Internal Medicine* 148 (1988): 1177–1181.

63. P. A. Shuler, *Homeless Women's Wholistic and Family Planning Needs: An Exposition and Test of the Nurse Practitioner Model,* unpublished dissertation, University of California at Los Angeles, 1991.

64. Shuler, Gelberg, and Davis, "Characteristics Associated with Unintended Pregnancy Among Urban Homeless Women"; and A. Burnam and P. Koegel, *The Course of Homelessness Among the Seriously Mentally Ill: An NIMH Funded Proposal* (Rockville, Md.: National Institute of Mental Health, 1989).

65. W. Chavkin, A. Kristal, C. Seabron, and P. E. Guigli, "The Reproductive Experience of Women Living in Hotels for the Homeless in New York City," *New York State Journal of Medicine* 87 (1987): 10–13.

66. Chavkin, Kristal, Seabron, and Guigli, "The Reproductive Experience of Women Living in Hotels for the Homeless in New York City."

67. Wright and Weber, *Homelessness and Health*; Shuler, Gelberg, and Davis, "Characteristics Associated with Unintended Pregnancy Among Urban Homeless Women"; Weitzman, "Pregnancy and Childbirth"; and C. M. Paterson and P. Roderick, "Obstetric Outcome in Homeless Women," *British Medical Journal* 301 (1990): 263–266.

68. Chavkin, Kristal, Seabron, and Guigli, "The Reproductive Experience of Women Living in Hotels for the Homeless in New York City."

69. Chavkin, Kristal, Seabron, and Guigli, "The Reproductive Experience of Women Living in Hotels for the Homeless in New York City."

70. Paterson and Roderick, "Obstetric Outcome in Homeless Women."

71. C. T. Mowbray, V. S. Johnson, A. Solarz, and C. J. Combs, *Mental Health and Homelessness in Detroit: A Research Study* (Detroit: Michigan Department of Mental Health, 1986).

72. Wright and Weber, *Homelessness and Health.*

73. L. Gelberg, L. S. Linn, and D. J. Rosenberg, "Dental Health of Homeless Adults," *Special Care in Dentistry* 8 (1988): 167–172.

74. Institute of Medicine, Committee on Health Care for Homeless People, *Homelessness, Health, and Human Needs;* Fischer, Shapiro, Breakey, et al., "Mental Health and Social Characteristics of the Homeless"; P. Koegel, M. A. Burnam, and R. K. Farr, "The Prevalence of Specific Psychiatric Disorders Among Homeless Individuals in the Inner-City of Los Angeles," *Archives of General Psychiatry* 45 (1988): 1085–1092; E. Bassuk, L. Rubin, and A. Lauriat, "Is Homelessness a Mental Health Problem," *American Journal of Psychiatry* 141 (1984): 1546–1550; J. M. Sacks, J. Phillips, and G. Cappelletty, "Characteristics of the Homeless Mentally Disordered Population in Fresno County," *Community Mental Health Journal* 23 (1987): 114–119; A. A. Arce, M. T. Tadlock, M. J. Vergare, and S. H. Shapiro, "A Psychiatric Profile of Street People Admitted to an Emergency Shelter," *Hospital & Community Psychiatry* 34 (1983): 812–817; E. M. Smith, C. S. North, and E. L. Spitznagel, "Alcohol, Drugs, and Psychiatric Comorbidity Among Homeless Women: An Epidemiologic Study," *Journal of Clinical Psychiatry* 54, 3 (1993): 82–87; and E. Susser, S. Conover, and E. Struening, "Problems of Epidemiologic Method in Assessing the Type and Extent of Mental Illness Among Homeless Adults," *Hospital & Community Psychiatry* 40 (1989): 261–265.

75. Institute of Medicine, Committee on Health Care for Homeless People, *Homelessness, Health, and Human Needs;* Fischer, Shapiro, Breakey, et al., "Mental Health and Social Character-

istics of the Homeless"; Koegel, Burnam, and Farr, "The Prevalence of Specific Psychiatric Disorders Among Homeless Individuals in the Inner-City of Los Angeles," 1085–1092; E. Bassuk, L. Rubin, and A. Lauriat, "Is Homelessness a Mental Health Problem," *American Journal of Psychiatry* 141 (1984): 1546–1550; J. M. Sacks, J. Phillips, and G. Cappelletty, "Characteristics of the Homeless Mentally Disordered Population in Fresno County," *Community Mental Health Journal* 23 (1987): 114–119; A. A. Arce, M. T. Tadlock, M. J. Vergare, and S. H. Shapiro, "A Psychiatric Profile of Street People Admitted to an Emergency Shelter," *Hospital & Community Psychiatry* 34 (1983): 812–817; E. M. Smith, C. S. North, and E. L. Spitznagel, "Alcohol, Drugs, and Psychiatric Comorbidity Among Homeless Women: An Epidemiologic Study," *Journal of Clinical Psychiatry* 54, 3 (1993): 82–87; E. Susser, S. Conover, and E. Struening, "Problems of Epidemiologic Method in Assessing the Type and Extent of Mental Illness Among Homeless Adults," *Hospital & Community Psychiatry* 40 (1989): 261–265; P. Koegel and M. A. Burnam, "Alcoholism Among Homeless Adults in the Inner- City of Los Angeles," *Archives of General Psychiatry* 45 (1988): 1011–1018; and E. Struening, D. Padgett, J. Pittman, et al., "A Typology Based on Measures of Substance Abuse and Mental Disorder," *Journal of Addiction and Disease* 11 (1991): 99–117.

76. Wright and Weber, *Homelessness and Health*; and Koegel, Burnam, and Farr, "The Prevalence of Specific Psychiatric Disorders Among Homeless Individuals."

77. L. Chafetz and S. M. Goldfinger, "Residential Instability in a Psychiatric Emergency Setting," *Psychiatric Quarterly* 56, 1 (1984): 20–34.

78. Bassuk, Rubin, and Lauriat, "Characteristics of Sheltered Homeless Families."

79. C. I. Cohen, J. A. Tersi, and D. Holmes, "The Physical Well-Being of Old Homeless Men," *Journal of Gerontology* 43 (1988): 121–128; M. J. Robertson, R. H. Ropers, and R. Boyer, *The Homeless of Los Angeles County: An Empirical Evaluation* (Los Angeles: Basic Shelter Research Project, UCLA School of Public Health, 1985); and Fischer, Shapiro, Breakey, et al., "Mental Health and Social Characteristics of the Homeless."

80. J. V. Martell, R. S. Seitz, J. K. Harada, et al., "Hospitalization in an Urban Homeless Population: The Honolulu Urban Homeless Project," *Annals of Internal Medicine* 116 (1992): 299–303.

81. J. T. Kelly and S. M. Goldfinger, *Homeless Inpatients: Medical, Surgical, and Psychiatric Problems* (San Francisco: University of California, San Francisco, 1985).

82. Fischer, Shapiro, Breakey, et al., "Mental Health and Social Characteristics of the Homeless."

83. P. W. Brickner, D. Greenbaum, A. Kaufman, et al., "A Clinic for Male Derelicts: A Welfare Hotel Project," *Annals of Internal Medicine* 77 (1972): 565–569.

84. P. W. Brickner and A. Kaufman, "Case Finding of Heart Disease in Homeless Men," *Bulletin of the New York Academy of Medicine* 49 (1973): 475–484.

85. J. McAdam, P. W. Brickner, R. Glicksman, et al., "Tuberculosis in the SRO/Homeless Population," in *Health Care for Homeless People,* eds. P. W. Brickner, L. K. Scharer, B. Conanan, et al. (New York: Springer, 1985), pp. 155–175.

86. Bassuk, Rubin, and Lauriat, "Is Homelessness a Mental Health Problem."

87. K. Kinchen and J. D. Wright, "Hypertension Management in Health Care for the Homeless Clinics: Results from a Survey," *Am J Public Health* 81 (1991): 1163–1165.

88. Fischer, Shapiro, Breakey, et al., "Mental Health and Social Characteristics of the Homeless."

89. Robertson and Cousineau, "Health Status and Access to Health Services Among the Urban Homeless."

90. Fischer, Shapiro, Breakey, et al., "Mental Health and Social Characteristics of the Homeless"; and Robertson and Cousineau, "Health Status and Access to Health Services Among the Urban Homeless."

91. Fischer, Shapiro, Breakey, et al., "Mental Health and Social Characteristics of the Homeless"; Koegel, Burnam, and Farr, "The Prevalence of Specific Psychiatric Disorders Among Homeless Individuals"; P. H. Rossi, J. D. Wright, G. A. Fisher, and G. Willis, "The Urban Homeless: Estimating Composition and Size," *Science* 235 (1987): 1336–1341; S. P. Segal, J. Baumohl, and E. Johnson, "Falling Through the Cracks: Mental Disorder and Social Margin in a Young Vagrant Population," *Social Problems* 24 (1977): 387–401; J. Kroll, K. Carey, D. Hagedorn, et al., "A Survey of Homeless Adults in Urban Emergency Shelters," *Hospital & Community Psychiatry* 37 (1986): 283–286; and L. Gelberg, L. S. Linn, and B. D. Leake, "Mental Health, Alcohol and Drug Use, and Criminal History Among Homeless Adults," *American Journal of Psychiatry* 145 (1988): 191–196; D. Roth, G. Bean, and P. Hyde, "Homelessness and Mental Health Policy: Developing an Appropriate Role for the 1980s," Community Mental Health Journal 22 (1986): 203–214.

92. Martell, Seitz, Harada, et al., "Hospitalization in an Urban Homeless Population."

93. Fischer, Shapiro, Breakey, et al., "Mental Health and Social Characteristics of the Homeless."

94. Gelberg, Linn, and Leake, "Mental Health, Alcohol and Drug Use, and Criminal History Among Homeless Adults."

95. Robertson, Ropers, and Boyer, *The Homeless of Los Angeles County: An Empirical Evaluation.*

96. Robertson and Cousineau, "Health Status and Access to Health Services Among the Urban Homeless"; and L. Gelberg and L. S. Linn, "Social and Physical Health of Homeless Adults Previously Treated for Mental Health Problems," *Hospital & Community Psychiatry* 39 (1988): 510–516.

97. Robertson, Ropers, and Boyer, *The Homeless of Los Angeles County: An Empirical Evaluation.*

98. D. Padgett, E. L. Struening, and H. Andrews, "Factors Affecting the Use of Medical, Mental Health, Alcohol, and Drug Treatment Services by Homeless Adults," *Medical Care* 28 (1990): 805–821.

99. Cohen, Tersi, and Holmes, "The Physical Well-Being of Old Homeless Men"; and Robertson and Cousineau, "Health Status and Access to Health Services Among the Urban Homeless."

100. Robertson, Ropers, and Boyer, *The Homeless of Los Angeles County: An Empirical Evaluation;* R. K. Farr, P. Koegel, A. Burnam, *A Study of Homelessness and Mental Illness in the Skid Row Area of Los Angeles* (Los Angeles: Los Angeles County Department of Mental Health, 1986); and Bassuk, Rubin, and Lauriat, "Is Homelessness a Mental Health Problem."

101. Fischer, Shapiro, Breakey, et al., "Mental Health and Social Characteristics of the Homeless"; and Miller and Lin, "Children in Sheltered Homeless Families."

102. P. Koegel and L. Gelberg, "Patient-Oriented Approach to Providing Care to Homeless Persons," in *Delivering Health Care to Homeless Persons: The Diagnoses and Management of Medical and Mental Health Conditions,* ed. D. Wood (New York: Springer, 1992), pp. 16–29.

103. Robertson and Cousineau, "Health Status and Access to Health Services Among the Urban Homeless."

104. F. J. Ball and B. E. Havassy, "A Survey of the Problems and Needs of Homeless Consumers of Acute Psychiatric Services," *Hospital & Community Psychiatry* 35 (1984): 917–921; Sacks, Phillips, and Cappelletty, "Characteristics of the Homeless Mentally Disordered Population in Fresno County"; and Gelberg and Linn, "Social and Physical Health of Homeless Adults Previously Treated for Mental Health Problems."

105. Koegel and Gelberg, "Patient-Oriented Approach to Providing Care to Homeless Persons."

106. Miller and Lin, "Children in Sheltered Homeless Families."

107. Robertson and Cousineau, "Health Status and Access to Health Services Among the Urban Homeless."

108. Wright and Weber, *Homelessness and Health*; and S. Crystal, "Homeless Men and Homeless Women: The Gender Gap," *Urban & Social Change Review* 17 (1984): 2–6.

109. Gelberg and Linn, "Social and Physical Health of Homeless Adults Previously Treated for Mental Health Problems"; and L. Gelberg and L. S. Linn, "Psychological Distress Among Homeless Adults," *Journal of Nervous and Mental Disease* 177 (1989): 291–295.

110. L. Bachrach, "Issues in Identifying and Treating the Homeless Mentally Ill," in *Leona Bachrach Speaks: Selected Speeches and Lectures*, by L. Bachrach, *New Directions for Mental Health Services* 35 (San Francisco: Jossey-Bass, 1987), pp. 43–62.

111. Roth and Bean, "New Perspectives on Homelessness."

112. Morse and Calsyn, "Mentally Disturbed Homeless People in St. Louis"; Gelberg, Linn, and Leake, "Mental Health, Alcohol and Drug Use, and Criminal History Among Homeless Adults"; Gelberg and Linn, "Social and Physical Health of Homeless Adults Previously Treated for Mental Health Problems"; and Crystal, "Homeless Men and Homeless Women."

113. L. Bachrach, "Issues in Identifying and Treating the Homeless Mentally Ill"; and Morse and Calsyn, "Mentally Disturbed Homeless People in St. Louis."

114. Baxter and Hopper, *Private Lives / Public Spaces.*

115. Wright and Weber, *Homelessness and Health*; and P. W. Brickner, T. Filardo, M. Iseman, et al., *Medical Aspects of Homelessness* (New York: Department of Community Medicine, St. Vincent's Hospital and Medical Center of New York, 1984).

116. J. D. Wright, P. H. Rossi, J. W. Knight, et al., *Health and Homelessness in New York City: Research Report to the Robert Wood Johnson Foundation* (Amherst: University of Massachusetts, 1985); and Brickner, Filardo, Iseman, et al., *Medical Aspects of Homelessness.*

117. Koegel and Gelberg, "Patient-Oriented Approach to Providing Care to Homeless Persons."

118. Koegel and Gelberg, "Patient-Oriented Approach to Providing Care to Homeless Persons"; and Brickner, Filardo, Iseman, et al., *Medical Aspects of Homelessness.*

119. Koegel and Gelberg, "Patient-Oriented Approach to Providing Care to Homeless Persons."

120. L. R. Stark, "Barriers to Health Care for Homeless People," in *Homelessness: A Prevention Oriented Approach*, ed. R. I. Jahiel (Baltimore, Md.: Johns Hopkins University Press, 1992).

121. R. I. Jahiel (ed.), *Homelessness: A Prevention-Oriented Approach* (Baltimore, Md.: Johns Hopkins University Press, 1992).

122. Stark, "Barriers to Health Care for Homeless People,"

123. J. B. Reuler, "Health Care for the Homeless in a National Health Program," *AJPH* 79 (1989): 1033–1035.

124. Brickner, Scharer, Conanan, et al., *Health Care of Homeless People.*

125. Baxter and Hopper, *Private Lives / Public Spaces.*

126. Koegel and Gelberg, "Patient-Oriented Approach to Providing Care to Homeless Persons."

127. Koegel and Gelberg, "Patient-Oriented Approach to Providing Care to Homeless Persons."

128. Stark, "Barriers to Health Care for Homeless People."

129. U.S. Department of Housing and Urban Development, *Priority: Home! The Federal Plan to Break the Cycle of Homelessness*, HUD–1454–CPD (Washington D.C.: U.S. Department of Housing and Urban Development, 1994).

130. National Association of Community Health Centers, *Opening Doors to Benefit Programs: A Medicaid Resource Guide for Health Programs Serving the Homeless* (Washington D.C.: National Association of Community Health Centers, 1990).

131. Jahiel (ed.), *Homelessness: A Prevention-Oriented Approach;* and Brickner, Scharer, Conanan, et al., *Health Care of Homeless People.*

132. J. J. O'Connell and J. Lebow, "AIDS and the Homeless of Boston," *New England Journal of Public Policy* 8 (1992): 541–556.

133. J. D. Wright and E. Weber, *Homelessness and Health* (New York: McGraw-Hill, 1987); and I.C.F. Lewin, *Health Needs of the Homeless: A Report on Persons Served by the McKinney Act's Health Care for the Homeless Program* (Washington, D.C.: National Association of Community Health Centers, 1989).

134. D. Mauch and V. Mulkern, "The McKinney Act: New England Responses to Federal Support for State and Local Assistance to Homeless Mentally Ill," *New England Journal of Public Policy* 8 (1992): 419–430.

135. Mauch and Mulkern, "The McKinney Act."

136. National Resource Center on Homelessness and Mental Illness, *National Organizations Concerned with Mental Health, Housing, and Homelessness* (Delmar, N.Y.: National Resource Center, Policy Research Association, Inc., 1995).

137. Center for Mental Health Services, *Making a Difference—Interim Status Report of the McKinney Demonstration Program for Homeless Adults with Serious Mental Illness* (Rockville, Md.: U.S. Department of Health and Human Services, 1994).

138. National Institute on Alcohol Abuse and Alcoholism, *Homelessness, Alcohol, and Other Drugs* (Rockville, Md.: National Institute on Alcohol Abuse and Alcoholism, 1989).

139. S. Kessler, "The Needs of Hartford's Homeless Mentally Ill," *New England Journal of Public Policy* 8 (1992): 703–713.

140. Kessler, "The Needs of Hartford's Homeless Mentally Ill."

141. Kessler, "The Needs of Hartford's Homeless Mentally Ill."

142. E. Nasper, C. Melissa, and E. Omara-Otunnu, "Aggressive Outreach to Homeless Mentally Ill People," *New England Journal of Public Policy* 8 (1992): 715–727.

143. J. T. Ungerleider, T. Andrysiak, N. Siegel, et al., "Mental Health and Homelessness: The Clinician's View," in *Homelessness: A National Perspective,* eds. M. J. Robertson and M. Greenblatt (New York: Plenum Press, 1992), pp. 109–116.

144. Nasper, Melissa, and Omara-Otunnu, "Aggressive Outreach to Homeless Mentally Ill People."

145. National Resource Center on Homelessness and Mental Illness, *National Organizations Concerned with Mental Health, Housing, and Homelessness.*

146. R. Rosenheck, C. A. Leda, and P. Gallup, "Program Design and Clinical Operation of Two National VA Initiatives for Homeless Mentally Ill Veterans, *New England Journal of Public Policy* 8 (1992): 315–337.

147. National Resource Center on Homelessness and Mental Illness, *National Organizations Concerned with Mental Health, Housing, and Homelessness.*

148. National Resource Center on Homelessness and Mental Illness, *National Organizations Concerned with Mental Health, Housing, and Homelessness.*

149. Robert Wood Johnson Foundation, *The Homeless Families Program* (Princeton, N.J.: Robert Wood Johnson Foundation, 1993).

150. B. Doblin, L. Gelberg, and H. E. Freeman, "Patient Care and Professional Staffing Patterns in McKinney Act Clinics Providing Primary Care to the Homeless," *Journal of the American Medical Association* 267 (1992): 698–701.

151. U.S. General Accounting Office, *Homelessness—McKinney Act Programs and Funding Through Fiscal Year 1993,* GAO/RCED–94–107 (Washington, D.C.: U.S. General Accounting Office, 1994).

152. Gelberg, Linn, and Rosenberg, "Dental Health of Homeless Adults."

153. Gelberg, Linn, and Mayer-Oakes, "Differences in Health Status Between Older and Younger Homeless Adults."

154. Stark, "Barriers to Health Care for Homeless People"; and J. Goetcheus, M. A. Gleason, D. Sarson, T. Bennett, P. B. Wolfe, "Convalescence: For Those Without a Home: Developing Respite Services in Protected Environments," in *Under the Safety Net*, ed. P. W. Brickner (New York: Norton, 1990), pp. 169–183.

155. Stark, "Barriers to Health Care for Homeless People."

156. Goetcheus and others, "Convalescence."

157. U.S. Department of Housing and Urban Development, *Priority: Home!*

158. Burt and Cohen, "America's Homeless."

159. U.S. Department of Housing and Urban Development, *Priority: Home!*

160. Doblin, Gelberg, and Freeman, "Patient Care and Professional Staffing Patterns in McKinney Act Clinics."

161. Koegel and Gelberg, "Patient-Oriented Approach to Providing Care to Homeless Persons," p. 23.

162. National Health Care for the Homeless Council, National Coalition for the Homeless, *Tis a Gift to be Simple: Homelessness, Health Care Reform, and the Single-Payer Solution* (Nashville, Ky.: National Health Care for the Homeless Council, 1994).

163. National Coalition for the Homeless, National Health Care for the Homeless Council, *Life and Death on the Streets: Health Care Reform and Homelessness* (Washington, D.C.: National Coalition for the Homeless, 1993).

164. Reuler, "Health Care for the Homeless in a National Health Program."

165. L. A. Aday, *At Risk in America: The Health and Health Care Needs of Vulnerable Populations in the United States* (San Francisco: Jossey-Bass, 1993).

166. National Health Care for the Homeless Council, National Coalition for the Homeless, *Tis a Gift to be Simple.*

167. Jahiel (ed.), *Homelessness: A Prevention-Oriented Approach.*

168. G. Blasi, "And We Are Not Seen—Ideological and Political Barriers to Understanding Homelessness," *American Behavioral Scientist* 37, 4 (1994): 563–586, pp. 563–564.

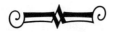

CHAPTER THIRTEEN

# HOSPITAL PRICE COMPETITION
# AND THE GROWTH OF MANAGED CARE

Glenn Melnick

Under President Clinton's plan for national health care reform, a managed competition system administered at the state level was to serve as the foundation for restructuring the nation's health care system. Through a combination of newly formed health alliances and competitive bidding by health plans, the incentives of the health care market would have been restructured to inject price competition into the health care market at both the health plan and provider levels.

With the failure to pass national health care reform legislation, the responsibility for restructuring the health care system to achieve the goals of universal coverage and cost containment falls primarily to the private sector and the states. To assist policy makers in both the public and private sector, this chapter provides a review and synthesis of the empirical literature on the effects of competition and managed care and discusses the implications of current trends, what we have learned to date, and some directions for future research.

## California: Laboratory for Evaluation of Competition and Managed Care

In June 1982, the California legislature adopted what was to become model legislation for the nation, designed to encourage price competition in the health care sector. The law explicitly permitted the formation of health plans that entered into contracts with selected or *preferred* providers. This legislation allowed the state's Medicaid program, known as MediCal, to contract with a subset of licensed hospitals to which it would channel its enrollees in return for signing participating contracts. Private insurance companies received the same privilege. The contracts often required price concessions and increased utilization review oversight aimed at controlling both price and utilization of health services. This law spawned the formation and growth of numerous preferred provider organizations (PPOs) and health maintenance organizations (HMOs), generically known as managed care plans, which offered a wide range of innovative arrangements in an attempt to identify those features that would be most attractive to consumers. In the early years following introduction of the law, the number of plans in California peaked at over one hundred. However, recent consolidation of plans has reduced the number substantially.

Enrollment in managed care plans in California grew dramatically during the 1980s. As can be seen in Figure 13.1, during the period 1980–1982 the percentage of the insured population enrolled in managed care plans was relatively sta-

## FIGURE 13.1. GROWTH OF ENROLLMENT IN MANAGED CARE PLANS, CALIFORNIA, 1980–1992.

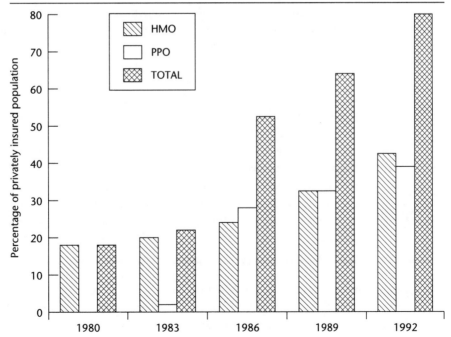

ble at slightly less than 20 percent. In fact, most of the managed care enrollment was in the Kaiser Permanente HMO. Early in 1983, immediately after the introduction of the law, enrollment in PPOs grew moderately. By the end of the period, however, PPO population experienced explosive growth. During this same period, enrollment in HMOs, particularly new HMOs competing with Kaiser, also experienced a rapid growth. By 1991, the insurance market in California had been transformed, with more than 80 percent of the insured population enrolled in PPOs and HMOs.

Because California is considered to be the most mature managed care market in the country, it can serve as a laboratory to inform policy makers on what might be expected in other parts of the country as managed care expands nationally. Such information will be useful both to state as well as national policy planners, who are in the process of designing competition-based health reform plans. For example, Florida has recently enacted health care legislation based on a competitive approach very similar to California's. In addition, other states, such as Illinois and New Jersey, are moving quickly to embrace a competitive approach to health care reform.

## Evolution and Development of Managed Care Markets

An essential element of the development of the managed care market is competition among health plans and the interaction between health plans and consumers. These interrelationships can have important implications for ongoing product innovation and the overall development of the managed care market in a state. To better understand this process, it is instructive to examine the evolution of the managed care market in California and its impact on the restructuring of California's health care system.

In the early 1980s, less than 20 percent of the insured population was enrolled in managed care plans (most of them being in the Kaiser Permanente HMO). With the passage of California's selective contracting law, health insurance plans had greater flexibility to develop alternative health insurance patterns and to test different design features to attract subscribers. This increased competition in the health insurance market led to a burst of innovation and a proliferation of choices available to consumers. For example, PPOs grew rapidly by offering a wide choice of providers in their networks. In addition, they combined this feature with lower monthly premiums (compared to prevailing standard fee-for-service indemnity plans) and financial incentives to use network providers, while still providing some financial coverage for out-of-network care. The number of people voluntarily selecting these plans and accepting some reduction in choice of provider grew dramatically. At the same time, innovations in the HMO market were being tested. The number of HMOs competing with Kaiser and with PPOs grew dramatically.

The new HMOs differed dramatically from Kaiser in ways that made them attractive to both providers and consumers. Physicians could join the HMOs either as individuals or as part of an independent practice association (IPA) or a group practice. Hospitals, likewise, could contract with the plans on a selective basis. Consumers had a wide choice of private providers in these plans and the monthly premium was generally less than conventional indemnity plans. During this same time period, employers began changing their fringe benefit contribution rates for health insurance, requiring employees to pay more from their monthly paychecks if they selected plans with higher premiums. The response of consumers to these changes has been remarkable. Voluntary enrollment in managed care plans grew so rapidly that within ten years a majority of the privately insured population had joined some type of managed care plan that offered lower monthly premiums in return for some restrictions on choice of provider. This shift from general indemnity health insurance to managed care plans requiring consumers to accept some restrictions on providers and hospitals was largely caused by market forces without the need for government action. The basis for this dramatic restructuring of the health care system is the increased role of price competition in the health care sector among providers and health insurance plans and more efficient pricing in the health insurance market.

As might be expected, the supply side of the health market has also undergone dramatic changes. As the number of people joining managed care health plans grew, health plans had to add capacity to their provider networks to handle the increased volume. Consequently, the percentage of physicians and hospitals who contract with managed care plans has increased substantially. The growth in enrollment in health plans provides the plans with greater bargaining power when negotiating with providers for participation in their networks. To counter this growing power on the part of health plans, providers have been consolidating to form their own networks. These networks allow for expanded primary care capacity within local areas as well as wider geographical coverage.

## Studies of Hospital Competition and Selective Contracting

In the traditional setting, hospitals competed on the basis of services, technology, and amenities to attract physicians and their patients.[1] Physicians' ability to deliver quality care and compete for patients depends in part on the range of services that they can provide. Hospitals partially control the range of available services by deciding what specialized equipment and staff to invest in. In negotiating with hospitals, physicians can increase their bargaining leverage by credibly threatening to shift their patients to another hospital. Hospitals, in turn, can remove admitting privileges from physicians who do not bring in many patients. Lack of admitting privileges to a highly regarded local hospital could put a physician at a competitive disadvantage.

## Nonprice Hospital Competition

The degree to which hospitals must increase the range of available services, technology, and amenities in order to attract more patients depends on the competitiveness of both the hospital and physician markets. The more competitive the hospital market, the easier it is for physicians to shift their patients to other hospitals when they become dissatisfied with a hospital. The essential insight of this amenity-based model of hospital competition is that the number of hospitals in an area serves as a good measure of the relative bargaining strength of hospitals and their medical staff. As the number of hospitals increases, hospitals must expend substantial resources competing for area physicians. A converse hypothesis would be that as physician markets become more competitive—as the number of physicians per capita increases—hospitals are not as dependent on any particular group of physicians for patients and can reduce the intensity of costly quality- or amenity-based competition.

Hospitals' desire to raise quality and offer greater amenities to attract more physicians and patients is constrained by the pressure imposed by insurers to contain costs. Under cost-based fee-for-service reimbursement, it is easy for hospitals to compete on the basis of quality, as they can recover their costs from third-party payers. However, the ability to compete on the basis of quality is restricted as insurers begin to exert their market power and limit payments through managed care techniques such as selective contracting.

## Introduction of Price Competition

The introduction of selective contracting and managed care risk contracts changes the economic incentives faced by both insurers and providers. The ability to assemble preferred provider networks endows insurers with the potential power to channel patients away from more expensive providers. Insurers, competing with one another for subscribers, have both a financial incentive and the benefit of scale economies to search the market for an optimal mix of high-quality and low-price providers. Under such conditions, insurance carriers can leverage excess capacity and competitive hospital market conditions to negotiate lower prices with health care providers. In theory, effective use of the selective contracting mechanism can generate savings for insurers, thereby leading to price advantages over other insurers. Such price advantages could be important in building or maintaining a subscriber base in competitive insurance markets. However, selective contracting plans operate under constraints that in all likelihood prevent them from selecting providers solely on the basis of price. If payers use only a price criterion in choosing providers, they may assemble too limited a network, thereby putting themselves at risk of diminishing their subscriber base because of unacceptable quality or access. Thus, payers must assess the relative attractiveness of individual hospitals to consumers before choosing which hospitals to exclude on the basis of high prices.

Providers, faced with the pressure to reduce prices or risk being locked out of an insurer's network, must also balance trade-offs in negotiating with selective contracting plans. They must assess their importance to the insurer's network, which determines the likelihood of being excluded should they refuse to grant requested price concessions. Their ability to retain patients should the contract not be offered influences their bargaining position.

## Hospital Costs and Revenues Under Price Competition

Previous research on the early effects of California's competitive approach indicates that restructuring the health care market can lead to increased price competition and lower cost growth. My colleagues and I found that increasing price sensitivity on the part of buyers has resulted in increased price competition among hospitals, leading them to offer price discounts to secure contracts with managed care plans.[2] Hospitals lowered their costs when faced with competitive pricing pressure exerted by managed care plans.[3]

Previously published studies showing that competition can lead to lower increases in hospital prices and costs have been limited in several ways. Because they were done soon after the introduction of price competition, they do not address the question of whether the cost containment effects can be sustained over a long period of time or if they are simply a one-time reduction followed by increases at previous rates.

A recently completed analysis addresses the question of whether price competition in California resulted in a long-term and sustained reduction in hospital expenditures.[4] This analysis consisted of a multivariate analysis of hospital net revenues. The data used in the multivariate analysis were drawn from three data sets created by the California Office of Statewide Health Planning and Development: a quarterly data set including total quarterly expenses, discharges, and visits for each hospital in California from the beginning of 1980 until the end of

1990; an annual disclosure data set containing detailed utilization, cost, revenue, and staffing data for each California hospital; and an annual discharge data set providing demographic and clinical information regarding each discharge from a California acute care institution that took place during the years 1983 to 1988. Census data provided demographic characteristics for each zip code area in California.

The multivariate analysis was designed to isolate and compare the effects of competition on hospital revenues prior to and following the growth of managed care plans. The dependent variable, total annual net revenue, is the total amount collected by the hospital from all sources during the year and as such represents total expenditures for hospital services.[5] It is important to note that total annual net revenue includes the revenues for providing both inpatient and outpatient services at the hospital. Thus, to the extent that hospitals have been shifting more of their activities to the outpatient side in response to competitive pressure, it is still captured in our measure of total net revenue. The measure of competition, the Hirschman-Herfindahl index (HHI), was constructed using the discharge data.[6] The multivariate regression model controlled for the other factors that might influence total annual net revenue, including output, input prices, case mix, teaching status and service breadth, demographic characteristics of the hospital's market, ownership, payer mix, financial impact of Medicare's prospective payment system (PPS) program, competitiveness of the physician market, and individual year effects.[7] The analysis included data for each acute care general hospital in California for which complete data were available for the period 1980 through 1990. A variance components model was estimated to correct for the correlation of residuals for individual hospitals.

The coefficients from the model were used to compare revenues for hospitals in highly competitive markets to those in uncompetitive markets, keeping all other factors constant. Hospitals in the most and least competitive market quartiles (as defined by quartile distribution) were identified and their net revenues were calculated for each year over the 1980–1990 period, controlling for all other factors. If competition were effective in controlling hospital expenditures, we would expect that revenues would be lower for hospitals in more competitive markets than for hospitals in less competitive markets after enactment of selective contracting legislation in 1982. The results of this simulation are presented in Figure 13.2.

As can be seen in Figure 13.2, in the period 1980–1982, before the introduction of price competition, hospital expenditures in the most competitive market quartile were 13.75 percent higher than those in the least competitive market quartile. Beginning in the years immediately following the introduction of California's procompetition law, the differences in hospital expenditures between hospitals in the highly competitive markets and least competitive markets began a

## FIGURE 13.2. EFFECT OF COMPETITION ON HOSPITAL TOTAL NET REVENUE, CALIFORNIA, 1980–1990.

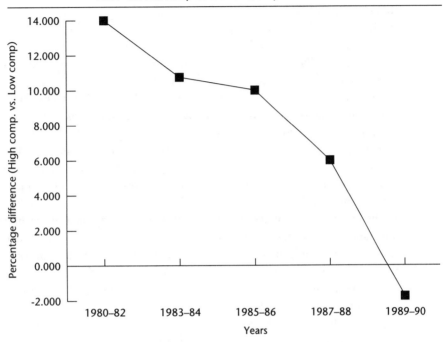

steady and sustained decline. In 1983–1984, hospitals in high-competition markets collected 11.13 percent more revenue than hospitals in the least competitive markets. The difference in net revenue between hospitals in the most competitive and least competitive markets continued to narrow in each subsequent year. Finally, by 1989–1990, the last years for which data are available, the difference in net revenues between hospitals in highly competitive compared with those in the least competitive markets had reversed its historical relationship. Hospitals in markets with the greatest competitive pressure now receive 1.62 percent less revenue per year than those facing least competitive pressure.

## Hospital Prices

Despite the rapid growth in health plans that feature selective contracting, there is very little empirical evidence in the literature concerning its effects on hospital prices. While the desired outcome is lower prices, some researchers caution that endowing insurers with substantial market power could have negative impact. For instance, Pauly suggests that in areas where an insurance carrier commands a large share of the health insurance market, it may exploit its position to gain greater discounts.[8] Hospitals in these areas may be so hampered by revenue constraints that serious reductions in quality of care could occur or financial losses could eventually threaten their viability.

Several articles in the *Journal of Health Economics* have addressed these issues both theoretically and empirically.[9] One of the best empirical tests of these issues to date was conducted by Staten, Umbeck, and Dunkelberg in a study the journal published in 1988. They evaluated the effects of hospital market structure and insurer market share on the discount rate that hospitals offered to gain acceptance into the newly formed Blue Cross of Indiana PPO. They compared historical charges with the initial proposed bid for each hospital to calculate the discount rate. These discount rates were regressed on two alternative measures of hospital market structure (sole hospital in the county or number of hospitals in the county) and two alternative measures of Blue Cross market share (Blue Cross share of the individual hospital's volume and Blue Cross share of the private market). The ratio of inpatient days per bed for a one-month period was included as a measure of capacity utilization. The study found that hospitals located in counties with more competitors offered greater discounts and that higher Blue Cross share at either the hospital or market level did not significantly lower the proposed discounts offered by hospitals.

While the paper by Staten, Umbeck, and Dunkelberg provided the first analysis of hospital prices under PPO arrangements, it has several important limitations. The dependent variable, the discount rate, was calculated using the initial bid proposed by the hospital and not the final price agreed upon between the PPO and the hospital. Our survey of hospital behavior under selective contracting in California indicates that substantial negotiation occurs between the first bid and the final agreed-upon price. The measure calculated by Staten, Umbeck, and Dunkelberg is likely to overestimate the final price agreed upon by hospitals in the PPO contract.

Staten, Umbeck, and Dunkelberg apply their analysis to a newly formed PPO. It is likely that both parties to a PPO negotiation exhibit a learning curve as they adjust their terms over time and become more astute at balancing the requisite trade-offs in an effort to improve their bargaining strength. Therefore, early experience in the life of a PPO may not reflect the long-run equilibrium.

The measure of market structure employed in the analysis may not be appropriate for all hospitals. Staten, Umbeck, and Dunkelberg define the hospital's geographical market as the county in which the hospital is located. For hospitals located in rural counties with no other hospitals, this may be a reasonable approximation (although there is probably some border crossing). For counties with more hospitals, however, the use of an arbitrary market definition, such as the county, becomes more problematic. For example, Los Angeles County contains over 120 hospitals. Our research based on actual patient flow data clearly shows that individual hospitals compete directly with only a small percentage of the total hospitals in the county.[10] In general, the use of county boundaries to delineate geographical market areas will tend to overestimate the actual degree of hospital competition.

More recently, my colleagues and I published a study of hospital prices that was designed to provide a better empirical test of these issues than has appeared in previous studies.[11] We used actual hospital price data from one of the oldest and largest PPOs in the country. The data set contained per diem prices paid by the PPO in 1987, which was nearly five years after the PPO's formation. By this time, the PPO and its hospital network had been involved in several rounds of negotiations, allowing provider membership in the PPO to solidify into a more-or-less stable network and the per diem contract prices to reflect a more stable pattern of relative price differences between facilities. In addition, our measure of hospital market structure is empirically derived from patient origin data.

Our findings indicate that prices paid to hospitals in the Blue Cross of California PPO network, after controlling for hospital product differences, are strongly influenced by the competitive structure of the hospital market.[12] Hospitals located in less competitive markets are able to secure higher prices. The estimated value of the coefficient for the HHI is 0.11 to 0.13. To illustrate the effect of the HHI on prices, consider a market where a merger leads to a reduction in the number of competitors from three to two. Assuming that the competitors have equal market shares, the HHI would change from 0.33 to 0.50, an increase of 50 percent. Such a reduction in the level of competition would lead, on average, to an estimated price increase of approximately 9 percent.

This is likely to be an underestimate of the price effects of competition. The HHI used in our analyses to measure the competitive structure of hospital markets is based on all admissions, while the dependent variable is the price paid by a single, albeit large, private insurance plan. As constructed in this study, the HHI measures the market's competitiveness with some error. It is intended to measure the presence in the market of alternative hospitals that could serve Blue Cross subscribers. For example, county-owned hospitals that primarily serve indigent patients tend to have a small Blue Cross patient base and so may not pose a competitive threat to nearby privately owned facilities. A better measure of market structure for our purpose would be to construct an HHI based on the discharges of privately insured patients. The error in the measurement of the HHI will tend to bias downward the estimated magnitude of its coefficient and the level of its significance, leading to an underestimate of the effects of competition on price.

Relative bargaining position was assessed in terms of both the importance of each hospital in the payer's network and the importance of the payer to each hospital's patient base. Hospitals that serve a larger share of the Blue Cross market in their area are in general able to negotiate higher prices—and those serving a larger share of Blue Cross patients in their market and located in less competitive markets are able to negotiate even higher prices. Our other measure captures the importance of the payer to each individual hospital and is intended to measure the monopsonistic effects of the insurer initially raised by Pauly.[13] In our data, the payer has on average only 2.6 percent of the patient days in its network hospitals, with a maximum of only 8.9 percent. Despite this low level, it appears that the payer is able to gain some price concessions from network hospitals as its importance to them increases. It is important to note that this finding is tentative because our measure is endogenous.

These two findings on the relative bargaining position of the hospital and the PPO provide some insight into payer strategies for network design and network pruning. They suggest that consolidating a payer's business in fewer hospitals produces offsetting price effects. The consolidation increases the importance of the PPO to the hospital, enabling the PPO to extract bigger price discounts. At the same time, however, the payer becomes more dependent on those hospitals and must eventually pay them higher rates.

High-occupancy hospitals in markets with little excess capacity receive much higher prices than expected. These results are particularly striking since neither hospital occupancy nor the average occupancy of the other hospitals in the market individually affects prices. Only a relatively small number of hospitals have high occupancy rates, defined as 75 percent or greater. Still, the results show how important the availability of excess capacity is to the PPO in maintaining a credible threat to move patients elsewhere. When this spare capacity becomes too small, the negotiated price paid by the PPO increases dramatically.

The findings on the percentage of a hospital's business represented by Medicare and MediCal are mixed. Only the estimated coefficient for the MediCal share of business is statistically significant and it is positive. There are two possible explanations for this result. One interpretation would be that hospitals that are already under pressure from MediCal to prune costs are unable to offer the level of discounts that other hospitals are able to offer. A positive coefficient may also represent cost shifting to more lucrative business areas.

Our final set of findings relate to the appropriate geographical area for market definition and price determination. Two approaches are compared: one based on hospital-specific markets and one based on the county as the geographical market. We calculate a measure of hospital market structure and a payer-specific measure of market share using both approaches. The estimated coefficients for the measures based on county-defined market areas are much smaller than those on the comparable measures for hospital-specific markets. Tested models, containing both sets of variables, show that it is the hospital-specific HHI that truly distinguishes competitive hospital markets.

The results show that the use of county boundaries to define hospital market areas leads to an underestimate of the price-increasing effects resulting from hospital mergers. This occurs for at least two reasons. First, the estimated coefficient on the county-based HHI is smaller, suggesting a smaller effect of market concentration on price than that obtained using empirically defined markets (there is a fivefold difference in the coefficients on the two HHI measures). Second, using the county as the basis to measure competitive structure will tend to underestimate the effects of a merger on the HHI itself. Since the county is generally larger than most empirically defined hospital markets, the increase in the HHI caused by the merger will be much lower in the county-based HHI than in the hospital-specific HHI.

The results illustrate some of the subtleties involved in developing hospital networks. In general, it pays for plans to contract with midsized hospitals where they can gain greater leverage with the same patient volume than in larger hospitals, which can absorb a greater number of Blue Cross patient days without becoming too dependent on a single payer. In addition, these findings suggest that increased consolidation among plans would lead to greater hospital cost savings since the importance of any single hospital diminishes with larger plan size. Factors other than minimum price are important for the PPO to consider in determining the configuration of its networks.

## Hospital Prices and HMOs

Kralewski and colleagues identified factors that affect the ability of HMOs to secure hospital discounts.[14] By analyzing hospital-HMO contracts, hospital operating characteristics, and market conditions, they identified that the level of risk sharing, the number of hospitals within a five-mile radius, the proportion of the population enrolled in HMOs, and the number of HMOs operating in the metropolitan statistical area were directly related to the ability of HMOs to provide discounts. Further analysis showed that higher cost sharing by enrollees, higher numbers of hospitals within a five-mile radius, and more HMOs operating within a metropolitan statistical area result in greater discounts. This suggests that competitive HMO markets do lead to price concessions for hospital services. Hospitals are using discounts as one way to attract HMO business and garner market share.

In addition, Feldman and colleagues found that hospitals in competitive health care markets have to compete with each other for managed care patients by providing discounts for inpatient services.[15] More specifically, staff and network model HMOs can extract larger discounts from hospitals compared to an IPA or a group model HMO because they usually have higher patient enrollment.

HMOs, however, do not always seek services of hospitals providing the lowest prices. Another study by Feldman and colleagues found that HMOs use different criteria in contracting with hospitals.[16] Low price is an important element, but is nonetheless only one aspect taken into consideration. Out of six HMOs reviewed in this study, four staff/network HMOs place price as the most important factor and intensely seek discounts. The two IPA-model HMOs focus more on other factors such as access and quality rather than seeking the lowest prices. As a result, their provider networks were larger and included more community hospitals.

## Conclusion

In summary, there is an emerging empirical literature providing strong evidence that competition in the hospital sector can lead to lower hospital costs and lower prices for major purchasers. Third-party plans that use selective contracting (PPOs and HMOs) can leverage competitive market conditions to negotiate lower prices with hospitals. However, the ways in which these insurance plans design and manage their hospital networks are important in determining the benefits ultimately derived by the consumers of health care services. The effectiveness of selective contracting as a cost and price control method is highly dependent on the existence of a sufficient level of competition in the market. This suggests that both third-party payers (through their contracting activities) and government agencies (through regulatory oversight) must ensure that market conditions remain competitive.

Given the rapid growth of managed care throughout the country, it is necessary that there be additional research into the various effects of the significant structural changes brought about by managed care. In addition to more analysis on costs, prices, and expenditures, it is necessary to conduct research into the quality and access implications of a competitive system. There has been almost no research on how managed care plans are able to achieve their cost savings and whether the savings come from increased efficiency or reduced quality. Further, recent findings from California indicate that increased price competition leads to a reduction in access to the uninsured population.[17] These findings underscore the importance of reforming the health insurance system to include everyone.

# Notes

1. J. P. Newhouse, "Toward a Theory of Non-Profit Institutions: An Economic Model of a Hospital," *American Economic Review* 60, 1 (1970): 64–74; M. V. Pauly and M. Redisch, "The Not-for-Profit Hospital as a Physicians' Cooperative," *American Economic Review* 63, 1 (1973): 87–99; J. Harris, "The Internal Organization of Hospitals: Some Economic Implications," *Bell Journal of Economics and Management Science* 8, 2 (1977): 467–482; and R. P. Ellis and T. G. McGuire, "Provider Behavior Under Prospective Reimbursement: Cost Sharing and Supply," *Journal of Health Economics* 5 (1986): 129–151.

2. Glenn Alan Melnick, Jack Zwanziger, Anil Bamezai, and R. Pattison, "The Effects of Market Structure and Hospital Bargaining Position on Hospital Prices," *Journal of Health Economics* 11 (1992): 217–233.

3. J. C. Robinson, "HMO Market Penetration and Hospital Cost Inflation in California," *Journal of the American Medical Association* 266 (1991): 2719–2723; and Glenn Alan Melnick and Jack Zwanziger, "Hospital Behavior Under Competition and Cost Containment Policies: The California Experience," *JAMA* 260 (1988): 2669–2675.

4. Jack Zwanziger, Glenn Alan Melnick, and Anil Bamezai, "Cost and Price Competition in California Hospitals, 1980–1990," *Health Affairs* 13 (1994): 118–126.

5. Total net revenue is equal to total gross charges less any contractual adjustments, such as the difference between charges and payments under the Medicare PPS program, and also less deductions for charity care and uncollectible accounts.

6. Construction of the HHI is described in detail in Melnick and Zwanziger, "Hospital Behavior Under Competition and Cost Containment Policies: The California Experience."

7. The structure of the model is essentially identical to that used in Melnick and Zwanziger, "Hospital Behavior Under Competition and Cost Containment Policies," but additional data were included to extend the analysis through the end of 1990.

8. M. V. Pauly, "Monopsony Power in Health Insurance: Thinking Straight While Standing on Your Head," *Journal of Health Economics* 6 (1987): 7–81.

9. Pauly, "Monopsony Power in Health Insurance"; M. V. Pauly, "Reply: A Response to Market Share/Market Power Revisited," *Journal of Health Economics* 7 (1988): 85–87; M. V. Pauly, "Market Power, Monopsony, and Health Insurance Markets, *Journal of Health Economics* 7 (1988): 111–128; M. W. Staten, W. Dunkelberg, and J. Umbeck, "Market Share and the Illusion of Power: Can Blue-Cross Force Hospitals to Discount?" *Journal of Health Economics* 6 (1987): 43–58; and M. J. Staten, J. Umbeck, and W. Dunkelberg, "Market Share/Market Power Revisited: A New Test for an Old Theory," *Journal of Health Economics* 7 (1988): 73–83.

10. Jack Zwanziger, Glenn Alan Melnick, and Joyce M. Mann, "Measures of Hospital Market Structure: A Review of the Alternatives and a Proposed Approach," *Socio-Economic Planning Sciences* 24, 2 (1990): 81–95.

11. Melnick, Zwanziger, Bamezai, and Pattison, "The Effects of Market Structure and Hospital Bargaining Position on Hospital Prices."

12. Melnick, Zwanziger, Bamezai, and Pattison, "The Effects of Market Structure and Hospital Bargaining Position on Hospital Prices."

13. Pauly, "Reply: A Response to Market Share/Market Power Revisited."

14. J. E. Kralewski, T. D. Wingert, R. Feldman, G. J. Rahn, and T. H. Klassen, "Factors Related to the Provision of Hospital Discounts for HMO Inpatients," *Health Services Research* 27 (1992): 133–153.

15. R. Feldman, H. C. Chan, J. Kralewski, B. Dowd, and J. Shapiro, "Effects of HMOs on the Creation of Competitive Markets for Hospital Services," *Journal of Health Economics* 9 (1990): 207–222.

16. R. Feldman, J. Kralewski, J. Shapiro, and H. C. Chan, "Contracts Between Hospitals and Health Maintenance Organizations," *Health Care Management Review* 15 (1990): 47–60.

17. Joyce M. Mann and Glenn Alan Melnick, "Uncompensated Care: Hospital Responses to Increased Price Competition and Medicare/Medicaid Payment Reform," *Health Affairs* 14, 1 (1995): 263–270.

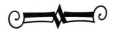

CHAPTER FOURTEEN

# REGULATORY APPROACHES

Gerald F. Kominski

Proposals for comprehensive health care reform at both the state and national level generally focus on two fundamental issues, namely, how society can increase access for those who are uninsured while improving the ability of the health care system to control the growth of health care expenditures. Although some analysts dispute the assumption that health care costs are rising too rapidly,[1] most proposals for reform attempt to address the issues of cost control and universal access either through explicit regulatory efforts or through market-based approaches, or some combination.[2] A great deal of research has been conducted during the past decade assessing the consequences of various regulatory efforts.[3] Nevertheless, policy makers and analysts still do not agree on the best mechanisms for controlling costs and expanding access, or on whether regulatory controls will be more effective than market-based approaches in achieving these goals in the future.

This chapter begins with a discussion of the research and policy issues related to two major regulatory approaches: price controls and global budgets. It presents a review of the important research findings of the past ten to fifteen years concerning these cost containment efforts, including the experience of four states with all-payer rate-setting systems and the Medicare program's efforts to regulate hospital and physician payments. These findings have often been overlooked or even misrepresented in the rhetoric surrounding alternative proposals for reform.

The major conclusion is that all-payer rate-setting programs have been successful in the United States in controlling costs while maintaining or improving access. Also, Medicare price controls have been successful in substantially slowing the growth in Medicare expenditures for hospital inpatient and physician services. Despite the success of these regulatory approaches, however, they are based on fee-for-service payment methods that are increasingly viewed as outdated because the market for private insurance is moving rapidly away from fee-for-service arrangements and toward managed care.[4] Therefore, future regulatory approaches are more likely to be directed toward addressing inequities in the market and achieving cost containment and universal access within a market-based, managed care environment.

After the defeat of national health care reform in 1994, any government effort in the near future to achieve universal access and cost containment, even through market-based reforms, is likely to face stiff political and ideological opposition—political opposition because the American public seems increasingly distrustful of government's effectiveness and unwilling to support government entitlement programs; ideological opposition because of the belief that private markets require minimal government intervention. The role of regulatory approaches in the future, therefore, may depend both on addressing these political and ideological concerns as well as on further research. The chapter concludes with a proposed research agenda for addressing some of the most salient policy and research issues related to future regulatory approaches, including their distributional consequences on households, employers, providers, and private and public insurers. It is to be hoped that this research agenda will be useful in shaping future proposals for health care reform and in overcoming some of the political and ideological opposition to government's role in the market for health care services.

# Policy and Research Issues

Regulatory efforts have generally been targeted to the supply side of the market for health care services.[5] Although a variety of efforts have been implemented over the years, price controls and global budgets are the two regulatory approaches that continue to receive serious attention as components of health care reform. The primary arguments in favor of price controls and global budgets are that they would be more effective than the current market in:

- Controlling the rate of growth in health expenditures
- Improving equity by reducing or eliminating financial barriers to care

- Eliminating cost shifting
- Expanding access for the uninsured

A number of analysts have proposed health care reform based on an expansion to all insurers of hospital and physician price controls developed during the past decade under the Medicare program, and have argued that such an expansion would achieve the listed goals.[6] Furthermore, the consequences and implementation issues related to an expansion of Medicare payment policies to private insurers has been rather extensively analyzed by relevant federal agencies.[7]

Even if one accepts these assumptions concerning the advantages of regulation, price controls and global budgets continue to face one significant limitation; namely, they are difficult to justify on theoretical grounds when compared to pure market competition. In fact, most analysts would agree that perfect competition could achieve the advantages identified above (with the possible important exception of expanded access) if health care markets in general and the market for health insurance in particular functioned under perfectly competitive conditions.[8]

Two major questions facing policy makers, providers, and researchers, therefore, are: Can the market for health care services be restructured to be truly competitive? and, if not, Are regulatory approaches merely a short-term, pragmatic solution to rising costs and inequitable access, or should they be viewed as a necessary, permanent intervention to address inherent structural problems in the market? Empirical evidence can be used to determine whether regulatory approaches are effective; the next section summarizes this evidence. Nevertheless, despite extensive experience with price controls and global budgets in other countries and the U.S. experience at the state and national level with price controls, regulatory approaches continue to be opposed primarily on theoretical or ideological grounds. Regulatory controls can be justified by examining some of the structural problems in the current market, however.

Price controls have been employed in health care markets because the classical conditions for competition, which lead to economic efficiency in the production of goods and services, are often not met in health care markets. Price competition is still rare in the market for health care insurance despite the growth of managed care plans and their potential for competing on the basis of price.[9] Price discrimination (that is, charging different prices for the same service to patients based on ability to pay or insurance status) is common and leads to cost shifting, with private insurers paying higher prices than public insurers for the same services. Uncertainty about the quality and in some cases the effectiveness of specific health services produces large variations in utilization rates. Although some analysts argue that these variations reflect patient preferences or that individuals may use ineffective services for other reasons,[10] the full costs of such preferences are not borne by the individuals using those services because of extensive insurance in the health care marketplace.

# Impact of Regulatory Efforts

Price controls have been used at the state level to set hospital payment rates for all insurers as part of all-payer rate-setting programs. At the federal level, price controls have been used under the Medicare program since 1983 for hospital payment and since 1992 for physician payment. Global budgets have not been used widely in the United States, with the exception of the Department of Veterans Affairs, but have been used in other industrial nations, most notably Canada and Germany. The remainder of this section reviews the research findings and experiences with these regulatory approaches.

## State All-Payer Programs for Hospital Care

During the 1980s, four states had all-payer programs for hospital care: Maryland, New Jersey, New York, and Massachusetts. These all-payer programs required all public and private insurers to use payment rates for hospital care established by a state rate-setting authority. In most cases, these programs established uniform payment rates so that public and private insurers paid the same price for the same unit of care (such as day or admission). To include Medicare in their all-payer systems, these states had to apply to the Health Care Financing Administration (HCFA) for waivers exempting them from Medicare's national payment rules. In granting these waivers, HCFA specified limits on the rate of growth in total Medicare inpatient payments, or in Medicare inpatient payments per case, under the all-payer programs.[11] Thus, when Medicare's prospective payment system (PPS) was implemented starting in October 1983, these states were originally exempted from PPS payment rules because of the waivers obtained for their all-payer systems.

As discussed below, the empirical evidence suggests that the all-payer systems in these states were successful in controlling hospital inpatient costs relative to other states. However, since 1985, these states, with the exception of Maryland, have either lost their waivers because expenditures increased more rapidly than specified in the waiver application, or did not reapply for new waivers. The reasons these states lost or abandoned their waivers reflect a complex interaction of political and fiscal concerns specific to those states, often involving conflict between state departments of health and state hospital associations. Ironically, one factor contributing to the financial pressure for these states to abandon their waivers was the implementation of PPS. Because payment rates during the first three years of PPS were a blend of hospital-specific and national payment amounts, these states experienced pressure from their hospital associations to abandon their waivers because hospitals could increase their Medicare revenue by joining PPS. For example, projections showed that New York hospitals could increase their Medicare revenue by as much as $500 million in the first year after joining PPS. New York allowed its waiver to expire on January 1, 1986. Similar analyses in Massachusetts showed that hospitals in that state could also increase their revenue by joining PPS. In Massachusetts, the waiver expired in October 1985.

New Jersey's Medicare waiver expired on January 1, 1989, although it continued to operate its diagnosis-related group (DRG)–based payment system for other insurers until January 1, 1993. In contrast to New York and Massachusetts, New Jersey's Medicare revenue declined after it joined PPS. Furthermore, because Medicare was no longer part of the payment system, it was no longer contributing its share to New Jersey's uncompensated care pool. This created substantial financial pressure on other insurers—who were paying a 19 percent surtax for uncompensated care—and contributed to the collapse of New Jersey's DRG-based payment system.

The design features of these state programs differed considerably. A brief description of each state's program follows, along with a summary of the effectiveness of each program in controlling hospital costs. In general, the rate of increase in hospital costs during the early 1980s, when these programs were in effect, was lower in these four states than in others without all-payer systems.[12]

*Maryland.* Maryland was the first state to adopt a per-case (that is, per-admission) system of hospital payment.[13] It began its all-payer system in 1974 using per-service payment rates. Beginning in 1976, hospitals could choose between per-service or per-case payment rates, and all hospitals have operated under a Medicare waiver since 1977. Per-case payment rates are adjusted for case mix, using patient service categories, broad diagnostic categories, or DRGs.[14] Maryland's system is more accurately defined as a provider-specific all-payer system. Each hospital has its own set of all-payer rates based on an initial detailed analysis of its budget and service volume compared to other hospitals in its peer group, conducted by the state's Health Services Cost Review Commission. This initial budget is then trended forward to determine future payment rates, adjusting for changes in input prices, projected volume, and projected payer mix. Budget shortfalls lead to higher payments in the next year to reflect unrecovered fixed costs, but hospitals are at risk for the shortfall in revenue related to variable costs. Payments in excess of the budget are discounted to reflect only the marginal cost of services. The hospital's entire budget, including outpatient and capital expenses, is factored into its payment rates.

Maryland hospital expenses have grown more slowly than the national average since its budget review–based all-payer system was implemented in 1974. Maryland's cost per admission declined steadily from 125 percent of the national average in 1976 to 92 percent in 1990, and per-capita expenditures remained below the national average as well.[15] Its rate of increase in cost per admission between 1982 and 1986 was well below the national average.[16] Hospital expenditures per capita also grew more slowly between 1979 and 1989 compared to the national average.[17] Maryland's program was the second most successful of the four waiver states in controlling hospital expenditures during the period from 1982 to 1986 when all were in operation.[18] This success appears to be due, at least in part, to the stringency of payment rates and the cost constraints associated with budget review of individual hospitals.[19]

***New Jersey.*** New Jersey was the first state to adopt an all-payer system that paid hospitals using per-case rates based on DRGs. Perhaps the most important feature of this system is that it was designed to use a single set of DRG payment rates for all insurers, with one exception. This feature was based on an analysis of resource use within DRGs that showed no significant difference between Medicare patients and patients from other insurers.[20] Blue Cross was the one major insurer successful in restoring a discounted price for its patients, but the size of the discount was considerably smaller than before the implementation of DRGs.[21]

New Jersey's program served as model for the Medicare PPS because of its use of DRGs as the basis for payment, but it differed from the PPS in many fundamental aspects.[22] Outpatient hospital services were included in New Jersey's system. Inpatients with unusually long or short lengths of stay (that is, outlier cases) were defined using extremely lenient criteria, allowing a substantial number of cases to fall outside the DRG payment rate.[23] While DRG payments were based on direct patient-care costs, additional indirect costs were added to the payments that had previously not been recognized as reimbursable, such as uncompensated care, capital facility and working capital allowances, and working cash infusions. These payment adjustments provided a redistribution of revenue to financially troubled hospitals.[24] Finally, payments were calculated using a blend of hospital-specific and statewide peer group costs that varied by DRG. The hospital-specific portion increased as the amount of cost variation within a DRG increased. This feature was designed to protect hospitals from the financial risks of heterogeneous DRGs.

New Jersey's program was effective in controlling increases in cost per admission and hospital expenditures per capita during the early 1980s, compared to national averages. These advantages seemed to have disappeared by the late 1980s, however. New Jersey was the least successful of the waiver states in controlling expenditures during the 1982–1986 period.[25] Furthermore, the savings from lower costs per admission were largely offset by increased admission rates.[26] Payment for bad debt and charity care appears to have helped financially distressed hospitals and to have improved access for the uninsured.[27]

***New York and Massachusetts.*** These states began their all-payer systems later than other states, and abandoned their Medicare waivers earlier. Both states employed a per diem rather than a per-case approach to rate setting.

Beginning in 1983, New York implemented a prospective payment system for three major payers: Medicare, Medicaid, and Blue Cross.[28] This system paid all hospitals in the state a fixed per diem rate, with the exception of hospitals in the Rochester area that were part of a separate rate-setting demonstration. Each hospital's per diem included components for operating costs and capital costs, as well as allowances for bad debt and charity care, financial distress, and discretionary expenses. Operating costs per day were adjusted for case mix using DRGs. Payment differentials between Blue Cross and other payers were permitted but were regulated.[29] Massachusetts began operation of its all-payer program in 1982. This program substantially reduced payment differentials among payers and provided for uncompensated care.

While each waiver state was successful during the period from 1982 to 1986 in controlling total hospital expenditures, Massachusetts experienced the greatest savings.[30] Evidence also suggests that payments for uncompensated care in New York were successful in increasing access to care for uninsured patients.[31] Thus, both New York and New Jersey were able to achieve what are often viewed as competing goals—namely, improving access while controlling costs.

## Hospital Payment: DRGs and the Medicare Prospective Payment System

Medicare has used a system of price controls for payment of hospital inpatient services since October 1983. Despite this extensive experience at the national level with price controls, proposals for comprehensive national health care reform have often ignored Medicare's experience or have recommended cuts in Medicare payment rates as a method of financing subsidies for the uninsured. When price controls were discussed as part of the national debate on health care reform during 1993 and 1994, most of the evidence focused on the negative consequences of price controls during the Economic Stabilization program of the Nixon era rather than the extensive recent experience under the Medicare PPS, which has had a considerable impact on the key participants in the health care system, including hospitals, other providers of health care services such as postacute care facilities and physicians, other payers for hospital services, Medicare beneficiaries, and the Medicare program. The major effects of PPS during the past decade are summarized below.

***Reduced Length of Stay.***  Average length of stay (ALOS) for Medicare patients declined sharply during the first two years of PPS, by a total of 9.2 percent.[32] This decline appears to have leveled off between 1986 and 1989, although recent research suggests that this was due to offsetting trends. The continuing decline in ALOS for most conditions was offset by a shift in hospital admissions toward more long-stay diagnoses.[33] The decline in Medicare length of stay was matched during the first two years of PPS by sizable declines in the ALOS of non-Medicare adult patients.[34] This suggests that PPS had a spillover effect on the treatment of all hospital patients, regardless of their insurance status.

***Site-of-Care Substitution.***  Hospital admissions also declined by a total of 8.8 percent during the first three years of PPS.[35] This decline in inpatient care was at least partly responsible for a substantial increase in outpatient care. Outpatient revenue, as a percentage of total hospital revenue, increased from 13.4 percent in 1983 to 25.4 percent in 1992.[36]

***Case-Mix Index Change.***  The Medicare case-mix index is a measure of the relative costliness of a hospital's mix of Medicare patients. Case-mix index change has continued to grow by about 3 percent annually since 1984.[37] This is a potential concern because hospitals can increase their payments under PPS by coding patients into higher-weighted DRGs. To date, however, studies of this increase suggest that it is mostly related to improvements in coding practice rather than true changes in the types of patients admitted to the hospital.[38] Between 1984 and 1993, payments per case increased by 28.4 percent due to changes in PPS payment rules, including updates to the payment rates, and by 28 percent due to case-mix index change.[39] This suggests that Medicare admissions continue to increase in average complexity.

This conclusion is supported by recent research indicating that about 36 percent of the increase in real cost per Medicare admission between 1984 and 1987 was attributable to the increased use of high-cost technologies within DRGs and the increased volume of high-cost DRGs related to new technologies.[40]

***Operating Margins.***  PPS operating margins (that is, PPS payments minus operating cost, divided by PPS payments) have declined considerably since 1984; average PPS operating margins have been negative since 1990.[41] Hospital total margins peaked in 1985, the second year of PPS, declined for several years, and have been increasing again since 1988.[42] This suggests that hospitals are subsidizing their operating losses under PPS with profits from other payers. In fact, the Prospective Payment Assessment Commission estimates that private insurance payments were equal to 131 percent of costs in 1992.[43] Furthermore, since 1986, the last year of large profits under PPS, cost shifting onto private insurers has almost doubled.[44]

***Impact on Other Providers.*** The impact on physicians has been difficult to measure because their fees are exempt from PPS. Nevertheless, the decline in average length of stay during the first two years of PPS did have an impact on the patterns of follow-up care provided to patients receiving surgery.[45] After PPS, surgical patients were more likely to receive follow-up visits from physicians other than their primary surgeon and to receive more visits after discharge from the hospital. This increase in outpatient follow-up care was offset by a substantial decline in visits billed while the patient was still hospitalized. Thus, PPS appeared to produce a savings in Medicare expenditures for physician services.

***Beneficiary Impact.*** Quality of care was a major concern during the implementation of PPS. To date, no study has found declines in quality of care under PPS. The RAND Quality of Care study[46] indicated that for five high-volume conditions, Medicare patients in the post-PPS period were more severely ill at admission, had better quality of care during the inpatient stay, were less stable at discharge, and had no significant change in outcomes. This study focused on the first two years of PPS, however, when hospital profits were at their highest. Concerns have been raised about the impact of PPS on quality in recent years as hospitals have experienced continued losses under PPS.

***Impact on Other Payers.*** Other payers clearly benefited from reduced lengths of stay for non-Medicare patients and may have experienced windfall profits because of lower expenses for hospital inpatient care during the early years of PPS. However, one continuing concern of other insurers is that declining Medicare operating margins may force hospitals to shift some of the costs of treating Medicare patients onto other payers. As discussed above, cost shifting has increased dramatically since 1986, with private insurers paying substantially more than their share of costs. A number of state Medicaid programs have adopted payment systems based on DRGs. Commercial insurers, however, have not followed.[47]

***Impact on Medicare Expenditures.*** According to the estimates of Russell and Manning,[48] PPS produced an estimated real savings of about 20 percent in Medicare hospital expenditures between 1983 and 1990. More importantly, they found that these savings were not offset by the increased outpatient expenditures that have occurred under PPS. Furthermore, since 1986, Medicare expenditures for hospital care have grown more slowly than expenditures by other payers. Therefore, PPS seems to have achieved one of its primary goals—to control expenditures under the Medicare program for hospital inpatient care.

## Physician Payment: RBRVS and the Medicare Fee Schedule

Medicare also implemented price controls and global expenditure targets for payment of physician services beginning in 1992. The Medicare Fee Schedule (MFS), based on the Resource-Based Relative Value Scale (RBRVS) developed at Harvard University, establishes limits on both Medicare payments and the amount of additional payment above the Medicare-allowed payment (that is, balance billing) physicians may seek from Medicare beneficiaries. The MFS will not be fully implemented until 1996, and only a few studies have been completed related to its initial impact. Nevertheless, simulations of its impact prior to implementation suggest that the MFS will have as substantial an effect on physicians as PPS has had on hospitals.

*Redistribution of Payments.* An explicit goal of the MFS is to redistribute payments from surgical to primary care services. As a consequence, the MFS will redistribute Medicare revenue from physicians in surgical specialties to those in primary care specialties. In addition, because of geographical adjustment factors applied to physician payments based on the relative practice expenses in different areas of the country (including malpractice), Medicare revenue will be redistributed from physicians in urban areas to those practicing in rural areas. In fact, two-thirds of the total redistribution in payments is expected to result from the use of the geographical adjustment factors rather than from the new physician work values developed as part of the RBRVS.[49]

*Volume Increases.* Because the MFS controls only unit prices, Medicare also adopted a form of expenditure targets (as opposed to global budgets) to control possible increases in Medicare expenditures related to volume responses on the part of physicians.[50] These targets, known as volume performance standards, take into account changes in population growth and technology and represent an allowed rate of growth in total expenditures. If actual growth exceeds the targets, the difference is subtracted from future updates to MFS payments. Separate standards apply to surgical procedures and nonsurgical services. Preliminary evidence from 1992, the first year of the MFS, indicates that the standards were effective in controlling expenditures, particularly for surgical services, which experienced a decline of 0.6 percent.[51]

***Beneficiary Access.*** A major concern is that the substantial payment reductions for many surgical services under the MFS will reduce access to those services for Medicare beneficiaries. A comprehensive theoretical model of physician response to changes in payment rates has been developed by McGuire and Pauly.[52] Preliminary evidence indicates that beneficiary access has not been compromised.[53] However, further reductions in payment rates may affect access in the future.

***Out-of-Pocket Expenses of Beneficiaries.*** By establishing explicit limits on balance billing, the MFS is expected to have a substantial impact in reducing out-of-pocket expenditures by beneficiaries, particularly those who have high utilization and no or minimal supplemental coverage. Early results indicate a 34 percent reduction in the total amount of balance billing.[54]

***Impact on Other Payers.*** Private insurers and state Medicaid programs have been quick to adopt RBRVS-based fee schedules. Private insurers are particularly concerned about avoiding the kind of cost shifting that has occurred under PPS.[55] At least one early study of Medicare payment reductions implemented just prior to the MFS indicates that physicians have increased their volume and prices for non-Medicare patients in response to Medicare fee reductions.[56]

## Global Budgets

Many analysts have proposed global budgets as an effective mechanism for controlling total health care expenditures.[57] The United Sates has no direct experience with global budgets except in the Veterans Affairs health system. Thus, most of the evidence concerning the effectiveness of global budgets and expenditure caps comes from other nations, such as Germany and Canada. The literature generally supports the conclusion that global budgets have been effective in these countries at the aggregate level.[58] One reason for the effectiveness of global budgets is reduced access to advanced (that is, high-cost) technologies due to strict controls on the diffusion of such services.[59] The distributional consequences of global budgets and technology controls on patients by age, clinical condition, and other relevant characteristics, as well as on providers and on payers, have not been well documented, however.[60]

Several states have considered health care reform initiatives in recent years based on expenditure targets or global budgets, but most of these efforts have been abandoned or repealed since the defeat of comprehensive national reform in 1994. Expenditure targets, based on volume performance standards, have been used since 1990 as part of physician payment under Medicare. Early experience indicates that Medicare expenditures for physicians' services have grown at a substantially lower rate since the adoption of volume performance standards.[61]

A number of significant policy and data collection issues need to be addressed before implementing global budgets at the state or federal level.[62] A fundamental policy issue is whether budgets should be based on historical per capita expenditure patterns, which differ substantially across geographical areas, or on risk-adjusted projected per capita expenditures. Another is how to handle the considerable fluctuations in annual expenditures at the state level. For example, Medicare expenditures for physician services vary substantially from year to year for individual states.[63] Finally, the absence of uniform patient-level encounter data is a major obstacle to implementing global budgets. Despite the growth of management information systems in health care organizations, the uniform data needed for developing and monitoring global budgets do not currently exist for most health care services. A substantial effort would thus be required to develop a national system of uniform encounter data. Although health services researchers clearly understand the value and significance of such a national database (independent of its use in establishing global budgets), there is little reason to believe that health plans or health care providers will voluntarily establish such a uniform database without government mandate.

## Policy Options and Future Research

As discussed previously, any proposal for comprehensive national health care reform, whether it is a regulatory, market-based, or combined approach, should be evaluated according to how well it controls the rate of growth in health expenditures, improves equity by reducing or eliminating financial barriers to care, eliminates cost shifting, and expands access for the uninsured.

Previous research on hospital price controls in all-payer rate-setting states suggests that these goals were achieved. Evidence regarding Medicare price controls indicates that expenditures can be brought under control without diminishing access, although cost shifting may increase. Because cost shifting offsets public savings with increased expenditures by private insurers, it represents a type of implicit taxation on private insurers that must be addressed in the future. Otherwise, access under the Medicare program may diminish as private insurers face more competitive pressures, thus reducing the opportunity for providers to subsidize losses under Medicare by charging higher prices to privately insured patients. These adverse consequences of Medicare price controls suggest that cost containment cannot be pursued effectively unless all payers and providers are included. They are also a primary reason why global budgets have been proposed as a mechanism for reducing or eliminating cost shifting across providers and across payers.

In addition to price controls, other regulatory approaches based on various types of mandates have been proposed in recent years at the state and federal levels. These mandates are usually combined with market-based reforms and are intended to address potential problems and inequities that are likely to arise in unregulated markets. They include mandates requiring employers to pay some portion of health insurance premiums, mandatory health care purchasing alliances, mandatory community rating, and caps on insurance premiums. Some of these approaches are being implemented at the state level. Evaluations of these state programs should provide valuable data in future debates over the direction of national health care reform, despite the limitation that state programs are often viewed as not generalizable.

Does the defeat of comprehensive national health care reform in the 103rd Congress mean that the goals of universal access and cost control are not viable? Perhaps for the immediate future, but the high proportion of uninsured citizens and continuing cost increases in both the public and private sectors are structural problems that still have not been adequately addressed. And although some analysts interpret the defeat of comprehensive reform as proof of underlying satisfaction with the status quo or at least majority support for a more incremental approach to reform,[64] other evidence suggests that health security, involving universal access at a reasonable cost, continues to have a powerful appeal for a majority in the United States.[65]

Assuming that managed care continues its rapid proliferation in both private and public markets, policy analysts and health services researchers might find it useful to have answers to the following questions before the next round of debate over comprehensive health care reform reemerges at the national level:

- What are the ongoing effects of the high rate of uninsurance?
- What are the aggregate and distributional consequences of current patterns of cost shifting, and what are the most effective ways of reducing or eliminating cost shifting?
- What are the effects of managed care on costs, quality, access, and outcomes, particularly for populations that traditionally have not been well served by private insurers?
- What are the expected effects of various types of mandates?
- What types of nationally representative databases are needed to evaluate costs, quality, access, and outcomes, particularly in an environment dominated by managed care plans?

These research questions assume that regulatory approaches to health care reform, at least for the immediate future, will only be feasible if proposed in combination with market-based approaches, that is, reforms based on a managed care model. Under this assumption, future research and policy analysis should focus on the distributional consequences of these issues on each major stakeholder in the health care system. Support for comprehensive reform depends in part on continuing to investigate how well the health care system is performing not just for most citizens but for all.

The remainder of this section discusses how future research can contribute to our understanding of the expected effects of regulatory approaches to health care reform, including those used in combination with market-based reforms, on the following major stakeholders in the American health care system: households, employers, providers, private insurers, and public insurers (that is, governments).

## Households

For households, a major consequence of any regulatory approach is the likely effect on expenditures for insurance premiums, cost sharing for covered services, and out-of-pocket expenses for services not covered by insurance. Another issue affecting families is the potential disemployment effect of employer mandates.

*Premiums.* One method of implementing global budgets is to regulate insurance premiums directly. Regulation of health insurance premiums would certainly change current patterns of cross-subsidization. Mandatory community rating without risk adjustment, for example, would most likely increase premiums paid by or on behalf of younger, healthier individuals and families. Therefore, further research on appropriate risk adjusters is essential. Also, very little is known about the impact of current premiums or experience rating on the magnitude of cross-subsidization in the current market for private insurance. Specifically, what portion of private insurance premiums currently goes to subsidize both uncompensated care and inadequate payment rates from public insurers? Further research on current premiums by family size, income, and characteristics of the employer will provide valuable baseline information for evaluating the impact of mandatory community rating.

Another method of regulating premiums is to establish mandatory purchasing alliances, which would effectively establish mandatory community rating. Mandatory alliances are likely to result in premium subsidies from rural to urban areas and from low-income to high-income families.[66] These redistributive consequences were not well understood when managed competition proposals based on mandatory purchasing alliances were first developed. Subsidies to low-income families and to small businesses could be used to offset this regressive aspect of mandatory alliances. Community rating in the small-group market, for example, through voluntary purchasing alliances, is likely to produce a similar but less pronounced pattern of redistribution, since higher-income families may remain outside the alliance.

Employer mandates also would have an impact on working households. The most obvious concern is the impact on low-wage individuals who might face unemployment as a result of such mandates. Hawaii, where employer mandates have been in effect since 1974, has not been studied extensively but may provide important empirical evidence related to this concern.[67]

***Cost Sharing and Out-of-Pocket Expenses.*** The RAND Health Insurance Study (HIS) provides the best estimates of the response of families to different levels of cost sharing, including how uninsured families are likely to respond to insurance coverage.[68] Key results from the HIS should continue shape the design of future reform proposals. For example, income-related cost sharing could be implemented to offset the adverse consequences of uniform cost sharing on low-income individuals and families.[69]

Another significant finding from the HIS is the substantial welfare loss (that is, additional expenditures for insured health services that would not be purchased in the absence of insurance) related to extensive health insurance coverage. Many economists have called for a cap on the tax-exempt status of employment-based health insurance premiums to address this issue. Further research estimating the impact on households of such a cap would be useful.

Out-of-pocket expenditures for some health services, such as nursing home care and pharmaceuticals, are likely to continue to be substantial for many households. Further research on the financial impact of expenditures for such non-covered services will be important in determining the effects of including these services as covered benefits in the future.

***Subsidies.*** One of the most contentious issues in developing proposals for national health care reform is how to provide subsidies to low-income families and individuals to purchase health insurance. Employer mandates would solve this problem for a substantial portion of the uninsured but with uncertain consequences for employers and employees in firms that currently do not provide insurance. This is one area where research could move future debates out of the realm of ideology alone and provide an empirical basis for determining whether the nation can afford health care reform.

***Access.*** An important goal of most proposals for health care reform is to increase access to health care services for those who are currently uninsured. In states that are undertaking efforts to expand coverage to the uninsured, a high priority for future research should be studies to examine how utilization of and expenditures for health care services change for previously uninsured and underinsured subpopulations, including the working poor and ethnic and racial minorities. Studies comparing changes in access (for example, provider availability), utilization, and expenditures among these groups should provide valuable information about whether particular reform efforts are improving access.

Another important issue for future research is to evaluate and monitor the ongoing impact of having a substantial portion of the population without health insurance. The cost of expanding health insurance coverage to the uninsured has been difficult to estimate because of the lack of reliable data on the current costs of providing care to the uninsured. An effective mechanism for conducting this research would be a regular survey of utilization and expenditures, such as the National Medical Expenditure Survey (NMES), modified to sufficiently oversample individuals from low-income, poor health status, and ethnic populations and conducted on a regular basis (perhaps biannually). In general, the 1993–1994 national debate exposed the inadequacies of existing databases for developing and evaluating the potential effects of alternative reform proposals.[70]

A related issue is the increased importance of accurate state- and market-level estimates of utilization and expenditures. Accurate state-level estimates are usually obtained by combining population characteristics from the Current Population Survey with utilization and expenditure data from NMES. Future research would be greatly enhanced by expanding the sampling frame of an existing survey, such as NMES or the National Health Interview Survey (NHIS), so that accurate state-level estimates, by population subgroups, could be developed.

## Employers

Most people in the United States continue to receive health insurance through their place of employment. A major concern related to regulatory approaches is how regulation might affect the current patterns of employment-based insurance. A particular concern is the potential impact of employer mandates on employers. There is a great deal of descriptive information about the types of firms that currently do not offer insurance to their employees but little information about how firms might respond to an employer mandate. Such a mandate, even with subsidies to small firms with low average wages, is viewed politically as detrimental to small businesses. Again, the one state that has an employer mandate—Hawaii—has not been studied thoroughly. Although its experience with mandates may not be applicable to other states, surprisingly little information is available in the research literature about the impact of mandates in Hawaii.

Employer mandates are often proposed along with subsidies to small businesses. Information on how new businesses develop could be used to target subsidies to the firm's stage of development or overall profits rather than average payroll. Research in this area will require better surveys of businesses, particularly small businesses. One such survey, the National Employers Health Insurance Survey (NEHIS), was conducted for the first time in 1994.

## Providers

As research on the appropriateness and effectiveness of medical practice and technology progresses, distributional issues can be addressed through targeted studies examining how providers respond to specific practice guidelines, new technologies, and information about inappropriate medical practices. One major research issue is whether certain subpopulations are more likely to receive new technologies, experience better outcomes, or receive inappropriate or poor quality care. A prerequisite for conducting such research will be an expanded effort to collect patient-specific utilization data from all privately insured patients, not just those who receive subsidies to purchase their insurance. Although billing claims may be irrelevant for most health plans and providers under health reform, research on effectiveness, appropriateness, quality, and outcomes will be extremely difficult and costly without some requirement for uniform reporting of utilization data.

Another major concern is how providers respond to changes in their payment rates. Continued cost shifting is likely to cause access problems for publicly insured patients, particularly for services where the payment differential between private and public insurance is substantial.

## Private Insurers

One major issue for insurers deals with how insurance premiums should be risk adjusted. The predictive power of most risk adjusters is still relatively poor, with some exceptions.[71] An important area for future research, therefore, is to identify and incorporate appropriate risk adjusters into premiums, particularly for capitated health plans.

Another major issue for private insurers is the extent to which cost shifting can continue. Private health insurance premiums currently include an implicit tax for costs not covered by other payers, primarily the costs of the uninsured and costs for the publicly insured that are not fully covered by public payers. Mandatory purchasing alliances and mandatory community rating are the most likely mechanisms to reduce or eliminate such cost shifting. Voluntary alliances should have less impact and may establish new patterns of cost shifting based on relative purchasing power. For example, large corporations may be more effective in negotiating discounts than smaller firms. If they are able to extract concessions on premiums even when per capita expenditures are increasing, those increased costs may be passed on to purchasers with less market power. Whether voluntary alliances are viewed by insurers as desirable, and thus capable of negotiating substantial discounts, remains uncertain. Because voluntary alliances are currently found in various markets throughout the United States, future research should focus on the factors leading to the development of these alliances as well as their effectiveness.

## Public Insurers

Regulatory approaches hold the promise of increasing access and controlling total health expenditures, but are subject to two major criticisms that are difficult to address through research alone. One concern is that further regulation of the health care market will preempt the ongoing development of market-based reforms. A related issue is that regulatory approaches may shift more control over expenditures from private to public decision makers. Both issues could derail future efforts at comprehensive health care reform. Thus, an important area for research and policy analysis in the immediate future will be defining the rights and responsibilities of private health plans that receive funding through public programs such as Medicare and Medicaid.

The relative contributions of local, state, and federal governments to health care financing under various proposals for health care reform are often not well understood. In recent years, rapid increases in Medicaid expenditures have placed demands on state budgets that are increasingly difficult to meet. National proposals usually include maintenance-of-effort provisions, which require states with generous Medicaid benefits to continue paying more per capita than states with less generous benefits. Recent proposals call for replacing Medicaid with block grants to states. Budgetary pressures to limit Medicaid expenditures are likely to place low-income families at greater financial and medical risk. In general, the patterns of financing under various reform proposals and their impact on state and local governments and on family expenditures will require ongoing analysis.

A related issue is how government expenditures would be controlled under various proposals. Some proposals would specifically target federal subsidies and limit their growth, but leave private expenditures to be controlled solely by market forces. By limiting public but not private expenditures, such proposals may subject low-income individuals and families to continuing political pressure against increased spending (that is, taxes) for subsidies, similar to that now experienced in many state Medicaid programs. Obviously, the distributional consequences would fall almost exclusively on low-income families and low-income states under such proposals. Evaluating expected and actual changes in the patterns of government financing under alternative reform approaches will thus continue to be a valuable research topic.

## Conclusion

As discussed earlier, political and ideological support for market-based reform is very strong and seems likely to remain that way for the foreseeable future. Does this mean that price controls, global budgets, mandates, or other regulatory approaches have no role in the future? As long as fee-for-service medicine continues, price controls based on an expansion of Medicare's payment methods to other payers are likely to play a role in future reform efforts. Global budgets are also likely to be viewed as essential for aggregate expenditure control. The potential effects of various mandates are less well understood, and thus should be subject to extensive additional study. Options for combining regulatory approaches with market-based reforms also need further development.

Empirical evidence from previous and current use of price controls in the United States indicate that they are effective in controlling expenditures, improving or maintaining access, and reducing or eliminating cost shifting when applied to all payers. Nevertheless, deep distrust of increased government intervention into the health care market poses a substantial barrier to proposals based on price controls, global budgets, or mandates. Furthermore, regulatory approaches do not have the theoretical appeal of approaches based on market competition. Health services research can make a valuable contribution to future debates concerning regulatory versus competitive strategies by focusing on the distributional consequences of different approaches on the major stakeholders in the health care system. This research may provide additional evidence that the empirical advantages of regulatory mechanisms outweigh the theoretical advantages of reforms based solely on market competition.

## Notes

1. Mark V. Pauly, "U.S. Health Care Costs: The Untold True Story," *Health Affairs* 12 (Fall 1993): 152–159.
2. Paul B. Ginsburg and Kenneth E. Thorpe, "Can All-Payer Rate Setting and the Competitive Strategy Coexist?" *Health Affairs* 11 (Summer 1992): 73–86.
3. The most comprehensive summary of research findings is found in Marsha Gold, Karyen Chu, Suzanne Felt, Mary Harrington, and Timothy Lake, "Effects of Selected Cost Containment Efforts: 1971–1993," *Health Care Financing Review* 14 (Spring 1993): 183–213.

4. See, for example, Gail R. Wilensky, "Incremental Health System Reform: Where Medicare Fits In," *Health Affairs* 14 (Spring 1995): 173–181.

5. Thomas Rice, "Containing Health Care Costs in the United States," *Medical Care Review* 49 (Spring 1992): 19–65.

6. Gerard F. Anderson, "All-Payer Rate Setting: Down but Not Out," *Health Care Financing Review* (1991 Annual Supplement): 35–41; Thomas Rice, "Including an All-Payer Reimbursement System in a Universal Health Insurance Program," *Inquiry* 29 (Summer 1992): 203–212; Ginsburg and Thorpe, "Can All-Payer Rate Setting and the Competitive Strategy Coexist?"; and Gerald F. Kominski and Thomas Rice, "Should Insurers Pay the Same Fees Under an All-Payer System?" *Health Care Financing Review* 16 (Winter 1994): 1–15.

7. Congressional Budget Office, *Universal Health Insurance Coverage Using Medicare's Payment Rates* (Washington, D.C.: Congressional Budget Office, December 1991); Prospective Payment Assessment Commission, *Optional Hospital Payment Rates,* Congressional Report C–92–03 (Washington, D.C.: Prospective Payment Assessment Commission, March 1992); Physician Payment Review Commission, *Optional Payment Rates for Physicians: An Analysis of Section 402 of H.R. 3626* (Washington, D.C.: Physician Payment Review Commission, 1992); and Congressional Budget Office, *Single-Payer and All-Payer Health Insurance Systems Using Medicare's Payment Rates* (Washington, D.C.: Congressional Budget Office, April 1993).

8. Advocates for market-based reform acknowledge that market forces alone will not produce universal access. See, for example, Alain C. Ethoven and Sara J. Singer, "Market-Based Reform: What to Regulate and by Whom," *Health Affairs* 14 (Spring 1995): 105–119.

9. Ethoven and Singer, "Market-Based Reform: What to Regulate and by Whom."

10. Roger Feldman and Bryan Dowd, "What Does the Demand Curve for Medical Care Measure?" *Journal of Health Economics* 12 (1993): 193–200; and Mark V. Pauly, "Editorial: A Reexamination of the Meaning and Importance of Supplier-Induced Demand," *Journal of Health Economics* 13 (1994): 369–372.

11. Karen Davis, Gerard F. Anderson, Diane Rowland, and Earl P. Steinberg, *Health Care Cost Containment* (Baltimore, Md.: Johns Hopkins University Press, 1990), p. 98.

12. James C. Robinson and Harold S. Luft, "Competition, Regulation, and Hospital Costs: 1982–1986," *Journal of the American Medical Association* 260 (November 11, 1988): 2676–2681.

13. David S. Salkever, Donald M. Steinwachs, and Agnes Rupp, "Hospital Cost and Efficiency Under Per Case Payment in Maryland: A Tale of the Carrot and the Stick," *Inquiry* 23 (Spring 1986): 56–66.

14. Fred J. Hellinger, "Recent Evidence on Case-Based Systems for Setting Hospital Rates," *Inquiry* 22 (Spring 1985): 78–91.

15. Anderson, "All-Payer Rate Setting: Down but Not Out," p. 36.

16. Kenneth E. Thorpe, "Does All-Payer Rate Setting Work? The Case of the New York Prospective Hospital Reimbursement Methodology," *Journal of Health, Politics, Policy, and Law* 12 (Fall 1987): 391–408.

17. Samuel A. Mitchell, "Response to: All-Payer Rate Setting: Down but Not Out," *Health Care Financing Review* (1991 Annual Supplement): 42–44.

18. Robinson and Luft, "Competition, Regulation, and Hospital Costs: 1982–1986."

19. Salkever, Steinwachs, and Rupp, "Hospital Cost and Efficiency Under Per Case Payment in Maryland: A Tale of the Carrot and the Stick."

20. New Jersey State Department of Health, "Fundamentals of Rate Setting" in *A Prospective Payment System for New Jersey Hospitals, 1976–78, Seventh Quarter Report* (Trenton: New Jersey State Department of Health, 1978).

21. Paul L. Grimaldi, *Setting Rates for Hospital and Nursing Home Care* (Jamaica, N.Y.: Spectrum, 1985), pp. 165–166.

22. William C. Hsiao, Harvey M. Sapolsky, Daniel L. Dunn, and Sanford L. Weiner, "Lessons of the New Jersey DRG Payment System," *Health Affairs* 5 (Summer 1986): 32–45.

23. Health Research and Educational Trust of New Jersey, *DRG Evaluation;* vol. 2: *Economic and Financial Analysis* (Princeton, N.J.: Health Research and Educational Trust, 1984).

24. Michael D. Rosko and Robert W. Broyles, "The Impact of the New Jersey All-Payer DRG System," *Inquiry* 23 (Spring 1986): 67–75.

25. Robinson and Luft, "Competition, Regulation, and Hospital Costs: 1982–1986."

26. William C. Hsiao and Daniel L. Dunn, "The Impact of DRG Payment on New Jersey Hospitals," *Inquiry* 24 (Fall 1987): 212–220.

27. Hsiao and Dunn, "The Impact of DRG Payment on New Jersey Hospitals"; and Michael D. Rosko, "All-Payer Rate Setting and the Provision of Hospital Care to the Uninsured: The New Jersey Experience," *Journal of Health, Politics, Policy, and Law* 15 (Winter 1990): 815–831.

28. New York State Department of Health, *New York's Prospective Hospital Reimbursement Methodology* (Albany: New York State Department of Health, 1983).

29. Thorpe, "Does All-Payer Rate Setting Work?"

30. Robinson and Luft, "Competition, Regulation, and Hospital Costs: 1982–1986."

31. Thorpe, "Does All-Payer Rate Setting Work?"

32. Prospective Payment Assessment Commission, *Medicare and the American Health Care System: Report to Congress, June 1993* (Washington, D.C.: Prospective Payment Assessment Commission, 1993), p. 80.

33. Gerald F. Kominski and Christina Witsberger, "Trends in Length of Stay for Medicare Patients: 1979–87," *Health Care Financing Review* 15 (Winter 1993): 121–135.

34. Prospective Payment Assessment Commission, *Medicare and the American Health Care System, 1993*, p. 80.

35. Prospective Payment Assessment Commission, *Medicare and the American Health Care System, 1993*, p. 80.

36. Prospective Payment Assessment Commission, *Medicare and the American Health Care System, 1993*, p. 67.

37. Prospective Payment Assessment Commission, *Medicare and the American Health Care System, 1993*, p. 49.

38. Grace M. Carter, Joseph P. Newhouse, and Daniel A. Relles, *How Much Change in the Case-Mix Index Is DRG Creep?* R–3826–HCFA (Santa Monica, Calif.: RAND, April 1990).

39. Prospective Payment Assessment Commission, *Medicare and the American Health Care System, 1993*, p. 47.

40. Thomas B. Bradley and Gerald F. Kominski, "Contributions of Case Mix and Intensity Change to Hospital Cost Increases," *Health Care Financing Review* 14 (Winter 1992): 151–163.

41. Prospective Payment Assessment Commission, *Medicare and the American Health Care System: Report to Congress, June 1994* (Washington, D.C.: Prospective Payment Assessment Commission, 1994), p. 56.

42. Prospective Payment Assessment Commission, *Medicare and the American Health Care System, 1994,* p. 40.

43. Prospective Payment Assessment Commission, *Medicare and the American Health Care System, 1994,* p. 44.

44. Prospective Payment Assessment Commission, *Medicare and the American Health Care System, 1994,* p. 29.

45. Gerald F. Kominski and Andrea K. Biddle, "Changes in Follow-Up Care for Medicare Surgical Patients Under PPS," *Medical Care* 31 (March 1993): 230–246.

46. William H. Rogers, David Draper, Katherine L. Kahn, Emmett B. Keeler, Lisa V. Rubenstein, Jacqueline Kosecoff, and Robert H. Brook, "Quality of Care Before and After Implementation of the DRG-Based Prospective Payment System: A Summary of Effects," *JAMA* 264 (October 17, 1990): 1989–1994.

47. Grace M. Carter, Peter D. Jacobson, Gerald F. Kominski, and Mark J. Perry, "Use of Diagnosis-Related Groups by Non-Medicare Payers," *Health Care Financing Review* 16 (Winter 1994): 127–158.

48. Louise B. Russell and Carrie Lynn Manning, "The Effect of Prospective Payment on Medicare Expenditures," *New England Journal of Medicine* 320 (February 16, 1989): 439–444.

49. Jesse M. Levy, Michael J. Borowitz, Stephen F. Jencks, Terrence L. Kay, and Deborah K. Williams, "Impact of the Medicare Fee Schedule on Payments to Physicians," *JAMA* 264 (August 8, 1990): 717–722.

50. Thomas Rice and Jill Bernstein, "Volume Performance Standards: Can They Control Growth in Medicare Services?" *Milbank Quarterly* 68 (1990): 295–305; William A. Glaser, "How Expenditure Caps and Expenditure Targets Really Work," *Milbank Quarterly* 71 (1993): 97–127; and M. Susan Marquis and Gerald F. Kominski, "Alternative Volume Performance Standards for Medicare Physicians' Services," *Milbank Quarterly* 72 (1994): 329–357.

51. Physician Payment Review Commission, *Annual Report to Congress, 1993* (Washington, D.C.: Physician Payment Review Commission, 1993).

52. Thomas G. McGuire and Mark V. Pauly, "Physician Response to Fee Changes with Multiple Payers," *Journal of Health Economics* 10 (1991): 385–410.

53. Physician Payment Review Commission, *Annual Report to Congress, 1993,* p. 99.

54. Physician Payment Review Commission, *Annual Report to Congress, 1993,* p. 105.

55. R. Jones, "Should Private Payers Adopt RBRVS Fee Schedules?" *Business and Health* 10 (November 1992): 24–26.

56. Sally Stearns, Thomas Rice, Susan DesHarnais, Donald Pathman, Michelle Brasure, and Ming Tai-Seale, "Physician Responses to Medicare Payment Reductions: Impacts on the Public and Private Sector," paper delivered at the American Economic Association Annual Meeting, Washington, D.C., January 1995.

57. Henry J. Aaron and William B. Schwartz, "Managed Competition: Little Cost Containment Without Budget Limits," *Health Affairs* (1993 Supplement): 204–215; Stuart H. Altman and Alan B. Cohen, "The Need for a National Global Budget," *Health Affairs* (1993 Supplement): 194–203; William A. Glaser, "How Expenditure Caps and Expenditure Targets Really Work," *Milbank Quarterly* 71 (1993): 97–127; and Paul Starr and Walter A. Zelman, "Bridge to Compromise: Competition Under a Budget," *Health Affairs* (1993 Supplement): 7–23.

58. Altman and Cohen, "The Need for a National Global Budget," and Klaus-Dirk Henke, Margaret A. Murray, and Claudia Ade, "Global Budgeting in Germany: Lessons for the United States," *Health Affairs* 13 (Fall 1994): 7–21.

59. Dale A. Rublee, "Medical Technology in Canada, Germany, and the United States," *Health Affairs* 8 (Fall 1989): 178–181.

60. Marquis and Kominski, "Alternative Volume Performance Standards for Medicare Physicians' Services," p. 330.

61. Physician Payment Review Commission, *Annual Report to Congress, 1993;* and Physician Payment Review Commission, *Annual Report to Congress, 1995* (Washington, D.C.: Physician Payment Review Commission, 1995).

62. Stephen H. Long and M. Susan Marquis, *Toward a Global Budget for the U.S. Health System: Implementation Issues and Information Needs,* RAND Issue Paper (Santa Monica, Calif.: RAND, July 1995); and Elizabeth Kilbreth and Alan B. Cohen, "Strategic Choices for Cost Containment Under a Reformed U.S. Health Care System," *Inquiry* 30 (Winter 1993): 372–388.

63. Physician Payment Review Commission, *Annual Report to Congress, 1990* (Washington, D.C.: Physician Payment Review Commission, 1990), pp. 186–191.

64. Wilensky, "Incremental Health Care Reform: Where Medicare Fits In."

65. Theda Skocpol, "The Rise and Resounding Demise of the Clinton Plan," *Health Affairs* 14 (Spring 1995): 66–85.

66. U.S. General Accounting Office, *Health Care Alliance: Issues Relating to Geographic Boundaries* (Washington, D.C.: U.S. General Accounting Office, April 1994).

67. U.S. General Accounting Office, *Health Care in Hawaii: Implications for National Reform* (Washington, D.C.: U.S. General Accounting Office, February 1994).

68. Willard G. Manning, Joseph P. Newhouse, Naihua Duan, Emmett Keeler, Bernadette Benjamin, Arleen Leibowitz, M. Susan Marquis, and Jack Zwanziger, *Health Insurance and the Demand for Medical Care: Evidence from a Randomized Experiment,* R–3476–HHS (Santa Monica, Calif.: RAND, February 1988).

69. Thomas Rice and Kenneth E. Thorpe, "Income-Related Cost Sharing in Health Insurance," *Health Affairs* 12 (Spring 1993): 21–39.

70. Linda T. Bilheimer and Robert D. Reischauer, "Confessions of the Estimators: Numbers and Health Reform," *Health Affairs* 14 (Spring 1995): 37–55; Len M. Nichols, "Numerical Estimates and the Policy Debate," *Health Affairs* 14 (Spring 1995): 56–59; John F. Sheils, "Need for Continued Refinement in Cost Estimations," *Health Affairs* 14 (Spring 1995): 60–62; and Kenneth E. Thorpe, "A Call for Health Services Researchers," *Health Affairs* 14 (Spring 1995): 63–65.

71. Barbara Starfield, Jonathan Weiner, Laura Mumford, and Donald Steinwachs, "Ambulatory Care Groups: A Categorization of Diagnoses for Research and Management," *Health Services Research* 26 (April 1991): 53–74.

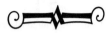

CHAPTER FIFTEEN

## LESSONS FROM OTHER COUNTRIES

Milton I. Roemer

Many concepts and practices in the organization and financing of health services can obviously be learned from other countries. Indeed, most of the policies implemented in the U.S. health system today were derived from experience in the older countries of Europe.

## Major Past Lessons

We may take note of several fundamental features of our health system adopted from elsewhere: training of physicians in universities, with clinical instruction in hospitals; professionalization of nursing through formal training in general hospitals; design and administrative structure of hospitals; construction and use of health centers for the care of ambulatory patients; organized preventive health services for babies and pregnant women; establishment of governmental public health agencies; occupational health services at workplaces; organized medical services for the poor; voluntary or nongovernmental insurance to pay for medical care; and mandatory government-controlled insurance for health services.[1]

Each of these policies and practices, originating in other countries, has been modified and adapted to the U.S. social environment. In the same broad components of the health system—its production of resources, its organization of programs, its financial support, and so on—many new lessons could be learned to improve the effectiveness of the U.S. health system or to heighten its economic efficiency.

# Innovations in Health Personnel Training

Several changes that emulated European patterns in the training of health personnel might improve quality of services or reduce costs, or do both.

Physicians in the United States typically study four years for a baccalaureate degree, followed by four more years for the M.D. degree. With more careful vocational guidance in secondary school, the European schedule of a continuous six-year sequence might well be adopted. Admittedly, this would reduce the time devoted to basic sciences, social sciences, and humanities, but these investments may be an extravagance in overall health system expenditures.[2]

Greater numbers of nurse practitioners might well be trained, to replace physicians in the delivery of primary medical care.[3] Such policies, however, would require that primary care be delivered in health centers, with organized teams of personnel, rather than in independent private offices.

Much greater numbers of midwives could be trained and used for handling normal childbirths in hospitals or—in most cities—in maternity institutions.[4] There might be one obstetrician available for every five to ten midwives. In smaller hospitals, nurse-midwives (registered nurses with special training in midwifery) would be most appropriate.

Specialization in medicine is excessive in the United States in relation to the need for primary care physicians. Counting general internists as well as specialists in family practice and noncertified general practitioners as primary care physicians, this group constitutes only 32 percent of our active office-based physicians as of 1989.[5] The comparable proportion in Europe and other continents is at least 50 percent, which corresponds much more closely to population needs.[6]

More reasonable personnel ratios could be achieved by national policy controlling hospital residencies. Maximum numbers of positions could be established in the various specialties, and financial inducements could be offered in primary care fields.

Regarding dental personnel, much greater efficiency could be achieved by use of "dental nurses," along the lines pioneered by New Zealand for school children.[7] Secondary school graduates can be trained for two years to do fillings and deciduous-tooth extraction as well as dental hygiene service under the general supervision of a dentist. Studies by the World Health Organization have shown the dental health of New Zealand children to be superior to that of children in Europe and the United States, and this was achieved at lower cost.

## Health Facility Innovations

Many more facilities should be established for the delivery of ambulatory health service, therapeutic and preventive, as in the Scandinavian countries.[8] The conventional setting for primary medical care should be a health center staffed with teams of personnel, as already noted. These facilities should be constructed and managed by local units of government.

Specialized services for the ambulatory patient should be available at the outpatient departments of general hospitals. If a hospital, however, is a long distance from the primary care units, it might establish extensions of its outpatient department in the form of polyclinics in rural regions. These would be staffed by hospital specialists periodically, as may be needed.

## Organization

Currently, the vast majority of personal health services are provided by private and independent practitioners of medicine. In the private-practice setting and especially in solo practice, there is no surveillance with respect to accepted medical standards, and the average patient may lack sound judgment concerning the appropriateness of specific treatments. This situation will probably continue for many years in the United States, but the work of those practitioners will be subject to a great deal of social organization. The objective will be to assure that everyone can reach good-quality preventive and treatment services on a regular basis.

Fortunately, there is a mounting U.S. movement toward the increased structuring of medical practice or toward various patterns of managed care. Since 1973, the federal government has established standards for health maintenance organizations (HMOs) and has provided grants for their promotion.[9] Organization must take account of the quantity of population and its geographical distribution. As a rule of thumb, a population of 50,000 would require one general health administrator for organized preventive and treatment services.[10] As of 1990, the United States had 2,932 local public health departments. Some are departments of county governments, some of city governments, some of multiple governments (involving more than one county or involving both city and county).[11]

Legal responsibility for all health services should be held by the principal health authority in each jurisdiction. This would be the fifty state governments and, within the states, the 2,932 public health agencies noted earlier. It is important that these state and local agencies, already directing organized preventive services, be assigned this responsibility, instead of setting up separate agencies for treatment services.

# Health Service Delivery

Preventive and health screening services should be provided aggressively as functions of the health centers. Rather than simply waiting for patients to appear, a schedule of regular visits should be arranged according to the age, sex, and health status of all persons in the catchment area of each health center. As early as 1945, I suggested a schedule for such screening examinations and preventive procedures, adjusted to the needs of different demographic groups.[12] Similar and more sophisticated schedules have been proposed in numerous reports in recent years.[13]

These periodic health visits should offer counseling on healthful life-style, along with arrangements for group sessions to cope with evident problems, such as smoking, excessive alcohol or drug consumption, obesity, or conspicuous signs of stress. The health professional mainly responsible for this counseling should be the primary care physician, although he or she may, of course, delegate the task to other primary health care personnel.

Every childbirth in the hospital should mean a signal to the local public health agency to send a public health nurse to the home of the newborn.[14] Here advice should be offered on infant care and feeding, immunizations, and regular attendance at infant health clinics. Postpartum attention should also be given to the mother. Advice can be offered, if necessary, on safe and sanitary arrangements for an infant bassinet. It is noteworthy that in France, the social security programs require that the mother take her infant for regular preventive services if she is to receive official family allowances for the child.[15]

Long-term care always presents special problems as average longevity increases. In every community, there should be personnel for visiting chronically disabled or frail patients in their homes. Such arrangements have been well developed by the local health authorities in Great Britain.[16] For frail or disabled elderly patients, who require assistance in activities of daily living, careful assessments are made and custodial facilities have been established by local governments in the Scandinavian countries.[17] The vast numbers of proprietary nursing homes of very uneven quality would not have developed throughout the United States, if local governments had taken this initiative as in Europe. The continuing trends toward women being engaged in full-time work and the declining size of families have inevitably increased the demand for care of the elderly in nursing homes and other forms of caring facility.[18]

Until this fundamental reform in the provision of long-term care can be achieved, the days of care provided in skilled nursing homes under the Medicare Law should be greatly extended. The current limitation to one hundred days following at least three days of hospital care is of relatively little value; indeed, the value was reduced further in 1990 by requiring the patient to pay up to $74 per day for the twenty-first up to the hundredth day of nursing home care.[19] For persons entitled to Medicaid support, the duration is now essentially without limit.[20] It should be similarly extended for other elderly persons on the basis of increased social security revenues to support Medicare.

Hospital services should be provided in facilities related to each other according to principles of regionalization.[21] Thus, relatively simple cases requiring hospitalization should be admitted to district general hospitals, with modest staffing and equipment. Only more complicated cases should be referred to larger provincial hospitals, with specialists in organ-specific fields. Technical consultation should be offered regularly by the more central to the more peripheral facilities, especially with the new telecommunication techniques becoming available.

Within hospitals, the organization of medical staffs in Europe and most of the world is quite different from the pattern most prevalent in the United States. The majority of U.S. general hospitals have open staff arrangements, whereby almost any qualified local physician can be appointed to the medical staff and admit private patients. The physician becomes subject to various medical staff policies and has certain obligations and responsibilities but still has a great deal of autonomy in managing the care of private patients.[22]

By contrast, medical staffs in general hospitals of Europe and the rest of the world are closed staff and much more highly disciplined.[23] A relatively smaller number of physicians work in the hospital on a full-time or major-time basis. They are organized typically into departments, with department heads and some sort of hierarchical structure. Each physician is ordinarily attached to one hospital, and multiple hospital appointments, commonplace in the United States, are rare in Europe.

On the other hand, doctors in the community providing ambulatory care are regarded as practitioners of primary health care, with different standards of merit. Their attachment is to families, and their counsel may be sought in general community problems—not necessarily medical in nature. They often have separate medical societies and special programs for continuing education.[24]

Trends in U.S. general hospitals are somewhat toward the European pattern of medical staff organization, with appointments of increasing numbers of physicians on some sort of contractual basis.[25] They may be paid by straight salaries, full-time or part-time, or they may share departmental income with the hospital in various ways. This arrangement is most common in supportive fields such as pathology or radiology, but it is extending to all specialized fields. Appointment of full-time heads of clinical departments in open-staff hospitals is becoming increasingly widespread.

The increasing structure of medical staffs (as well as general operations) in hospitals and the implementation of regionalization in geographical areas suggest an overall framework of U.S. hospitals that will be much more organized than it was before World War II. These arrangements, however, are only evolving gradually, in tandem with the growth of programs of insurance to support health care costs. When and if legislation is enacted to mandate health insurance coverage for every U.S. resident, the entire health care system will mature.[26]

Health insurance organizations (or plans), to one of which every person would be required to become affiliated, would naturally seek to purchase the "best buys" for their members. Nearly always this would lead to choice of a delivery pattern in which physicians and allied health personnel work together in an organized framework.[27] Enrollment of persons in health insurance plans would have to be subject to regulations, which would prevent cream skimming (the selective enrollment of persons with predictably lower risk of need for medical care). Since payment to the providers would be made on a capitation (per capita) basis, there would be no incentive for excessive use of hospital or other ancillary services. Reasonable use of such extra services would be motivated by concern for good patient outcomes. Underuse of appropriate diagnostic or treatment procedures would also have to be subject to surveillance, to protect quality.

## Economic Support

As noted earlier, the costs of this program of health services would be borne mainly by funds derived from mandatory insurance. This is the mechanism used in Germany,[28] France,[29] and many other countries. At the present time, the great majority of U.S. residents are already insured for most medical and hospital expenses through their employment, with typically most of the premiums being paid by the employers. Such health care insurance is weakest or totally lacking among persons employed by small firms (under fifty employees) and among the self-employed.[30] In recent years—since about 1990—moreover, the proportion of the population without insurance protection has been rising, as individuals change their employment and as health insurance premiums have risen.

The costs of medical care are largely covered by government programs for certain sections of the population not covered by private insurance. Almost all persons over sixty-five years of age are socially insured for hospital and physician care through the U.S. Medicare law, enacted in 1965; this program also covers the totally disabled. This amounts to thirty-four million people.[31] In addition, indigent persons under age sixty-five (in certain demographic categories) are provided health service by the federal-state program known as Medicaid, which applies to another twenty-two million.[32] Altogether, government finances medical care for these fifty-six million people. It is widely recognized, however, that many of these people, especially the poor, have limited access to medical care, since certain physicians do not accept them as patients.

Subtracting the privately insured and the governmentally protected people from the total U.S. population leaves about thirty-eight million people (or some 15 percent of our total) without health insurance protection. A great deal of political debate has been concerned with how these people should be provided with health insurance protection.[33] A recent report, in 1995, estimates that forty-one million citizens are lacking health insurance protection.[34]

A system of universal health care coverage often advocated for the United States is that found in Canada. Here, the national government and each of the ten provinces pay for the hospital care of every resident.[35] More precisely, like Canada, we would have to channel all hospital insurance premiums to a state fund, from which all hospitals would be financed by paying *prospective periodic amounts*, based on a *global budget* approved for each hospital. At the year's end, any justified shortfall would be made up with a supplemental allotment, while a surplus (if not excessive) would be retained by the hospital.[36] Such prospective global budgetary payments are used for payment of public hospitals in Europe—both in the programs financed through social insurance and those financed wholly from general revenues.

Social insurance derived from mandatory employee and employer contributions is the principal source of health care funds in Germany, France, and other countries of continental Europe.[37] In Great Britain and the Scandinavian countries, financial support has been shifted almost entirely to general revenues.[38] The German and French policies would be more realistic politically in the United States.

## Health Expenditure Trends

Whatever may be the principal source of health system financing, the trend of expenditures—as a proportion of gross national product (GNP)—has been upward. Between 1960 and 1990, this share rose in France from 4.2 percent to 8.8 percent, in Norway from 3.3 percent to 7.4 percent, in Canada from 5.5 percent to 9.5 percent, and in the United States from 5.2 percent to 12.2 percent (and further to 14.3 percent in 1992).[39] Even in developing countries, where the proportion of GNP spent on health tends to be much lower, similar increases have been occurring; in the Philippines it rose between 1970 and 1976 from 1.9 percent to 2.2 percent, and in Sri Lanka between 1970 and 1982 from 3.0 percent to 5.1 percent.[40]

The health expenditures of other countries have also become more heavily governmental. Those of the Netherlands were only 33.3 percent public in 1960, rising to 78.3 percent public in 1984. The same governmental trend in Japan showed a rise from 60.4 percent in 1960 to 72.1 percent in 1984, and in Norway from 77.8 to 88.8 percent. Public-sector health spending in the United States rose from 24.7 percent of the total in 1960 to 41.4 percent in 1984. The expanding role of government has clearly promoted the distribution of health services to the lower income groups.[41]

Evidence for improving equity in U.S. health services is strikingly shown in data trends between 1930 and 1981. The incidence of illness was greater among the poor than among the affluent sixty years ago, and this is still true. However, household surveys in 1930 showed 1,900 patient-doctor contacts per 1,000 persons per year among the poorest fifth of the population, compared with 4,700 such contacts among the richest fifth.[42] In 1980, this relationship had become reversed, so that the poorest fifth had 5,600 contacts per 1,000, while the richest fifth had 4,400.[43] The same sort of reversal occurred for general hospital admissions—much lower for the poor in 1930 and much higher for the poor in 1981. The U.S. federal and state programs of public welfare have indeed created much greater health care equity.

## Cost Containment

With respect to cost containment, the payment of hospitals through prospective global budgets has been noted. Another important strategy, when physicians are paid by the fee-for-service method, is the negotiation of fee schedules, which usually is carried out between the health authority and the medical association. Sometimes such negotiations must be carried out with separate associations for general practitioners and various types of specialists.[44]

Control of pharmaceutical costs has been much more direct in European countries and Japan, where maximum prices for drugs are established nationally.[45] Drug control in the United States has become increasingly rigorous with respect to drug safety, advertising, production, and efficacy—but not at all on prices.[46] In spite of exceptionally high profits earned by the U.S. pharmaceutical industry, pricing is left entirely to market forces.[47]

Perhaps the most effective control on expenditures for hospital care in countries throughout the world has been governmental constraints on the construction of new hospital bed capacity. This is the general policy applied by ministries of health in Europe with respect to both public and private hospitals.[48] In developing countries, it is applied to public hospitals, but there are virtually no controls on the establishment of private hospital beds, aside from their being required to meet technical standards.[49] In most industrialized countries, there are also constraints on the acquisition of high-cost technology in public hospitals, to prevent excessive fixed costs and overutilization.[50]

Provisions for malpractice insurance are much more centralized in other industrialized countries than in the United States. Here, such insurance is mainly carried by individual doctors and hospitals through commercial insurance companies. To avoid litigation, which might result in very high awards for the plaintiff, insurance companies have a strong tendency to settle claims with relatively large financial sums. In most other industrialized countries, however, the medical association maintains a central defense fund against malpractice suits. Any claims are carefully investigated and, when reasonable, the accused doctor is rigorously defended. As a result, malpractice insurance premiums are much lower than in the United States.[51]

In two countries, Sweden and New Zealand, malpractice insurance is combined with social insurance for other types of accident on a no-fault basis. This results in larger numbers of awards of smaller average amounts of money. There are savings, of course, from the avoidance of the costs of litigation.[52]

## General Health Policy Lessons

The broad thrust of health policy in the major industrialized countries of the world has been the development of health protection as an entitlement of citizenship and even of simple residence in the country. This is not the same as a right to health, because a state of good health is determined by many influences that are stronger than personal health care. It does mean, however, that social actions must be taken to assure the resources necessary for providing health care and to assure people access to them under all circumstances.

Both the provision of resources and their use require planning, economic support, education, management, and many social strategies to coordinate all the components of national health systems. The demography of the population and the technology of health service are constantly changing so that the details of health policy must also change.[53] Strategies must always focus on the welfare of individuals as members of population groups.

Inevitably, there are limitations and constraints in any society for achieving ideal health policy goals at all times and places. In arriving at decisions, leaders must be guided by consideration of how best to achieve the greatest good for the greatest number of people. In reaching such judgments, there must be the broadest possible participation of all people, including both the recipients and the providers of health services.

# Notes

1. Milton I. Roemer, *An Introduction to the U.S. Health Care System*, 2nd ed. (New York: Springer, 1986).

2. Elizabeth Purcell (ed.), *World Trends in Medical Education* (Baltimore, Md.: Johns Hopkins University Press, 1971).

3. Vernon W. Lippard and Elizabeth F. Purcell (eds.), *Intermediate-Level Health Practitioners* (New York: Josiah Macy, Jr. Foundation, 1973).

4. Barbara Brennan and Joan R. Heilman, *The Complete Book of Midwifery* (New York: Dutton, 1977).

5. U.S. Department of Health and Human Services, *Health United States, 1991*, DHHS Pub. No. (PHS) 92–1232, (Washington, D.C.: Public Health Service, 1992), p. 246.

6. Steven A. Schroeder, "Reform and the Physician Work Force," *Domestic Affairs* 2 (Winter 1993–94): 105–131.

7. John I. Ingle and Patricia Blair (eds.), *International Dental Care Delivery Systems* (Cambridge, Mass.: Ballinger, 1978).

8. National Board of Health and Welfare, *The Swedish Health Services in the 1990s* (Stockholm: National Board, 1985).

9. Harold S. Luft, "Assessing the Evidence on HMO Performance," *Milbank Quarterly* 58, 4 (1980): 501–536.

10. This assumption was made in 1945; see Haven Emerson, *Local Health Units for the Nation* (New York: Commonwealth Fund, 1945), p. 2.

11. National Association of County Health Officials, *National Profile of Local Health Departments* (Washington, D.C.: National Association of County Health Officials, July 1990).

12. Milton I. Roemer, "A Program of Preventive Medicine for the Individual," *Milbank Quarterly* 23 (1945): 209–226.

13. For example, see Michael A. Stoto, Ruth Behrens, and Connie Rosemont (eds.), *Healthy People 2000: Citizens Chart the Course* (Washington, D.C.: Institute of Medicine, 1990); U.S. Department of Health and Human Services, *Prevention '91–'92 Federal Programs & Progress* (Washington, D.C.: U.S. Government Printing Office, 1992); and U.S. Department of Health and Human Services, *The 1990 Health Objectives for the Nation: A Midcourse Review* (Washington D.C.: U.S. Government Printing Office, 1986).

14. George A. Silver, *Child Health: America's Future* (Germantown, Md.: Aspen, 1978).

15. Ministère de la santé publique et de la population, *Protection de la santé publique en France* (Paris: Ministère de la santé publique et de la population, 1957), p. 58.

16. D. Boldy and R. Canvin, "Community Care of the Elderly in Britain: Value for Money," *Home Health Care Service Quarterly* 5 (1984–1985): 109–122.

17. Marilynn M. Rosenthal, "Beyond Equity: Swedish Health Policy and the Private Sector," *Milbank Quarterly* 64, 4 (1986): 592–621.

18. Miriam J. Hirschfeld and Rachel Fleishman, "Nursing Home Care for the Elderly," in *Improving the Health of Older People—A World View*, eds. Robert L. Kane, J. Grimley Evans, and David MacFadyen (Oxford, England: Oxford University Press, 1990), pp. 473–490.

19. U.S. Department of Health and Human Services, Health Care Financing Administration, *The Medicare Handbook*, HCFA Pub. No. 10050 (Washington, D.C.: U.S. Department of Health and Human Services, 1990).

20. E. Friedman, "Medicare and Medicaid at 25," *Hospitals* 64 (August 1990): 38–54.

21. Ernest W. Saward, *The Regionalization of Personal Health Services,* rev. ed. (New York: Prodist, 1976).

22. Milton I. Roemer and Jay W. Friedman, *Doctors in Hospitals: Medical Staff Organization and Hospital Performance* (Baltimore, Md.: Johns Hopkins University Press, 1971).

23. Milton I. Roemer, "General Hospitals in Europe," in *Modern Concepts of Hospital Administration,* ed. J. K. Owen (Philadelphia: Saunders, 1962), pp. 17–37.

24. Milton I. Roemer, "American Hospital System Is Moving Toward the European Pattern," *Modern Hospital* (October 1962): p. 6 ff.

25. Milton I. Roemer, "Medical Staff Organization in General Hospitals of the U.S.A.: The Influence of Contractual Physicians," in *Epidemiology Reports in Research & Teaching,* ed. J. Pemberton (London, Oxford University Press, 1963), pp. 307–313.

26. White House Domestic Policy Council, *The President's Health Security Plan* (New York: Random House, 1993).

27. John B. McKinlay (ed.), *Health Maintenance Organizations: Milbank Reader 5* (Cambridge Mass.: MIT Press, 1981).

28. Donald W. Light and Alexander Schuller, *Political Values and Health Care: The German Experience* (Cambridge, Mass.: MIT Press, 1986).

29. Jonathan E. Fielding and Pierre-Jean Lancry, "Lessons from France—'Vive la Difference': The French Health Care System and U.S. Health System Reform," *Journal of the American Medical Association* 270, 6 (August 11, 1993): 748–756.

30. Thomas Rice, E. Richard Brown, and Roberta Wyn, "Holes in the Jackson Hole Approach to Health Care Reform," *JAMA* 270, 11 (September 15, 1993): 1357–1362.

31. U.S. Department of Health and Human Services, *Health United States, 1992,* DHHS Pub. No. (PHS) 93–1232 (Washington, D.C.: Public Health Service, 1993), p. 185.

32. U.S. Department of Health and Human Services, *Health United States, 1992,* p. 188.

33. Steffie Woolhandler, David U. Himmelstein, and Quentin Young, "High Noon for U.S. Health Care Reform," *International Journal of Health Services* 23, 2 (1993): 193–211.

34. American Medical Association, "Over 41 Million Now Uninsured," *AMA News* (February 13, 1995), p. 3.

35. Malcolm G. Taylor, *Insuring National Health Care: The Canadian Experience* (Chapel Hill: University of North Carolina Press, 1990).

36. Richard Kirsch and Aviva Goldstein, *Hospital Global Budgeting: A Key to Health Care Reform* (Albany: Public Policy and Education Fund of New York, July 1993).

37. William A. Glaser, *Health Insurance in Practice: International Variations in Financing, Benefits, and Problems* (San Francisco: Jossey-Bass, 1991).

38. Ruth Levitt, *The Reorganised National Health Service* (London: Croom Helm, 1976).

39. U.S. Department of Health and Human Services, *Health United States, 1992,* p. 161.

40. David de Ferranti, *Paying for Health Services in Developing Countries* (Washington, D.C.: World Bank, 1985).

41. Organization for Economic Cooperation and Development, *Financing and Delivering Health Care* (Paris: Organization for Economic Cooperation and Development, 1987), p. 55.

42. I. S. Falk, Margaret C. Klem, and Nathan Sinai, *The Incidence of Illness and the Receipt and Costs of Medical Care Among Representative Families,* No. 26 (Chicago: Committee on the Costs of Medical Care, 1933), p. 110.

43. Avedis Donabedian, Soloman J. Axelrod, Leon Wyszewianski, and Richard L. Lichtenstein, *Medical Care Chartbook,* 8th ed. (Ann Arbor, Mich.: Health Administration Press, 1986), p. 53.

44. Milton I. Roemer, *The Organization of Medical Care Under Social Security* (Geneva, Switzerland: International Labour Office, 1969).

45. Albert I. Wertheimer (ed.), *Proceedings of the International Conference on Drug and Pharmaceutical Services Reimbursement,* Pub. No. (HRA) 77–3186 (Washington, D.C.: U.S. Department of Health, Education, and Welfare, 1977).

46. World Health Organization, *The World Drug Situation* (Geneva, Switzerland: World Health Organization, 1988).

47. Ned McCraine and Martin J. Murray, "The Pharmaceutical Industry: A Further Study in Corporate Power," *International Journal of Health Services* 8, 4 (1978): 573–588.

48. World Health Organization, Regional Office for Europe, *Health Planning and Organization of Medical Care* (Copenhagen, Denmark: World Health Organization, 1972).

49. Howard Barnum and Joseph Kutzin, *Public Hospitals in Developing Countries* (Baltimore, Md.: Johns Hopkins University Press, 1993).

50. David Banta and C. Behney, "Policy Formulation and Technology Assessment," *Milbank Quarterly* 59 (1981): 445–479.

51. F. Sloan and R. Bovbjerg, *Medical Malpractice: Crises, Response and Effects* (Washington, D.C.: Health Insurance Association of America, 1989).

52. C. Ham, R. Dingwall, P. Fenn, and D. Harris, *Medical Negligence: Compensation and Accountability* (London: King's Fund Institute, 1988).

53. Elizabeth Fee and Roy M. Acheson, *A History of Education in Public Health* (New York: Oxford University Press, 1991).

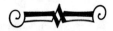

CHAPTER SIXTEEN

# THE ROLE OF PREVENTION

Charles E. Lewis

For those looking for challenging health policy issues, prevention is currently a gold mine—but it was not always so.

Greek mythology has it that Chiron, a centaur, taught Aesculapius, a son of Apollo, the art of healing. Aesculapius has become well known, but few are aware of his mythical fate. As his healing powers became more renown, so did the challenges presented to him. Finally, he restored life to the dead, and for this interference with fate he was struck dead by a thunderbolt from Zeus.[1] (One need not expand on this as a parable for modern technology and the medical profession.)

Aesculapius had several children, including two daughters, Panacea (about whom little is known) and Hygia, the goddess of health. In early drawings and friezes, Hygia and Aesculapius are often pictured together. Only recently has the separateness or political coolness between curative medicine and hygiene, or health promotion and disease prevention, become apparent.[2]

With time and the growth of the science and technology base in each area, they have been recognized as relatives—and frequently competitors for resources. The resolution of unnecessary competition between them and the prescription for a balance between the two present both challenges and opportunities to frame a comprehensive health care policy for the United States.

This chapter will focus on the answers to three groups of questions. First, What is preventable? In well-designed studies, what interventions have been shown to work? These data lead to our present recommendations for preventive care services.

Second, What are the problems associated with applying our knowledge to the care of individuals and populations in the real world? We may know the risk factors for a condition and the biological changes that must be reversed or terminated, yet we may not be able to prevent the condition. We know more than we are able to do because many of our treatments require major changes in human behavior or changes in society. Scholars have created theoretical models for these changes, enumerating key independent variables.[3] However, skilled practitioners concerned with behavioral changes may find the theoretical models less than helpful. Also, some potentially effective treatments are not currently socially acceptable to society as a whole.

The third and final group of questions is, What value does society place on prevention? What are we, as a nation, willing to do to eliminate certain causative agents or change our environment to remove certain hazards? How much are we willing to invest in something so that it will never occur? We may know what to do to prevent $X$ and how to do it, but still lack the collective will to take the actions necessary to prevent $X$, even though the consequences of this inaction are obvious.

The future-oriented and value-laden nature of prevention must be recognized by those who would teach, promote, or practice it. From a cognitive developmental perspective, this requires that the recipient be in what is termed a *formal stage of operation*.[4] That is, the target must be able to recognize the causal relationship between actions taken today and their delayed preventive effects tomorrow (or believe unquestioningly in the recommendations or mimic the actions of others). Individuals, therefore, must believe in tomorrow and place a value on their future.

Those professionals who are prepared to provide preventive services certainly are able to understand the causal chain of events and have reason to be future oriented. However, practicing prevention requires the ability to forgo the satisfaction of doing something that has a more immediate and visible effect (even if it is untoward) and to imagine the consequences of failure to prevent. A successful day in the practice of prevention could be seen as a series of zeros, or investments in the future, with nothing tangible to show for today's work.[5]

## Recent History

Pioneers in public health, many of whom were concerned with environmental hygiene, provided statistical support for the maternal admonitions "Always wash your hands" and "Cleanliness is next to godliness." Florence Nightingale made sound recommendations to the British Army, even though she never accepted the germ theory.[6] Public health principles form the basic tenets of the practice of prevention. Over the past several years, the relative roles of the individual, the professions, and the government in public health activities have changed. It has long been accepted that individuals must accept responsibility for their health behaviors, which supports our common practice of blaming the victim for ill health and other misfortunes. However, individuals have the right to expect that health care providers will recommend preventive services to them that are appropriate for their age and risk factors, and provide these services when professional intervention is required, as with immunizations and screening tests such as mammograms.

The role of public health agencies, while formerly limited to the provision of such services to special population groups, has grown to include the provision of leadership in terms of planning strategic objectives in prevention for the entire nation. In the process, public health practitioners have assumed a critical role in defining and answering the questions posed earlier.

The American Medical Association (AMA) proposed the annual physical examination as a method for maintaining health in 1922. Despite growing awareness that preventive services on an annual basis were not clinically effective, the AMA did not change its recommendation until 1983, when it issued a policy statement that withdrew support for the annual physical examination and instead focused on an individualized periodic health visit.[7]

Despite the progress made in other fields of medical science, it was more than fifty years after the AMA advocacy of an annual preventive examination that a formal commission was established by the Canadian Government to examine the scientific literature, and to bring forth a series of data-based recommendations for the practice of clinical prevention.[8]

Shortly afterward, the most significant event in the history of prevention in the United States occurred. In 1977, the Department of Health, Education, and Welfare published *Healthy People—The Surgeon General's Report on Health Promotion and Disease Prevention*.[9] This landmark work spelled out overall goals for five age groups, defined two examples for special focus within each, and defined four types of objectives to be accomplished for each: public and professional awareness, surveillance and evaluation, services improvement, and risk reduction. It also named a federal public health agency to lead the work on each specific objective. Thus it began to spell out the relationships between the private and public sectors and defined the players in the game of prevention. As suggested earlier, while the individual must be involved or feel empowered to take certain actions, these actions must be encouraged, recommended, and in some cases administered by health professionals. The public and the professions must know the threats to health and what is available to reduce the risks to an individual.

Primary prevention is obviously the prevention mode of choice. However, except under those circumstances in which immunizing agents have been developed, primary prevention involves the efforts of a variety of individuals to undo those learned life-style behaviors that are hazardous to health. As is evident in several studies, this is possible—but requires considerable effort.

Subsequently, the federal government established the U.S. Preventive Services Task Force, which further contributed to our knowledge of what is worth doing.[10] The task force echoed the findings of the Canadian group that many screening tests designed to detect disease at an early stage often produce large numbers of false positive results, leading to unnecessary subsequent diagnostic assessment. The task force reiterated the point that in examining proposals for secondary prevention (defined later), screening tests, or those used to detect health problems early, must be accurate and reliable. Here are some definitions basic to prevention through early detection:

*Accuracy* refers to the sensitivity, specificity, and positive predictive value of a test.

*Reliability* means the ability to produce the same result on repeated occasions (whether it is valid or not).

*Sensitivity* means the ability to detect individuals who have the condition targeted by the screening procedure. (A test with low sensitivity will fail to detect a number of individuals with the condition, producing a high number of false negative values.)

*Specificity* means the ability to differentiate individuals who have the condition targeted by the screening procedure from the rest of the population. (A test with poor specificity will result in a number of unaffected individuals being included in the group alleged to have the condition, producing a high number of false positive values.)

*Positive Predictive Value* (PPV) means the ability of a test to produce reliable values for population screening. It is a function of the prevalence of the target condition in the population being tested as well as of the sensitivity and specificity of a test. A test with high sensitivity and specificity can still generate more false positives than true positives when it is used to screen for a relatively rare condition. Table 16.1 shows what happens when a test that is 99 percent sensitive and 99 percent specific is used to screen for a condition with a prevalence of 0.1 percent in a population of 100,000 individuals.

The PPV is the value that results from dividing the number of *true positive* individuals by the total number of those with positive test results. In this illustration, the 99 true positives represent 9 percent of the total of 1,098. If one is only con-

### TABLE 16.1. HYPOTHETICAL TEST RESULTS.

| Test Is: | Condition Is: | | Totals |
|---|---|---|---|
| | Present | Absent | |
| Positive | 99 (true positive) | 999 (false positive) | 1,098 |
| Negative | 1 (false negative) | 98,901 (true negative) | 98,902 |
| Totals | 100 | 99,900 | 100,000 |

cerned about the consequences of missing actual cases, the 99 percent capture rate looks great. However, if one is concerned with the consequences of falsely labeling individuals—for example, telling healthy people they have HIV infection—the 9 percent PPV is unnerving. It indicates that roughly ten times as many persons are falsely labeled as having the condition in question as are truly identified. In addition to the psychological hardship thus imposed, a low PPV entails substantial additional expense for further evaluation and testing (necessary for all positive test results) of individuals who should have been properly identified initially.

Among the other critical issues considered by the task force was lead time bias; that is, whether early detection actually extends length of life or merely advances the diagnosis to an earlier date, with the patient dying at about the same time anyway. The gaps in evidence needed to answer the first question (What is worth doing?) were identified by the task force and suggested an enormous research agenda for preventive medicine.

Perhaps the most important contribution of the task force was the creation of a rating guide by which all preventive practices could be graded.[11] The ratings are based on strength of recommendation as well as quality of the evidence. The grading system is as follows:

*Recommendations*

A. There is *good* evidence to support the recommendation that the condition be specifically considered in a periodic health examination.
B. There is *fair* evidence to support the recommendation that the condition be specifically considered in a periodic health examination.
C. There is *poor* evidence to support the recommendation that the condition be specifically considered in a periodic health examination.
D. There is *fair* evidence to support the recommendation that the condition be *excluded* from consideration.
E. There is *good* evidence to support the recommendation that the condition be *excluded* from consideration.

Good, Fair, and Poor are defined by examining the burden of suffering created by the condition, and the nature of the intervention (cost/simplicity, etc.).

The *quality* of evidence is rated as follows:

I. Evidence is obtained from at least one properly designed *randomized* clinical controlled trial (RCT).

II-1. Evidence is from at least one well-designed controlled trial, without randomization.

II-2. Evidence is from at least one well-designed, cohort-case controlled analytic study.

II-3. Evidence is from a multiple time series design, with or without the intervention, in populations. All of the Type II evidence comes from quasi-experimental designs.

III. Evidence is based upon opinions of respected authorities, their clinical experience, descriptive studies, etc.

Thus, rating the recommendation for an annual mammogram in women over fifty years of age *IA* describes the quality of the evidence to support it, that is, the evidence comes from a randomized controlled trial.

## Concepts Underlying Prevention

Before pursuing the health policy issues facing decision makers in the health care system of tomorrow, it is important to understand certain terms or concepts drawn from epidemiology that underlie the practice of prevention.

The *natural history of a phenomenon* views a disease, illness, or threat to health as beginning at some point in time (often at birth) and increasing over time in terms of its degree of severity or impairment of functioning of a molecular system, an organ, or an individual. This history may be relatively long, as in the case of coronary heart disease, or it may be relatively short, as in the case of Hepatitis B.

For example, at birth there is little evidence of the presence of atherosclerosis. However, with the passage of time and depending on genetic influences, diet, physical activity, and other factors, arterial vessels such as the coronary arteries narrow due to the development of atheromas or lipid-laden plaques. Eventually, the condition *breaks the clinical horizon*. That is, the individual ceases to be asymptomatic and the problem manifests itself in the form of physical evidence or symptoms, such as chest pain on exertion or myocardial infarction.[12]

The most important derivative of the natural history of a disease is that diseases or disorders can be present at a subclinical stage, at which point they may be detected with appropriately sensitive and specific tests applied to those in whom a test is clinically indicated. From this perspective, we derive definitions of the *level of prevention*.

*Primary preventive services* are those activities or procedures that maintain the health of the individual. *Secondary prevention* refers to the early detection of a problem through the use of a variety of screening techniques. This means identifying the presence of the problem before it breaks the clinical horizon and becomes symptomatic. In the case of coronary artery disease, for example, data on some risk factors associated with the onset of the disease—lipid profile, history of smoking, lack of exercise—may be obtained very easily. Such data can indicate the desirability of a more expensive test, a stress electrocardiogram, that can reveal diminished blood flow to the heart. When positive, this test lowers the clinical horizon and advances the point in time at which a diagnosis is made. Then the question facing those concerned with prevention is, Can the individual be persuaded to alter those behaviors that led to the development of the condition?

Finally, although it may seem internally contradictory, *tertiary prevention* is defined as efforts to maintain existing levels of functioning in an individual once afflicted with a problem, as with the maintenance of residual musculoskeletal function after a cerebrovascular accident.

*Host-agent interaction* is a basic epidemiological concept that views phenomena threatening health in terms of the interactions among an agent (chemical, biological, or physical), a host (the individual), and the environment in which both exist. Both causes and means of prevention can be assessed in terms of these interactions

The epidemiological basis for prevention is quite simple. Hosts can be altered, that is, they can be changed immunologically through vaccination with biological agents, thus rendering them resistant to a specific agent in the environment. (There are no general panaceas.) Host behavior leading to increased risk of a disease (and there are many such behavior patterns) can be altered through counseling with regard to risk, if the individual can be persuaded of the importance of behavior change. Clearly, the most effective prevention is accomplished when the host is completely passive in the prevention process (does not have to think or change), as when the local water system employs fluoridation. Unfortunately, such examples are rare.

With regard to causative agents, they may be either eliminated, reduced in concentration, or altered. Smallpox has been eliminated from the globe. A variety of public health measures make our water free of bacteria, and we have substituted less toxic materials for things like asbestos that were once widely used in dwellings.

Changes in the environment can be accomplished by removing the agents, the hosts, or both from a threatening environment, or by affecting or attenuating their interactions. Legislatures often attempt to change the environment—for example, by mandating smog control devices or other physical measures. However, policy decisions leading to legislative changes in the environment through the elimination of certain agents are often difficult to achieve. Many agents have very strong support from interest groups of their own—only consider the efforts of the tobacco industry or the National Rifle Association.

# Policy Questions for Prevention

As suggested in the initial section, this chapter will discuss issues related to prevention in our current health care system. First, What is worth doing? How do we know? A derivative of this question is, Who must be involved or responsible if prevention is to occur?

In the United States, other issues have clearly become of considerable policy importance. These relate to our concerns with costs and overall resource allocation. One of these is, Who shall pay (and how much)? What is it worth (to whom) to prevent $X$? As noted earlier, this is not a purely cognitive endeavor. Values are associated with prevention, thus the subquestion, Whose values shall prevail?

We shall pursue these questions, not in an encyclopedic fashion but by focusing on certain targets for prevention that illustrate the barriers faced by those concerned. These targets are infectious diseases in childhood, pulmonary and cardiovascular diseases associated with cigarette smoking, and deaths due to firearms. In each case, preventive procedures or maneuvers advocated for each will be listed, and potential barriers to their accomplishments will also be reviewed. To do this, let us go back to the literature.

## What Do We Know and How Do We Know It?

The 1979 Surgeon General's Report listed one of the basic objectives as "surveillance and evaluation." Two years later, the Centers for Disease Control and Prevention (CDC), in collaboration with state health departments, initiated an ongoing system of telephone surveys designed to provide data on the prevalence of certain behaviors at a state level, to track the progress of programs designed to affect health behaviors.

In 1982, twenty-five state health departments conducted telephone surveys using CDC training and standardization methods.[13] In 1984, these activities evolved into the Behavioral Risk Factor Surveillance System (BRFSS), which was also designed to support major public health initiatives in prevention, such as legislation concerning cigarette taxation and mandatory seat belts. The system employs the Waksberg Method of random-digit dialing and a multistage cluster design to select random samples of noninstitutionalized adults for telephone interviews. Two sets of questions are asked: a core set of questions asked by all states, including standardized questions developed by the CDC, and a set of whatever questions the individual states develop to meet specific objectives.

The BRFSS provides estimates of a variety of important measures in the adult population, including prevalence of being overweight, leading a sedentary lifestyle, smoking, or avoiding seat belts. For weight, the survey used the Body Mass Index (BMI), defined as weight in kilograms divided by height in meters squared. In 1988, BRFSS data indicated that 20.9 percent of the population exceeded the recommended BMI for their age. Sedentary life-style was defined as fewer than three sessions per week of twenty minutes or more leisure physical activity; here the average was 58 percent. Cigarette smoking got a 24.7 percent yes rate, and seat belt nonuse got 30.1 percent. Several other factors were also queried, but this is enough for present purposes.[14] Data are reported by age group and gender; those cited in this paragraph are for the entire adult population of the United States.

A considerable volume of literature exists on what should be done, presenting evidence to support these recommendations. To examine this in one volume, the reader is referred to *A Guide to Clinical Preventive Services*.[15] This guide reviews the evidence on more than a hundred interventions to prevent sixty different illnesses and conditions. The latter are grouped as in a traditional medically oriented systems review. There are also chapters on counseling and immunizations. Each chapter cites the relevant literature available at the time of publication leading to a specific recommendation.

As indicated, the appointment of the task force was preceded by *Healthy People* (1979), which provides a litany of the health problems affecting the U.S. population. Subsequently, a series of similar reports (*Healthy People 1990* and *Healthy People 2000*) has marked our progress (or, in many cases, lack thereof) toward the goals. In each of these reports, a voluminous literature is cited.[16]

The latest version of this prescriptive effort is part of an initiative, Put Prevention into Practice (PPIP), announced in fall 1994 by the Secretary of Health and Human Services, Donna Shalala. The centerpiece of this effort is the *Clinician's Handbook of Preventive Services*.[17] It is divided into sections covering preventive services for children and adolescents, adults, and older adults, with appendices that include risk factor tables. The PPIP Kit includes the handbook *A Personal Health Guide,* designed to help people work with their doctors and other health care providers. It provides a reminder of recommended immunizations and screening tests, as well as spaces for recording the dates on which interventions are provided. In addition, the PPIP Kit includes reminder stickers for appointments, flow charts for office use, and other tools that have been shown to facilitate the provision of preventive services.

In addition to the BRFSS data on self-reported risk factors, the National Health Interview Survey (NHIS) provides data on the prevalence of abnormal physical, mental, and (recently) social health disturbances as determined by laboratory and clinical examination. NHIS tracks hypertension, body mass, anthropomorphic measurements, and serum cholesterol, all done in the field.

The extrapolation of these data to the United States population requires that clinical and laboratory examinations be performed by special teams of examiners on individuals carefully selected from the U.S. population in surveys designed by epidemiologists and statisticians. As suggested, both types of surveys involve random samples of the U.S. population, stratified in such a way as to permit estimates with stated confidence limits.

The United States Public Health Service (USPHS) has a long history of providing such population-based data. Initially, this was done by the free-standing National Center of Health and Vital Statistics, and that agency has continued to report such data following its administrative transfer to the CDC.[18] This transfer has not diminished the quality of its efforts. Also, the *Morbidity and Mortality Weekly Reports (MMWR)* of the CDC are a rich source of summaries of these data from surveillance and evaluation activities conducted by the federal government.[19]

## Community-Oriented Prevention

The majority of descriptive or analytical studies dealing with the efficacy of an intervention are based upon the study of individuals where an intervention, *X,* is provided by *Y* (where *X* and *Y* are highly specified). However, in the past two decades there has been an increase in the number of studies concerned with the possibility of applying a public health model to prevention; that is, a community intervention as it relates to the prevention of specific diseases (or the reduction in risks in the population related to those diseases). In addition to offering mass screening or immunization campaigns, these provide an intervention through the mass media and campaigns involving various civic and employer groups. These studies have, in general, shown some positive impact, but have not provided the level of change anticipated.[20] As a result, they have begged the question for policy makers: How should we invest or divide our resources—via community efforts or individualized clinical intervention? A recent editorial headed "Tribulations and Trials—Intervention in Communities"[21] appeared with two reports of the results of the Take Heart and COMMIT (smoking cessation) community trials. The Take Heart effort produced nothing but null results; the COMMIT trial had one modest, positive outcome.

In addition to the previously described efforts to provide preventive services in the public and private sectors, many private corporations have discovered the commercial benefits of organizing preventive services for their employees. Studies have shown such activities (exercise facilities at work, stress reduction classes, smoking cessation programs) result in reduced absenteeism, higher employee morale, and increased productivity.[22]

While the process of the review of scientific experimentation extends the frontiers of knowledge about prevention, it is based on available studies. It is likely that certain studies that would be important to policy makers will never be done because of the ethical consequences of the randomization of populations (specifically the disadvantaged) to treatment and control groups and the costs of some longitudinal studies. An example of this was reported by Lewis and colleagues in a recent report of the termination of a randomized controlled trial of asthma education for poor Latino children.[23]

## Three Examples of Prevention

Following are three examples of preventive practices, concerning infectious diseases in children, smoking, and gunshot wounds.

### Example 1: Prevention of Infectious Diseases in Childhood

Immunization is one of the greatest triumphs of science in the prevention of disease. It is now possible to protect children from almost all nonviral infections of early childhood. Mass vaccination programs have resulted in declines exceeding 97 percent in the incidence of diphtheria, mumps, measles, polio, and rubella. This is not the same as eradication, however, and the potential still exists for epidemics among nonprotected children.

Eighteen separate objectives for childhood immunization were set forth in the *1990 Health Objectives*. Some were rather rigorous: nationally, fewer than five hundred cases of measles, fewer than one thousand cases of mumps, and fewer than one thousand cases of pertussis. All of these seem unlikely to be achieved.[24] Most localized epidemics of measles have been traced to populations of unimmunized immigrant children or inadequately immunized teenagers.[25] In some instances, measles has been imported into the United States by those initiating these epidemics.[26] Similarly, the goal for a reduction in cases of tetanus will not be achieved; a significant proportion of cases occurs among adults over fifty years of age who were never protected or whose protection has lapsed.[27]

However, recent programs such as the Vaccine for Children Program, which is part of the Childhood Immunization Initiative (CII), has made immunizing agents available free in a variety of health care settings.[28]

Recently, the Immunization Practices Committee of the Public Health Service has added Hemophilus Influenza B (HIB) and Hepatitis B due to a virus (Hep B) to the list of recommended immunizations for this age group.[29] The current goal of CII is to increase, by 1996, the vaccination levels among children under two years of age to the coverage of 90 percent of children having the following: one dose of measles/rubella vaccine, three doses of diphtheria/tetanus and pertussis (DPT), three doses of oral polio vaccine, three to four doses of HIB vaccine, and three doses of Hep B vaccine.

In 1993, the NHIS indicated only 16 percent of children under thirty-five months of age had received the three doses of Hep B, while 88.2 percent had received three doses of DPT.[30] These aggregate data disguise major differences in socioeconomic groups. For example, among children from families with income below the poverty level, only 80.6 percent had received three doses of DPT, compared to 90.8 percent of those at or above this income level. The data also fail to reveal racial/ethnic differences—in Los Angeles, for example, 42 percent of Hispanic children were fully vaccinated by two years, compared to 25 percent of African Americans, despite the fact that the Hispanic families had lower annual incomes and less education.

This adds to the literature that suggests reducing financial barriers to access to preventive and other services does not solve the problem.[31] While the levels of immunization among certain groups of society must be improved, professionals are aware of immunization requirements. A surveillance system is in place. However, despite efforts to improve the availability of services, risks of infection still exist in certain subgroups. Nevertheless, while these diseases produce temporary disability, they seldom kill under modern conditions—in 1992, there were only twenty-seven deaths reported from measles in the United States.[32] Having achieved certain objectives, what more can we do? How many of our resources should be placed in this specific effort?

## Example 2: Prevention of Cardiopulmonary Diseases Attributable to Cigarette Smoking

The impact of cigarette smoking on health status is enormous. It is the primary cause of premature death in the United States.[33] Since the initial Surgeon General's report on smoking over thirty years ago,[34] people in the United States, as a group, have been gradually withdrawing from the addiction to nicotine produced by smoking. The CDC has developed software to estimate the smoking-attributable mortality of any population group, and to project years of life lost due to smoking.[35]

A variety of efforts have been mounted over the past thirty years to reduce the prevalence of smoking. Something is working, but slowly. The prevalence of smoking has fallen 0.5 percent per year over the period 1965–1985 and, more drastically, 1.1 percent per year, for the period 1986–1989. However, the most recent data suggest the prevalence of smoking among adolescents is increasing.[36]

Prevention efforts to reduce the unnecessary carnage attributable to tobacco use have followed the four objectives originally defined in 1979:

- *Increase awareness.* Recent studies indicate a growing awareness of the risks associated with smoking, especially amongst physicians.[37]
- *Monitor results.* Surveillance and evaluation systems are in place, including a "Teenage Attitudes Toward Smoking" system.[38]
- *Reduce risk factors.* Risk factor reduction is occurring with the decreasing prevalence of smoking.
- *Improve service.* Service improvement is represented by increased attention to the problem in all health care settings.

About 25 percent of all adults are still addicted smokers. The prevalence of smoking is inversely associated with years of education. Among those with twelve or fewer years of education, 32 percent are smokers versus 13.6 percent of those with sixteen or more years of education.[39]

A variety of programs have been designed to target the young, including legislation prohibiting the sale of cigarettes to minors from vending machines in forty-four states. A growing number of public places, restaurants, and workplaces have been declared no-smoking zones by local or state ordinances. The number of places where one can conveniently light up is shrinking. One U.S. airline recently declared that *all* its flights, including international ones, would be non-smoking.[40]

Other proposed efforts, such as increases in the taxes imposed on cigarettes, are gaining support. Recent hearings involving the Food and Drug Administration (FDA) and tobacco manufacturers have revealed a promising strategy.[41] Manufacturers have been accused of spiking their cigarettes with extra nicotine to enhance their addictive capacity. If cigarettes were to be considered a drug because of the presence of nicotine, they would fall within the jurisdiction of the FDA and thus be subject to regulation.

Despite these consumer-oriented prevention programs, there have been fewer serious attempts to affect the providers or growers of the agent (tobacco). The tobacco industry is large and powerful; growing the agent also represents the only means of economic survival for many farmers.

Given the slow reduction in the prevalence of smoking and the many programs designed to prevent teenagers from becoming addicted, the United States needs to address a major question. We seem to have reached a point where further reduction in tobacco consumption, especially among the young, is difficult to achieve. This begs the question, Should we continue to devote all efforts to reducing tobacco consumption while ignoring or even encouraging tobacco production? How much would it cost to buy out those commercial interests who currently work to maintain a cadre of nicotine-addicted individuals doomed to suffer the morbidity and mortality associated with their habit? How do we compare the relative value of twenty-seven deaths per year from measles to four hundred thousand deaths per year from tobacco-related disease?

## Example 3: Deaths Due to Gunshot Wounds

The magnitude of this problem has been described in many publications. Since 1960, more than five hundred thousand people in the United States have died from firearm injuries.[42] It is labeled a problem because it involves one common agent—the availability of a gun, usually a handgun—that binds together a heterogeneous group of specific disorders. However, as with the treatment of a medical symptom, such as a headache, it is necessary to establish a diagnosis (in this case, to define more clearly the problem) before prescribing a treatment or preventive intervention. The total of over thirty-one thousand deaths due to gunshot wounds reported in 1990 includes about nineteen thousand cases of suicide—over 60 percent. Another two thousand were accidental deaths, mainly children who discovered a loaded gun unsafely stored and killed themselves, and over eleven thousand were cases of homicide. Of the latter, most shootings (52 percent) were not done in the course of a crime; they were done by acquaintances or relatives of the victim as a result of escalating interpersonal conflict.[43]

As suggested, each shooting occurs because of the availability of a gun, and each case generates its own group of survivors who seek to prevent another similar episode (although the root cause is quite different). One of the main problems faced by all these advocacy groups of survivors is that the use of guns has been associated in the media with crime, when in fact, shootings associated with felonies represent only a fraction of all deaths due to guns.[44]

The history of efforts to regulate guns in the United States is a comedy with tragic results. This includes federal initiatives (now under the purview of the Bureau of Alcohol, Tobacco and Firearms) and a variety of community and state laws that have done little to stem the proliferation of handguns in the United States. It is estimated that there are currently two hundred million working firearms owned by U.S. citizens.[45]

## A Comparison

The problems created by tobacco are secondary to the effects of inhaled smoke and the development of a physical dependence due to addiction to nicotine. The problems associated with the existence of handguns are secondary to a psychological and cultural dependence—a need fostered by popular myths.

Both tobacco and handgun use are supported by large lobbying forces that have, to date, outsmarted governmental public health groups. For example, in 1994, the California Legislature passed 1,349 new laws; at least five specifically relate to gun control. These laws prohibit gun sales to minors, prohibit sale of ammunition to anyone under eighteen years of age, require gun dealers to make records of their sales available to law enforcement officials, prohibit anyone under a restraining order for domestic violence from owning a gun while the order is in effect, and suspend a minor's driver's license if the minor is apprehended for motor vehicle violations while carrying a concealed weapon.[46] All chip away at the central issue—the existence and ready availability of guns. All fail to recognize that the epidemic of homicide—the primary cause of death among African American young men—has grown with the availability of guns to this population. Those who have studied this subject feel these agents *must* be eliminated from the environment.[47] All the existing laws (such as the Brady Bill) are primarily focused on changing the environment to make guns harder to obtain, not on removing guns already in private hands. This could have some effect—a waiting period *may* reduce the number of suicides from gunshot wounds among those who do not have ready access to firearms at the peak of their depression—but barely touches the main issue.

The popular image of the usefulness of guns in self-protection against criminals is furthered by the advertising practices of gun manufacturers. They clearly have recognized the importance of creating a new market by suggesting in advertisements the value of handguns in self-protection among women. A recent study of trauma center workers in Alabama revealed that 74 percent of women (mostly nurses) employed in these centers owned a gun, and 45 percent carried loaded guns in their cars.[48]

What are the options for policy makers? Do they understand the epidemiology of firearm deaths? How will they limit the number of guns in the United States in the face of a strong constituency that believes ownership of guns is a right provided by the Second Amendment to the Constitution. Perhaps in no other area of prevention are values so evident and so powerful. Our inaction suggests that we do not understand, or we do not care, or both. How can policy makers introduce rationality into this discussion?

# Conclusion

Our three examples have one thing in common; all are due to agents—infectious, chemical, or physical. In the first instance, science has produced preventive measures (vaccines) that are socially acceptable; only a small segment of the population is unaware of or does not use or value these measures. The other two examples are different: one is associated with chemical addiction to nicotine, and the other is a product of cultural dependence. Both have powerful lobbies that have sought to confuse the public. One of them (smoking) is slowly being reduced at great public expense. The third is still called a symptom by those who deny that the real problem is the agent itself. One can only remember the *Surgeon General's Report* of 1979, noting that public and professional awareness and surveillance and evaluation must precede the reduction in risk factors and the improvement of services.

Where should we invest? It seems clear that among these three examples, *values* (confounded with economic interests), not lack of knowledge, are the primary obstacles in two. Policy makers reviewing other targets for prevention listed in *Healthy People 2000* should count the number for which we know what to do but fail to do. Answers to the second question—What *can* we do?—reveal how many health problems are not preventable because of our inability to apply existing knowledge. Finally, when we examine our values, we find the cause for our limitations.

# Notes

1. J. Schouten (ed.), *The Rod and the Serpent of Aesculapius, Symbol of Medicine* (New York: Elsevier, 1969), p. 260.

2. M. Susser, "The Bell Tolls for a School of Public Health—And for Thee?" (editorial), *American Journal of Public Health* 83, 11 (1993): 1524–1525.

3. M. H. Becker (ed.), *The Health Belief Model and Personal Health Behavior* (Thorofare, N.J.: Slack, 1974).

4. G. Lupin, J. Magyar, and M. Poulsen (eds.), *Proceedings Fourth Interdisciplinary Seminar: Piagetian Theory and the Helping Professionals* (Los Angeles: University of Southern California, February 15, 1974).

5. C. E. Lewis, "The Untimely Death of Preventive Medicine: The 1988 Duncan Clark Lecture," *American Journal of Preventive Medicine* 5, 1 (1988): 52–54.

6. E. Cook, *The Life of Florence Nightingale,* vol. 1 (London: Macmillan, 1913), pp. 1820–1861.

7. Council on Scientific Affairs, "Medical Evaluations of Healthy Persons," *Journal of the American Medical Association* 249 (1983): 1626–1633.

8. La Londe Commission, *A New Perspective on the Health of Canadians* (Ottawa, Canada: Minister of Health and Welfare, April 1975).

9. Public Health Service, *Healthy People: The Surgeon General's Report on Health Promotion and Disease Prevention,* DHEW-PHS Pub. No. 79–55071 (Washington, D.C.: U.S. Department of Health, Education and Welfare, 1979).

10. U.S. Preventive Services Task Force, *A Guide to Clinical Preventive Services: An Assessment of the Effectiveness of 169 Interventions* (Baltimore, Md.: Williams & Wilkins, 1989).

11. U.S. Preventive Services Task Force, *A Guide to Clinical Preventive Services.*

12. A. D. Giorci and M. L. Weisfeld, "Acute Myocardial Infarction," in *The Principles and Practices of Medicine,* eds. A. M. Harvey, R. J. Johns, V. A. McKusick, A. H. Owens, and R. S. Ross (East Norwalk, Conn.: Appleton & Lange, 1988), pp. 99–110.

13. "CDC—The Behavioral Risk Factor Surveillance, 1994" *MMWR* 39, 552 Surveillance Seminar (June, 1990): pp. 1–22.

14. "CDC—The Behavioral Risk Factor Surveillance, 1994" *MMWR.*

15. U.S. Preventive Services Task Force, *A Guide to Clinical Preventive Services.*

16. U.S. Department of Health and Human Services, Public Health Service, Office of Disease Prevention and Health Promotion, *Prevention, 1989–1990: Federal Programs in Progress* (Washington, D.C.: U.S. Government Printing Office, 1990); and U.S. Department of Health and Human Services, Public Health Service, Office of Disease Prevention and Health Promotion *Prevention, 1991–1992: Federal Programs in Progress* (Washington, D.C.: U.S. Government Printing Office, 1992).

17. U.S. Department of Health and Human Services, Public Health Service, Office of Disease Prevention and Health Promotion, *Clinician's Handbook of Preventive Services* (Washington, D.C.: U.S. Government Printing Office, 1994).

18. "Centers for Disease Control: The Nation's Prevention Agency," *MMWR* 41 (November 6, 1992): 833.

19. Centers for Disease Control, *Mortality and Morbidity Weekly Reports.* These reports are published by the Massachusetts Medical Society, Waltham, Massachusetts.

20. J. F. Farquhar, P. D. Wood, H. Bretrose, et al., "Community Education for Cardiovascular Health," *Lancet* (1977): pp. 1192–1195.

21. M. Susser, "Tribulations and Trials—Intervention in Communities," *American Journal of Public Health* 85 (1995): 156–158.

22. R. C. Jones, J. L. Gly, and J. E. Richardson, "A Study of a Worksite Health Promotion Program and Absenteeism," *Journal of Occupational Medicine* 32 (1990): 95–99.

23. M. A. Lewis, G. Rachelefsky, C. E. Lewis, et al., "The Termination of a Randomized Clinical Trial for Poor Hispanic Children," *Archives of Pediatric and Adolescent Medicine* 148 (1994): 364–367.

24. U.S. Department of Health and Human Services, Public Health Service, Office of Disease Prevention and Health Promotion, *1990 Health Objectives for the Nation: A Midcourse Review* (Washington, D.C.: U.S. Government Printing Office, November, 1986).

25. "Assessment of Under-Vaccinated Children Following a Mass Vaccination Campaign," *MMWR* (August 12, 1994): 572–574.

26. "Measles in the United States—The First 26 Weeks," *MMWR* (September 23, 1994): pp. 673–676.

27. "Tetanus—Kansas, 1993," *MMWR* (May 6, 1994): pp. 309–311.

28. "Vaccination Coverage of Two-Year-Old Children—The United States, 1992–1993," *MMWR* (April 22, 1994): pp. 282–283.

29. "Standards for Pediatric Immunization Practices," *MMWR* RR5 (April 23, 1993): 1–13. Note that these standards were recommended by the National Vaccine Advisory Committee and approved by the U.S. Public Health Service.

30. "Vaccination Coverage of Two-Year-Old Children—United States, 1993," *MMWR* 43 (October 7, 1994): 705–708.

31. S. J. Katz and T. P. Hofer, "Socioeconomic Disparities in Preventive Care Persist Despite Universal Coverage—Breast and Cervical Cancer Screening in Ontario and the United States," *JAMA* 272 (1994): 530–534.

32. "Summary of Notifiable Diseases—United States, 1993," *MMWR* 42 (October 21, 1993): 53.

33. "Cigarette Smoking Among Adults—United States, 1991," *MMWR* 42 (April 12, 1993): 230–233.

34. U.S. Department of Health, Education, and Welfare, Public Health Service, *Smoking and Health: Report of the Advisory Committee to the Surgeon General,* PHS Report 641103 (Washington, D.C.: U.S. Government Printing Office, 1964).

35. "Cigarette Smoking Among Adults—United States," *MMWR.*

36. U.S. Department of Health and Human Services, *Health United States, 1994,* DHHS Pub. No. (PHS) 95–1232 (Hyattsville, MD.: U.S. Department of Health and Human Services, Public Health Service, CDC, 1995).

37. "Smoking Control Among Health Care Workers: World No-Tobacco Day," *MMWR* 42 (May 21, 1993): 365–367.

38. "Changes in the Cigarette Brand Preferences of Adolescent Smokers—United States, 1989–1993," *MMWR* 43 (August 19, 1994): 577–581.

39. "Cigarette Smoking Among Adults in the United States—1992, and Changes in the Definition of Current Cigarette Smoking," *MMWR* (May 20, 1994): 42–47.

40. Delta Airlines Television Commercial, January 1995.

41. David A. Kessler, Commissioner on Food and Drugs, statement on nicotine-containing cigarettes to the House Committee on Health and the Environment, Washington, D.C., March 25, 1994, as reported by CBS News.

42. G. C. Wintemute, "Firearms as a Cause of Death in the United States: 1920–1982," *Journal of Trauma* 27 (1987).

43. J. Sugarman and K. C. Rand, *Cease Fire: A Comprehensive Strategy to Reduce Firearms Violence* (Washington, D.C.: Violence Policy Center, 1994).

44. Sugarman and Rand, *Cease Fire.*

45. G. Wintemute (ed.), *Ring of Fire—The Handgun Makers of Southern California* (Sacramento, Calif.: Violence Prevention Research Program, 1994).

46. "California Laws, '95," *Los Angeles Times* ( January 12, 1995): sec. 2A.

47. S. P. Teret and G. C. Wintemute, "Policies to Prevent Firearm Injuries," *Health Affairs* (Winter 1993): pp. 96–107.

48. C. A. Fargason and C. Johnston, "Gun Safety Practices of Trauma Center Workers in a Southern City," *Southern Medical Journal* 4, 87 (1994): pp. 964–970.

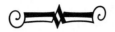

CHAPTER SEVENTEEN

# PUBLIC HEALTH AND PERSONAL HEALTH SERVICES

Lester Breslow and Jonathan E. Fielding

In our current effort to reform the organization, delivery, and financing of what is commonly called health care but which is more aptly described as personal health services or medical care, the broad questions of how providers of these services contribute to the public health goals for our country receive little consideration. Most of the debate about personal health services has focused on how to control the enormous and continually escalating costs of medical, hospital, and other services, and how to overcome the access barriers that arise due to lack of health benefits, inadequate ability to receive needed care, discrimination, poor distribution of providers, and other problems. In deciding how these medical care system problems should be addressed, what is the role, if any, of public health agencies?

Neglect of that question probably derives from the common view that public health is concerned only with disease control by such means as environmental measures, immunization, and health education. The purpose of this chapter is to delineate the appropriate roles for public health in the personal health services system.

For perspective on that role, it may be useful to start with public health's mission. According to the Institute of Medicine, National Academy of Sciences, that mission is "fulfilling society's interest in assuring conditions in which people can be healthy."[1] Public health thus concerns itself with the health of the entire population and how that may be enhanced by improving the health-related conditions in which people live. Public health efforts are directed at modifying three kinds of conditions that can contribute to population health: environmental, behavioral, and medical.

The environment, the physical aspects of people's surroundings, profoundly affects their health. The well-known impact of working conditions, food handling, and exposure to fluoride—among myriad other living circumstances—illustrates that point. Therefore, from its outset, public health has directed substantial effort toward assuring a safe environment, at first mainly focused on microbial threats to health but increasingly aimed more broadly at the whole physical milieu.

With the twentieth-century transition from communicable to noncommunicable diseases as the predominant health problem, evidence has grown that people's behavior—for example, with respect to tobacco and alcohol—largely determines the time and disease mechanisms of death. The Public Health Service has estimated that half of the premature deaths in the United States are due to the choices that people make in their everyday activities.[2] McGinnis and Foege, in explicating the actual causes of death rather than the disease mechanisms involved, assert that almost two-fifths of deaths are attributable to tobacco, diet and activity patterns, and alcohol.[3] Table 17.1 sets out their conclusions concerning 46 percent of all causes of death in the United States.

The third condition that contributes to health, besides environmental and behavioral influences, is the availability and quality of personal health services, that is, medical care. Extensive achievements in that field during recent decades—in

## TABLE 17.1. ACTUAL CAUSES OF DEATH IN THE UNITED STATES, 1990.

| Cause | Estimated Number | Percentage of Total Deaths |
|-------|------------------|----------------------------|
| Tobacco | 400,000 | 19 |
| Diet/activity patterns | 300,000 | 14 |
| Alcohol | 100,000 | 5 |
| Toxic agents | 60,000 | 3 |
| Firearms | 35,000 | 2 |
| Sexual behavior | 30,000 | 1 |
| Motor vehicles | 25,000 | 1 |
| Illicit use of drugs | 20,000 | <1 |
| Total | 970,000 | 46 |

*Source:* J. Michael McGinnis and William H. Foege, "Actual Causes of Death in the United States," *Journal of the American Medical Association* 270 (1993): 2208. Reprinted by permission.

surgery, biochemistry, radiation, and related medical sciences—have increased the possibility of longer and healthier lives. The dramatic impact that these achievements sometimes make on individual situations, however, creates a tendency to overestimate their overall health significance. Bunker and colleagues attribute only five years of the thirty-year increase in life expectancy of U.S. residents during this century to the work of the medical care system.[4]

Public health has generally operated inconspicuously, identifying and implementing means to improve all three kinds of conditions that can advance health and incorporating those advances into the context of life. Credit is rarely given for what has been accomplished through public health initiatives. Thus, we take for granted that water from the tap is safe to drink and, more recently, that automobiles have seat belts and public buildings are largely smoke free.

Given public health's history and orientation, what are appropriate public health roles related to personal health services? Reasons for involvement may be summarized as follows:

- Public health measures are becoming increasingly effective as a means of improving health.
- Substantial proportions of the population either do not have access to personal health services under current arrangements or may lose access with changes in living circumstances such as job moves.
- Much of the available personal health service suffers from deficiencies in quality.
- The recent spiral in medical care costs has absorbed a disproportionate share of the social resources that can be made available for all health activities, thus reducing the amount available for public health services.

Thus, examining public health's role in personal health services has become important. However the balance among the various means for achieving and maintaining health may be corrected, the question of how public health agencies should relate to personal health service remains.

## Public Providers of Personal Health Services

Public health departments, of course, have long administered certain personal health services aimed toward health promotion and disease prevention, such as prenatal care and childhood immunization. They have often provided such services directly, particularly for those segments of the population that the private health care system seldom reaches effectively. In addition, they have helped mobilize resources such as clinicians in the community for this purpose. Also, in many states and communities, public health departments have assumed responsibility for a broader array of personal health services for people with low incomes. For example, some departments carry responsibility for Medicaid and local indigent care programs. In fact, the latter duty has in some jurisdictions become so burdensome that it jeopardizes the conduct of other activities with a potentially greater impact on health.

Historically, involvement in personal health services emerged initially as a critical aspect of public health's original task, communicable disease control. During the early part of the century, when the struggle against infectious diseases extended beyond environmental action to include developing personal immunity in individuals, health departments undertook mass smallpox vaccinations and subsequently other immunizations. More substantial engagement in personal health services by public health expanded with maternal and child health activities during the 1920s, based on the growing conviction that such services could reduce the excessively high maternal and infant death rates recognized as prevailing at that time. Then came certain diagnostic procedures, especially as technology for communicable disease control advanced. For example, tuberculin testing of tuberculosis patients' contacts and x-raying positive reactors became an accepted public health practice. Further, health department laboratories offered communicable disease diagnostic services to physicians in their communities. Subsequently, these expanded into other realms such as screening for diseases due to congenital and environmental causes.

Advances in clinical science and corresponding improvements in medical care necessitate greater public health attention to them as a means of improving health. Widespread recognition of their potential for protecting and enhancing health has led to establishing large-scale public programs of medical care for people identified as having an unmet personal health service need, filling substantial gaps in the delivery system.[5] In other cases, this lack of availability of health care in defined populations has been met by providing payment for personal health services to individuals meeting specific eligibility requirements, as in Medicaid programs. In addition, the government may provide financial incentives for private organizations to finance or provide care to populations unable to afford it. The traditional tax-exempt status of nonprofit organizations and voluntary private hospitals requires that they use some of their resources to meet the health care needs of the poor.

In 1992, about 8 percent of all hospital beds in the United States were under federal auspices, 70 percent of these under the Department of Veterans Affairs. In that year, this department operated 171 medical centers, 128 nursing units, 35 domiciliary care units, and 191 outpatient clinics and other outpatient facilities. Inpatient services were provided to 1,053,238 inpatients, and there were 22,788,431 outpatient visits. The agency employed 204,489 full-time equivalent employees and the total federal government cost (called *obligations*) of operating the system was $14 billion.[6]

The Indian Health Service as of 1993 was operating or funding the operation by Indian tribal government of 52 hospitals, 282 health centers and stations, and 179 other types of ambulatory care units. In fiscal 1992, it provided 93,000 hospital admissions: 71,000 directly through its own facilities and 22,000 through contracts with community hospitals. It also provided 5.7 million outpatient visits (almost all in its own facilities). These health care operations were almost entirely paid for by a $1.4 billion 1992 federal appropriation for providing care to approximately 1.3 million Indians and Alaskan natives.[7]

A third federal government-run health delivery system is the Armed Forces Medical System, which included more than 160 hospitals and clinics at a cost of over $5 billion.[8]

States have traditionally directly supported and provided hospital care for patients with conditions that the private sector preferred to avoid, such as patients with tuberculosis and mental illness. As of 1992, 274 state hospitals with 125,000 beds were still providing (mostly long-term) care mainly to the mentally ill, despite the massive deinstitutionalization that has significantly contributed to increased homelessness around the country. The average total daily census in fiscal 1992 was 107,000 patients.[9]

Local government maintained 1,332 hospitals in 1992 with a total number of 146,000 beds. These were mostly for acute care and served an average daily census of 101,000 patients. These facilities constituted 55 percent of all government hospitals and about one-eighth of all hospitals in the United States. They were vastly underfunded and generally in poor physical condition and understaffed. Services were largely limited to emergency, secondary, and tertiary care, in response to the visibly most urgent needs of those without other access to personal health care services.[10]

These institutions often link with medical schools, with medical school faculty directing care in exchange for the opportunity to train medical students, residents, and fellows.

## Core Public Health Responsibilities

While the public health care system delivers substantial amounts of care, particularly for the economically disadvantaged and the chronic severely mentally ill and developmentally delayed, this role is not necessarily central to the broad public health mission. In fact, local fiscal authorities have often diverted what resources are appropriated for public health core functions into personal health services for the poor, usually secondary and tertiary services. This reflects the strain of 40 million people without health benefits, a number that has every likelihood of continued growth in the absence of national sentiment that health care should be the right of every citizen, and given the failure of national health reform in 1994. However, the other consequence of allocating money to what appears to be the most pressing priority—sick people without other sources of emergency medical services—is that these funds are not available for community-oriented prevention activities. Thus, public health has a diminished ability to respond to serious public health threats, such as the resurgence of tuberculosis and measles, or to AIDS, the greatest new health threat of the century.

The growing perception that our nation had lost sight of its public health goals, allowing the public health infrastructure to fall into disarray, led to the Institute of Medicine report cited earlier.[11] Defining the mission of public health as "assuring conditions in which people can be healthy," the report identified three principal core functions for public health: assessment, assurance, and policy development.

## Assessment

An indispensable role for each public health agency is to assess the opportunities to improve the health of the population in its area. In so doing, the public health agency needs sophistication in assessing the contributions of the various determinants of health to the population burden of ill-health. An essential initial step is to collect (directly or through analysis of external databases) a health and disease profile of the population. Traditionally, assessments have targeted the major causes of morbidity, mortality, and more recently, disability. In addition, health can be measured as a set of positive attributes based upon the more expansive definitions of health adopted by public health bodies nationally and internationally. In *Healthy People 2000: National Health Promotion and Disease Prevention Objectives*, this perspective on the meaning of health is well captured: "Health is . . . best measured by citizens' sense of well-being."[12] Health promotion is one of three categories under which priority areas are subsumed in that volume.

At the state and local levels, an ideal assessment would be to array the major causes of morbidity, disability, mortality, and lack of well-being for major segments of the population defined by age, gender, and geography and possibly also by race or ethnic identity. Traditionally, these have been arrayed by type of ill-health— cancer, heart disease, arthritis, and so on. However, as McGinnis and Foege have proposed, a possibly better way to consider health improvement opportunities is to focus on eight common factors (shown in Table 17.1) that underlie many of the most burdensome health conditions. At least seven of these eight factors have in common their ameliorability through individual behavior change.

In analogous fashion, how might we judge the potential contribution of health services to potential health improvement in the overall population of a defined area and in different population subgroups? The point of departure for such an exercise is determination of the percentage of the population variance in key health measures due to health services. As a hypothetical example, for acquired heart disease, health services might be found to account for 10 percent of the variance in mortality and disability rates. The next step would be to determine the characteristics of health service systems that are reproducibly associated with the best outcomes and with the worst outcomes.

To the degree possible, differences between the best and worst outcomes would be partitioned into problems of access to services, over- and underutilization of appropriate services, poor coordination of care, and poor technical quality of services. Although the development of databases that would permit this degree of problem definition is at an early stage for most health conditions, a substantial investment in quality indicators, practice guidelines, and outcomes measurement should in time provide sufficient tools for public health departments to assume leadership in assessment of the problems in the organization and delivery of personal health services by both private and public providers.

A related role is to identify the characteristics of populations that are not receiving adequate care by virtue of diminished access, poor quality of available services, or lack of financial resources. Traditionally, public health organizations have taken the lead in pointing out that there is a substantial segment of our population (40 million, including 10 million children) that do not have access to any organized source of continuing medical care or payment for such care.[13] These people are largely dependent on so-called emergency services that state and local governments may require local institutions to offer. In addition, many millions work in precarious job situations where they are at risk of both job loss and loss of health benefits provided by or through their employer. Although individuals losing their jobs can continue to receive the same health benefits under COBRA for up to eighteen months if their employer had twenty or more employees, many employees cannot afford to bear the entire cost and allow health benefits to lapse.

Public health agencies should become the most trusted source for information on unmet service needs, the nature of quality assurance practices utilized by providers, health outcomes, and the health status of different subpopulations within their territory. They should also systematically assess the degree of integration of health services with other government and private-sector services such as education, social services, and welfare.

Tools are available to help public health agencies in the overall assessment and planning process. APEX (Assessment Protocol for Excellence in Public Health) and PATCH (Planned Approach to Community Health) provide stepwise guides to assessing community health needs. While neither of these tools focuses primarily on personal health services, assessment of these needs can and should be built into an overall community assessment. APEX includes a three-stage process, with the last stage, policy development and assurance activities, intended to ensure implementation of the organizational action plan.[14] PATCH, developed by the Centers for Disease Control and Prevention as a community health promotion tool, also emphasizes community mobilization.[15] Many health departments are using *Healthy Communities 2000: Model Standards,* a guidebook to marrying the national objectives in *Healthy People 2000* with local needs and priorities.[16]

## Assurance

The Institute of Medicine report stressed "assurance . . . [to] constituents that services necessary to achieve agreed-upon goals are provided, either by encouraging actions by other entities (private or public sector), by requiring such action through regulation, or by providing services directly. [Public health agencies should involve] key policymakers and the general public in determining a set of high-priority personal and communitywide health services that governments will guarantee to every member of the community. This guarantee should include subsidization or direct provision of high-priority personal health services for those unable to afford them."[17]

Health assurance is a central function of public health. In proposing plans to improve the health of their populations, departments of public health should ensure that all groups have access to a minimum set of high-quality personal health care services. The plans should also set expectations for the performance of health care systems and health care providers.

The development of large managed care organizations with broad responsibility for the health care of a defined population of enrollees provides a natural point of leverage for assuring adequate performance of the health care system. Large managed care organizations are developing clinical data systems that generate databases amenable to analysis of outcomes of care and of the types of services provided to individuals and groups defined by disease (for example, adult onset diabetes mellitus), age group (for example, infants newborn to one year), income level, or geography. In addition, quality has become a basis for competition in the market for personal health services. Therefore, health department leadership should include helping to define the kinds of outcomes that organizations should be able to show based on best practices observed in the literature. Health departments have expertise in setting expectations for outcomes in clinical preventive services (such as age-specific immunization rates, mammography rates by age, and so on) and in monitoring these rates. However, monitoring the results of services provided when disease states are present is of equal importance. Thus, public health agencies should also participate in setting expectations for disease and procedure outcomes such as mortality rates for cardiovascular disease and complication rates for endoscopies or angioplasty. Further, they may suggest the specifications and dissemination plans for report cards that are increasingly required of health care providers, as these reports can identify problems with access and quality.

Most health departments currently have no jurisdiction over the organizations delivering comprehensive care except for licensing institutions and sometimes provider groups. In some areas, particularly large cities, health departments may also deliver clinical services—presenting a potential conflict of interest in setting standards or expectations for results. Nonetheless, there are existing levers that can be used to help assure good outcomes from the delivery of personal health care services. Health departments can help to establish local coalitions of private and public health benefit purchasers that set requirements for both services to be provided and the quality and service data that plans and providers must make available in standard formats. Health departments can also take the lead in disseminating information on what should be contained in a required core of preventive services,[18] such as those developed by the U.S. Preventive Services Task Force. They can also publicize the practice guidelines being developed through both public and private processes and can urge consumers to ask questions about outcomes, both in general and for conditions about which they are particularly concerned, before selecting choices under employer-sponsored health benefit plans.

Public health agencies should make it a central function to receive, analyze, and report on the results of quality assurance efforts in personal health services delivery. They can use their role as guardian of the public health to publicize both problems and progress to the public, as well as to inform providers and professional organizations about opportunities for improvements in efforts to assure both access and quality.

## Public Policy

A number of assurance functions are accomplished through informing the development of public policy. Some access, data, and quality assessment requirements are being incorporated into laws or administrative regulations. Public health, as an agent of the public with the responsibility of "fulfilling society's interest in assuring conditions in which people can be healthy,"[19] should be proactive in suggesting where and what regulation is appropriate and in commenting on proposals advanced by others.

An important public policy role is to underscore the large number of uninsured people and the continuing growth of this population. Policy makers need to be shown that the uninsured populations are much less likely to receive preventive care, to seek care for serious symptoms, to have continuing sources of care, and to have problems diagnosed at an early and more treatable stage. They need to understand that providing health benefits to the uninsured will be even more important as public systems to deliver health services atrophy under challenge from the private sector, reducing the availability of services for those who cannot afford to pay.

Identifying the opportunity to improve some health outcomes through broader health benefit coverage is part of a larger need to educate the public and policy makers on the key determinants of health and how different policy options can affect these factors. In this context, almost all careful studies of determinants of health have found that personal health care services make a difference in health, but this difference accounts for a small fraction of the variance in health among populations—overall and for specific health conditions. Determinants with generally larger contributions to variance include genetics, income distribution, social factors, environmental exposures, and health behaviors. Although health habits have received the most attention in recent years, the other contributors to common diseases also often display strong effect sizes. For example, in acquired cardiovascular disease, the degree of social isolation gives rise to risk gradients and effect sizes of about the same order of magnitude as behavioral risk factors.[20] For most disease categories, and certainly for quality of well-being, poverty is a quantitatively more important risk factor than access to health care services or the quality of those services in describing differences in health between populations. In addition, economic, community, social, and political factors are the primary contributors to major societal problems of ill-health such as child abuse, spousal abuse, other violence, and birth outcomes.

As part of their educational mission, public health departments can provide data that the current level of investment in health care services is disproportionate to their ability to alter the population burden of ill-health. Whether the data are used to argue for additional resources or for reallocation of existing resources to address the other causal factors, the rhetoric is not likely to strike a responsive chord unless health departments can make a convincing case about the types of investments that are likely to achieve greater societal returns. For example, would after-school programs for youth in areas of high risk for school dropout and gang membership be a better investment than a higher density of MRI machines or expanding preventive services under Medicare? Would a uniform home prenatal and postnatal home visiting program for lower-income pregnant women yield a better health return than routinely providing amniocentesis as a covered health benefit? Would a social marketing campaign to encourage youth to drink nonalcoholic beverages have more impact on alcoholism than more or better alcohol rehabilitation facilities?

While unequivocal answers are not available to most of these questions, the process of asking them could lead to a different type of policy analysis and a better balanced research agenda.

## Expertise and Capacity

What is the expertise and capacity of public health agencies at the state and local level to assume the set of responsibilities outlined above? The Institute of Medicine report and strong efforts by the Centers for Disease Control and Prevention, the American Public Health Association, and national and local health officer associations to define core public health functions have raised consciousness of the role public health should play in health promotion at the community level.[21] Barriers to assuming these central roles include restricted flexibility in use of funds (often channeled from categorical programs), mismatch of skills and interests between existing personnel and new priorities, and outside perception of a more limited role for public health agencies. For example, a survey of thirty-two health departments and districts in Washington State found that the self-assessed strengths of most were program management and direct provision of service. The departments and districts felt that most lacking were the assessment functions and utilization of data to guide community and program planning and policy.[22] If public health is to assure the health of populations, establishment of its expertise and credibility as the pathfinder organizer and lead planner must be accorded a high priority.

## Notes

1. Institute of Medicine, *The Future of Public Health* (Washington, D.C.: National Academy Press, 1988), p. 7.
2. U.S. Department of Health and Human Services, Public Health Service, *For a Healthy Nation: Returns on Investment in Public Health* (Washington, D.C.: U.S. Government Printing Office, 1994).
3. J. Michael McGinnis and William H. Foege, "Actual Causes of Death in the United States," *Journal of the American Medical Association* 270 (1993): 2207–2212.
4. John P. Bunker, Howard S. Frazier, and Frederick Mosteller, "Improving Health: Measuring Effects of Medical Care," *Milbank Quarterly* 72 (1994): 225–258.

5. Abdelmonem A. Afifi and Lester Breslow, "The Maturing Paradigm of Public Health," *Annual Review of Public Health* 15 (1994): 223–235.

6. U.S. Department of Veterans Affairs, *Annual Report of the Secretary of Veterans Affairs/Department of Veterans Affairs* (Washington, D.C.: U.S. Department of Veterans Affairs, 1994).

7. U.S. Department of Health and Human Services, Public Health Service, *Trends in Indian Health—1994* (Washington, D.C.: U.S. Department of Health and Human Services, 1994).

8. William Shonick, *Government and Health Services* (New York: Oxford University Press, 1995).

9. American Hospital Association, *Hospital Statistics, 1993–1994* (Chicago: American Hospital Association, 1995).

10. American Hospital Association, *Hospital Statistics, 1993–1994.*

11. Institute of Medicine, *The Future of Public Health*, p. 7.

12. U.S. Department of Health and Human Services, *Healthy People 2000: National Health Promotion and Disease Prevention Objectives*, DHHS Pub. No. (PHS) 91–50212 (Washington, D.C.: U.S. Government Printing Office, 1990), p. 6.

13. Fernando M. Trevino and Jeff P. Jacobs, "Public Health and Health Care Reform: The American Public Health Association's Perspective," *Journal of Health Policy* 15 (1994): 397–406; and U.S. Bureau of the Census, *March 1993 Current Population Survey* (Washington, D.C.: U.S. Government Printing Office, 1993).

14. National Association of County Health Officials, *Assessment Protocol for Excellence in Public Health (APEX/PH)* (Washington, D.C.: National Association of County Health Officials, 1991).

15. U.S. Department of Health and Human Services, Centers for Disease Control and Prevention, *Planned Approach to Community Health (PATCH)* (Atlanta, Ga.: Public Health Service, 1992).

16. American Public Health Association, *Healthy Communities 2000: Model Standards*, 3rd ed. (Washington, D.C.: American Public Health Association, 1991).

17. Institute of Medicine, *The Future of Public Health*, p. 8.

18. U.S. Preventive Services Task Force, *Guide to Clinical Preventive Services: An Assessment of the Effectiveness of 169 Interventions* (Baltimore, Md.: Williams & Wilkins, 1989).

19. Institute of Medicine, *The Future of Public Health*, p. 6.

20. Robert G. Evans, Morris L. Barer, and Theodore R. Marmor (eds.), *Why Are Some People Healthy and Others Not? The Determinants of Health of Populations* (Hawthorne, N.Y.: Aldine de Gruyter, 1944).

21. Mark W. Oberle, Edward L. Baker, and Mark J. Magenheim, "Healthy People 2000 and Community Health Planning," *Annual Review of Public Health* 15 (1994): 259–275.

22. Oberle, Baker and Magenheim, "Healthy People 2000," p. 270.

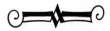

CHAPTER EIGHTEEN

# THE CONTINUING ISSUE OF MEDICAL MALPRACTICE LIABILITY

Ruth Roemer

Part of the national debate on health care reform in 1994 involved the contentious issue of medical malpractice liability and the tort system for addressing it. Despite the failure of health care reform in the 103rd Congress, the issue of medical malpractice liability continues to provoke debate and alternative proposals for modifying the tort system for handling it. Several reasons make this issue an aspect of any major change in the health system, whether brought about by legislative or voluntary action. First is the charge that high medical malpractice insurance premiums and the practice of defensive medicine are major contributors to escalating health care costs. Second is the concern that changes in the health care system, particularly increased use of managed care, will compromise the quality of care and lead to increased medical malpractice litigation. Third is the long dissatisfaction with the tort system of handling medical malpractice for its failure to compensate many victims of malpractice and its failure to deter negligent practice.

With respect to the first allegation, the evidence does not support the charge that medical malpractice litigation is a major cause of the rising cost of health care. On average, physicians pay less than 4 percent of annual practice receipts for malpractice insurance. This represents less than 1 percent of total U.S. health expenditures and therefore cannot be a primary cause of the growth in expenditures.[1] With respect to the impact of defensive medicine, although some procedures may be unnecessary, others may be beneficial and part of cautious, conservative medical practice.[2] Moreover, some precautions may prevent mistakes, making the net economic impact of defensive medicine unclear.[3] The Office of Technology Assessment (OTA) concludes, "Overall, a small percentage of *diagnostic* procedures—certainly less than 8 percent—is likely to be caused primarily by *conscious* concern about malpractice liability."[4] Much of the increased spending on health care can more reasonably be explained by expanding and proliferating medical technology rather than by the practice of defensive medicine.[5]

With respect to the second allegation—that changes in the health care system, particularly use of managed care, will affect the quality of care adversely and lead to increased malpractice litigation—recent evidence is not available. We do not know whether individual physicians in health maintenance organizations and preferred provider organizations have any higher incidence of malpractice settlements or judgments against them than physicians in solo practice. Data from 1972 indicate that health maintenance organization (HMO) malpractice experience was comparable to that of the general community.[6] Some evidence, however, points to an increase in claims against health maintenance organizations due to cost containment measures.[7]

With the growth of managed care and the increase in capitation payment of physicians, the incentive for cost containment may well reduce the practice of defensive medicine, which, despite criticism, provides some protection against lawsuits.[8] Two other features of managed care plans raise the concern of increased liability for the physician, the health plan, or both. First, both managed care and the general contemporary medical climate create incentives to reduce unnecessary care. While managed care plans are developing organizational, financial, and clinical strategies to monitor the adequacy and quality of care, a question of liability may arise when the physician is following the plan's guidelines and an adverse outcome occurs. Secondly, the practice of primary care physicians is changing. The number of patients that each physician must see under managed care is increasing, with a consequent decrease in the time available for each patient visit. Moreover, a plan's restrictions on referral to specialists means that primary care physicians must see more patients and more varied types of illness before making a referral. Both these features of managed care put the physician at risk even in the absence of any negligence.[9] Advocates of enterprise liability, discussed below, see the risk for gatekeeper primary care physicians as justifying a shift in liability from the individual physician to the institution or the health plan.[10]

While these factors raise the possibility of an increase in medical malpractice claims under managed care, it is also possible that malpractice claims will decline under a health care system with increased managed care plans. Most malpractice claims arise out of hospital practice, where high-risk procedures are performed,[11] and health maintenance organizations have a lower rate of hospitalization than the national average because of their generous use of ambulatory care and prudent use of hospitalization. These factors may militate against an increase in malpractice claims involving HMOs and perhaps managed care plans generally.

The third concern is dissatisfaction with the tort system on the grounds that it costs too much; is an erratic, unpredictable, and inefficient method of compensating persons injured by substandard care; and fails to deter negligent practice.[12] Despite extensive state legislation designed to curb malpractice suits, the question is still unresolved as to whether the present tort system of handling medical malpractice liability meets the objectives of fairly and adequately compensating persons injured by substandard care and of deterring negligent practice.

To examine the options available for addressing the issues concerning the medical malpractice liability system, it may be helpful first to review the medical malpractice insurance crises of the 1970s and 1980s and their sequelae, looking at the causes of these crises, the state legislative responses that ensued, and evaluations of these legislative actions. Then, we turn to alternative proposals that have been advanced. Finally, some comments are offered on how best to compensate victims of substandard medical care and how best to deter negligent medical practice—a question that may become urgent with legislative or voluntary reform of the health system.

# Medical Malpractice Insurance Crises of the 1970s and 1980s

In the 1960s and early 1970s, the frequency and severity of medical malpractice claims increased dramatically. Claim frequency increased nationally at an average annual rate of 12.1 percent, and paid claim severity increased at a rate of 10.2 percent. In some states, the increases were even greater. In California, both frequency and severity increased between 1969 and 1974 at an average annual rate of nearly 20 percent.[13] Throughout the 1970s, awards rose at a rate in excess of the general rate of inflation and of the cost of medical care. Between 1970 and 1975, the average malpractice award increased from $11,518 to $26,565—an average annual rate increase of 18 percent. By 1978, the average award had increased to $45,187, representing a cumulative increase of 70 percent for the three years 1976–1978.[14]

Because of this escalation in numbers of malpractice claims filed and in the size of awards, the premiums for malpractice liability insurance rose astronomically, by as much as 500 percent in some states.[15] In 1974, several important insurers withdrew from the market.[16] Thus, the crisis of the 1970s was not because

large numbers of patients were injured but because of the breakdown in the malpractice insurance market.[17]

As a result, many physicians without adequate insurance coverage avoided
high-risk cases, limited their practices in other ways (for example, obstetrician-gynecologists limited their practices to office gynecology), withdrew from emergency
service or from practice altogether, or practiced without insurance coverage or
with lowered coverage.[18]

The problems with availability and affordability of malpractice insurance led
to the formation of compulsory pooling arrangements—joint underwriting associations—to compel insurers to provide insurance for malpractice as a condition of writing other insurance.[19] These joint underwriting associations were
formed to assure insurance coverage for physicians who could not obtain insurance, by requiring insurance companies offering property and casualty insurance
to underwrite insurance for a physician who could not obtain liability insurance.
Patient Compensation Funds, funded by a surcharge on all insurers, were established in nine states to settle catastrophic claims up to a certain limit. Some physicians formed their own insurance companies. These physician-owned firms
currently insure about 60 percent of U.S. physicians and are represented by the
Physicians Insurers Association of America.[20]

In response to this crisis, many states formed commissions to investigate and
report on the medical malpractice insurance crisis in their states. In nearly every
state, new statutes were enacted to restrain medical malpractice suits by restricting the scope of liability, limiting the size of awards, reducing the statute of limitations, limiting contingent fees of attorneys, and introducing pretrial screening
panels or arbitration to discourage frivolous suits.[21] These measures are discussed
below.

After 1976, the frequency of claims leveled off, but the severity of awards continued to increase.[22] By 1985, when the second malpractice insurance crisis occurred, rates for malpractice insurance premiums were again rising. From 1981
to 1986, malpractice insurance premiums rose 75 percent, according to the 1983
Physicians' Practice Costs and Income Survey and the 1986 Physicians' Practice
Follow-Up Survey.[23] Claim frequency was rising by more than 12 percent after the
increase in the 1970s that led to the 1975 crisis. Between 1975 and 1984, average
medical malpractice verdicts increased at nearly twice the rate of the consumer
price index. These events led a leading authority on medical malpractice to say,
"the fact that claim frequency and severity have continued to rise tends to confirm
that the reforms enacted in response to the last crisis did not radically change
the malpractice system."[24]

Causes of the medical malpractice insurance crises have been ascribed to
medical factors, legal factors, and insurance practices. The medical factors include

greater utilization of health services because of the enactment of Medicare and Medicaid and the growth of voluntary insurance; increased use of advanced medical technology with greater risks; and the fact that the practice of medicine is inherently a high-risk undertaking with a certain number of adverse outcomes, regardless of negligence. Also contributing to malpractice claims are heightened expectations on the part of consumers (the "every couple expects a perfect baby" syndrome) and changes in the doctor-patient relationship as medicine has become more highly specialized and technical, with resulting depersonalization of health services.[25]

Legal factors have also contributed to the increase in claims. Abolition or modification of the locality rule, making the acceptable standard of practice a state or national standard, tends to increase claims and make expert witnesses more available. The abolition of the charitable immunity rule that formerly insulated voluntary hospitals from suits was a factor that favored plaintiffs' suits. Another contributing factor was the expansion of the scope of informed consent, requiring a subjective scope of disclosure of the risks of a procedure as needed by a particular patient rather than the objective scope of disclosure provided by what a reasonably prudent physician practicing in the same or similar circumstances would disclose. Similarly, expansion of the doctrine of *respondeat superior,* which imposes responsibility on an employer for an employee's wrongdoing, contributed to claim increases. States that abolished or expanded the locality rule, abolished charitable immunity, and adopted broadened informed consent and *respondeat superior* doctrines were found to have claim costs twice as high as states that made none of these changes.[26]

Insurance experience and practices also contributed to the crisis. In the mid 1970s, a decline in the stock market reduced capital and earnings on the investments of the insurance companies. Since most companies wrote *occurrence* policies, that is, policies stating that the insurance company would be responsible for future claims as long as the incident on which the claim was based occurred in a year for which the insurance was purchased, insurance companies had to maintain large reserves in order to cover the *long tail* of future claims (the period from the occurrence of the incident to the eventual claim and its disposition). After the 1975 crisis, insurance companies generally wrote *claims made* policies, in which the physician was covered for the year for which the policy was written, leaving the long tail of uninsured liability for the physician.[27] To cover claims that arise after a claims made policy has expired, health care providers can purchase insurance known as *tail* coverage.[28] As a result of these experiences and practices, although insurance was available in the 1980s, it was more expensive and less coverage was provided, largely because of increasing loss payments, declining interest rates, and tightening of the reinsurance market and also because of increasing awards and uncertainty about the tort system.[29]

While the medical malpractice insurance crises created problems in the medical, legal, and insurance sectors of society, the main losers were consumers. The major part of the cost of these premium increases was paid neither by physicians nor by hospitals but was passed on to third-party payers as part of the cost of medical and hospital service.[30]

# State Legislative Reforms

Following the medical malpractice insurance crisis of the 1970s, most states enacted various laws to restrain malpractice suits. These changed laws have been grouped as those relating to filing claims, defining standards of medical care or burden of proof, determining the amounts recoverable, and providing alternatives to court resolution of claims.[31]

## Filing Claims

In this category are the following types of statutes:

• *AD DAMNUM clause reform.* This legislation prohibits the plaintiff from stating the amount sought to be recovered, as is traditional in the pleadings, although some statutes permit the plaintiff's attorney to request a specific sum at the trial. The justification for this reform is the belief that publication of large claims is prejudicial to defendants and inappropriately influences juries.

• *Limitation on attorneys' fees.* Most commonly, attorneys in medical liability cases are paid a fee contingent on the outcome of the case—35 percent to 50 percent of any award made to the plaintiff plus the expenses of litigation, rather than an hourly rate. Legislative reforms establish a sliding scale, with the percentage declining with the size of the award, or provide for a reasonable amount as approved by the court.[32]

Contingent fees are supported on the ground that they provide an incentive for lawyers to take cases that have a reasonable likelihood of success and to refuse those in which the plaintiff is unlikely to prove that the doctor was negligent. Theoretically, contingent fees allow recourse to the courts for low-income persons, but in reality, lawyers will not take a case unless a substantial award is likely.[33] Thus, the contingent fee system tends to screen out frivolous cases, but it also denies recourse for minor injuries or for injuries to the elderly, which do not promise large awards. The exclusion of small cases from the court system, however, may be due to high fixed costs of suit, including the costs of expert witnesses, not to contingent fees.[34]

Contingent fees are prohibited in England and Canada, which have historically had a lower rate of malpractice litigation than the United States, although the frequency of litigation has been increasing in these countries recently.

In the United States, the Federal Tort Claims Act limits contingent fees to 25 percent, and state workers' compensation laws also regulate contingent fees. Opposition to contingent fees is urged on the ground that they stimulate excessive litigation, create a conflict of interest between attorney and client, and impede settlement of claims.[35] About half the states specify a limit on attorneys' fees or authorize the courts to set fees.[36] From a public policy point of view, limitation of the plaintiff's attorney's fee is prejudicial to claimants when defendants (physicians, hospitals, and insurers) may spend unlimited amounts for the most skilled defense. In a dissenting opinion in a case holding constitutional the California Medical Injury Compensation Reform Act (MICRA), which provides for a sliding scale of contingency fees, Chief Justice Rose Bird of the California Supreme Court stated that the act "prohibits severely injured victims of medical negligence from paying the general market rate for legal services, while permitting defendants to pay whatever is necessary to obtain high quality representation."[37]

• *Preventing frivolous suits.* Legislation to discourage claims without legal merit requires the losing party in malpractice cases to reimburse the opposing party for costs if the suit is fraudulent or in bad faith. About fifteen states have such laws. Alternatively, a state may require a certificate of merit by an affidavit of an expert before a suit is filed.

• *Pretrial screening panels.* Legislation to offer mandatory or voluntary screening of malpractice cases as a prerequisite to trial is intended to discourage nonmeritorious claims. The panel's decision is not binding and does not prevent the plaintiff from filing a lawsuit. The argument in favor of pretrial screening panels is that the number of claims going to trial will be reduced. In opposition is the contention that these panels add an extra step in the resolution of claims and do not reduce the number of suits.[38] OTA identified twenty-two states with some form of pretrial screening.[39]

The constitutionality of pretrial screening panels has been challenged as a violation of due process and equal protection, denial of a jury trial in violation of the Seventh Amendment to the Constitution, and improper delegation of judicial authority. Generally, the legislation has been upheld as a valid exercise of the police power, but in six states such statutes have been declared unconstitutional.[40]

• *Statutes of limitation.* Many states have shortened the time within which a medical malpractice claim must be filed after an injury occurs or should have been discovered. States have also limited the latest age at which a child may bring an action or have specified that a statute would be suspended only until a child reached a certain age. California sets a limit of three years from the time of the injury or one year from discovery, whichever is earlier. For minors, the rule is three years or the eighth birthday, whichever is later. Longer deferred statutes of limitation are designed to protect victims of latent injuries, but some late claims may be suits to recover by retroactive application of new standards, adding to the costs of the tort system. Instead, an authority in this field recommends a short statute of limitations with additional time for discovery, as in California; to offset the incentive to conceal injuries, physicians should be required to pay an uninsurable fine for fraud or concealment of a negligent injury.[41]

## Defining Standards of Care and Burden of Proof

In this category are the following types of statutes:

• *Standards of care.* Statutes specifying the applicable standard of care in malpractice suits, whether community, state, or national, were passed as the old locality rule has been replaced by state or national standards. One of the reasons for changing the strict locality rule was the difficulty in finding physicians willing to testify against their local colleagues, so that expanding the locality rule enabled plaintiffs to engage national experts.[42]

• *Qualifications of expert witnesses.* Some statutes specify the qualifications for an expert witness. For example, Ohio requires that an expert witness spend 75 percent of his or her professional time in the active practice of his or her specialty.[43]

• *Clinical practice guidelines.* Many specialty boards have developed clinical practice guidelines, and the Federal Agency for Health Care Policy and Research also has guidelines. Since such guidelines represent professional consensus on appropriate procedures, they may be applicable in medical malpractice cases, despite the possibility that courts may exclude them as hearsay evidence or admit them only as part of expert testimony.

Three states—Maine,[44] Minnesota, and Vermont—have passed legislation that permits guidelines to be used as a defense in malpractice litigation under certain circumstances. Both Maine and Minnesota bar the plaintiff from introducing the guidelines as evidence that the physician failed to meet the standard of care. Vermont permits guidelines to be admitted in evidence by either the plaintiff or defendant in mandatory malpractice arbitrations. Concern is expressed that guidelines may not reflect changes in medical practice promptly, that there is a potential for conflict among national, state, and institutional guidelines, and that these conflicts may hinder rather than help the solution of issues in medical liability.[45]

- *Informed consent.* The expansion in the 1970s of the doctrine of informed consent to a more patient-oriented standard, mentioned earlier, has led some states to enact legislation specifying what information must be provided to the patient or specifying professional or customary standards of disclosure as a defense.[46]
- *RES IPSA LOQUITUR.* The legal doctrine of *res ipsa loquitur* (the thing speaks for itself) was expanded in the 1970s from an inference of negligence to a presumption of negligence, which shifts the burden of proof from the plaintiff to the defendant and requires the defendant to show that the injury did not result from the defendant's negligence. This expanded application was found to place defendants at a disadvantage with the result that some states have prohibited or limited the use of the doctrine.[47]

## Determining Amounts Recoverable

In this category are the following types of statutes:

- *Joint and several liability.* About two-thirds of the states have modified the rule on joint and several liability, a rule that allows the plaintiff to sue all defendants responsible and recover from each in proportion to his fault *(joint liability)* or to sue any one defendant and recover the total amount, with that defendant able to recover from the other defendants for their shares *(several liability)*. In some states, several liability was abolished. More commonly, the statutes limit several liability depending on the degree of the defendant's or plaintiff's fault or the ability of other defendants to pay the claim. For example, in Iowa, a defendant who is less than 50 percent responsible for all damages is liable only for a proportionate share of the damages, while a defendant who is more than 50 percent responsible can be held severally liable for the entire amount of the damages.[48]
- *Collateral source offsets.* The collateral source rule is a rule of evidence that prevents the introduction of evidence that the plaintiff has health or disability insurance covering the same injury. This rule originated at a time when individuals privately provided such coverage, and the view was that the prudent person should not be penalized and the wrongdoer should not be relieved of liability because this would negate the deterrent effect of the penalty. The rule is opposed on the ground that recovery from multiple sources provides a windfall for the plaintiff, although in reality most health and disability policies require the plaintiff to reimburse the insurer for any payments received from the tort system.

At least thirty states have modified the collateral source rule either to require juries to be informed about payments from other sources or to mandate an offset from the award for all or some of the collateral benefits. Also, a statute may provide an exception to modification of the collateral source rule, allowing exclusion of collateral source benefits where the health care insurer has the right of *subrogation,* that is, the right to recover payments from an award in a tort action.[49]

• *Itemized jury verdicts.* Requiring juries to itemize the various components of an award for damages instead of issuing a lump sum figure is designed to promote more objective and realistic awards by juries and to permit subsequent analysis of verdicts.[50] Thus, with itemized jury verdicts, the economic components of an award—past and future medical expenses, past and future income losses—and noneconomic components—pain and suffering, bereavement, loss of consortium, loss of parental or filial support, and punitive damages—are clearly set forth.

• *Caps on damages.* Caps on damages may set a limit on noneconomic damages such as pain and suffering or put a total cap on both economic and noneconomic damages.

Fourteen states place some limit on noneconomic damage awards. These limits range from $250,000 to $1 million, and some states specify exceptions. For example, the Michigan cap does not apply to cases in which the patient has an injury to the reproductive system or has lost a bodily function.[51] Since no clear guidelines exist for assessing compensation for pain and suffering, proposals have been made to provide specific guidelines based on the age of the victim and the severity of the injury.

Only eight states have a cap on total damages—both economic and noneconomic damages. Permitted damages in these states range from $500,000 to $1 million. Four of these states have patient compensation funds.[52]

Statutory limits on damage awards are the subject of controversy and constitutional challenge. State supreme courts in fifteen states have held caps on damages unconstitutional as a denial of due process and equal protection, but in other states they have been upheld.[53]

• *Punitive damages.* Punitive damages may be imposed in cases of intentional, gross, or egregious negligence. Those who favor punitive damages in malpractice actions emphasize their deterrent effect; those who oppose punitive damages state that allegations of gross negligence are used for bargaining in settlement negotiations and that such conduct is more appropriately regulated by licensing bodies, institutional review committees, or the criminal justice system.[54] Some reformed statutes abolish punitive damages in suits for compensation for negligence; others limit punitive damages in various ways, for example, by limiting the amount, paying the punitive damage award to the state instead of permitting a windfall to the plaintiff, or restricting the contingency fee on a punitive damage award in order to reduce the incentive for pursuing such claims.[55]

• *Periodic payments.* In 1987, twenty-one states had enacted periodic payment provisions requiring or allowing periodic payments of an award.[56] Periodic payments benefit defendants and insurers by reducing the cost of large awards and permitting modification of the award in the event the injured person dies, thus eliminating a windfall to his beneficiaries. Periodic payments benefit the injured person by assuring the availability of funds and avoiding the risk of mismanagement of a large lump sum.

## Evaluations of State Legislative Reforms

To the ordinary observer, the increase in frequency and severity of medical malpractice claims in the 1980s after the malpractice insurance crisis of the 1970s and the state legislative reforms that followed would seem to indicate that these reforms were not effective. But one does not have to rely on this crude observation.

A number of studies have examined the effects of the various reforms described in the previous section. Of these, the Office of Technology Assessment selected six principal empirical studies that examined the impacts of tort reform in two or more states to ascertain whether these reforms reduced the frequency of medical malpractice claims, the size of awards or payments, or the levels of medical malpractice insurance premiums, collectively called *malpractice cost indicators*.[57] OTA has performed a valuable service in excerpting from its meta-analysis the principal lessons for policy makers.

Here I summarize the OTA evaluation of the various reforms, based on the six empirical studies in its meta-analysis.

- Only caps on damage awards and collateral source offsets reduced one or more of the malpractice cost indicators.
- Damage caps were found to reduce payment per claim paid in three studies. OTA concluded that caps on damages are effective in lowering payment per paid claim and therefore malpractice insurance premiums.
- With respect to collateral source offsets, the studies differed. Two studies found that mandatory collateral offsets had no effect on claim frequency. Danzon, however, examined discretionary and mandatory offsets and found a significant reduction in claim frequency and in amount of payment per paid claim.
- No significant effects of limits on attorneys' fees were found on frequency of claims, payment per claim paid, or insurance premiums.
- With respect to voluntary, binding arbitration, the findings differed. Danzon found that arbitration increased frequency and reduced payment per claim paid. Zuckerman, Bovbjerg, and Sloan found no significant impact of preinjury arbitration agreements on frequency, amount paid, or level of insurance premium.

- No significant effect of restricting the use of the *res ipsa loquitur* doctrine was found.
- One study found a greater number of malpractice claims from using the expanded, patient-oriented standard of informed consent. Another study found that statutory limits on the type of information that must be disclosed to the patient did not have a significant impact on payment per paid claim or on the probability that a claim would result in payment.
- Two studies found no significant impact of mandatory or discretionary periodic payments on payment per paid claim, and one study found no impact on malpractice insurance premiums.

The Office of Technology Assessment concluded that two reforms significantly reduced one or more of the malpractice cost indicators: caps on damage awards and mandatory collateral source offsets.

The following reforms showed no significant impact: limits on attorneys' fees, mandatory or discretionary periodic payments, and restricting the use of *res ipsa loquitur.*

Other reforms that were found to have mixed effects (some positive findings and some negative) or isolated effects (only one significant result) are restricting statutes of limitation, establishing pretrial screening panels, limiting the doctrine of informed consent, and allowing costs awardable in frivolous suits.

Since methods of alternative dispute resolution (ADR) have not been used extensively, no evaluation of the impact of these methods (neutral evaluation, court-annexed arbitration, summary jury trials, and mediation) was made. OTA comments that the reluctance to use ADR when it is voluntary and questions about its constitutionality when it is mandatory indicate that binding ADR is unlikely to have much impact on malpractice costs.[58]

As for use of practice guidelines as the standard of care, OTA predicts that practice guidelines may not be appropriate as a means of tort reform but that their development may be important in determining the standard of care under the existing tort system.

In its 1994 report on defensive medicine, OTA offers further evaluation of various strategies on malpractice reform, particularly with respect to their impact on the practice of defensive medicine. OTA concludes that tort reforms that tinker with the current system retaining personal liability of the physician are likely to be more successful in limiting the direct costs of malpractice—claim frequency, payment per paid claim, and insurance premiums—than in altering physician behavior. Use of practice guidelines, although not a panacea, OTA states, may reduce defensive medicine by providing guidance for the courts on standard of care. Alternative dispute resolution has the advantages of providing greater technical expertise in malpractice than a lay jury, and the process may be quicker, but it may increase the number of claims and strengthen the link between malpractice claims and professional licensing. Enterprise liability offers the advantages of reducing administrative costs associated with multiple defendants, of providing better quality control systems, and of removing the personal liability of the physician, but the physician is still likely to be called as a witness if the case goes to trial. Selective no-fault, an administrative system compensating patients who experience an *accelerated compensation event*—that is, an injury that is generally avoidable in good medical care—may limit physicians' involvement in the claims process, but the idea of personal responsibility may remain and thus may make unlikely any change in the practice of defensive medicine.[59]

An earlier review of four published studies evaluating the effectiveness of tort reform in reducing claim frequency and severity concluded that piecemeal reforms have varied widely in measurable effects.[60] After summarizing the findings of these studies, Halley refers to Professor Law's characterization of tort reform as "consumer hostile."[61] Pointing out that these piecemeal measures make recovery by an injured person more difficult and restrict the awards obtained, Halley writes:

> In this view, tort reform compounds the other undesirable features of the tort approach: the lottery effect, yielding overcompensation to a few injured patients, and undercompensation or no compensation to a larger number; long delays for those finally obtaining compensation; great system expense, since attorneys for the plaintiffs and the defense and insurers receive the major share of the premium dollar; and the increasing hardships of adversarial tort litigation [footnote omitted]. As a consequence, there has been considerable interest in new approaches, although none of these has obtained widespread support, and the level of such interest has always been crisis-driven.[62]

## Alternatives to the Tort System

An important criticism of the tort system of handling medical malpractice is the small fraction of the premium dollar that reaches the injured person. In 1976, a landmark report of the Special Advisory Panel on Medical Malpractice of the State of New York found that of total medical malpractice premiums, only 25 percent to 40 percent goes to the claimant and that most of this payout goes to claimants with large claims.[63] In 1977, Munch (later Danzon) estimated that only 40 to 50 cents of the premium dollar reaches the injured person—much less than the 62 cents for workers' compensation and 80 cents for first-party health insurance.[64]

Another criticism is the small proportion of injured patients who are compensated. In 1985, Danzon reported that the incidence of malpractice is much greater than the frequency of claims.[65] In 1990, the Harvard Medical Practice Study found that not more than 6.25 percent and possibly fewer than 1 percent of those injured receive compensation for medical injuries. Most victims of relatively minor injuries and most victims of even severe injuries who are over sixty-five receive no compensation.[66] The universe of injuries includes those due to adverse outcomes of the disease or medical procedures and those due to negligence. For those due to negligence, only a small proportion of patients injured sue; of those who sue, a smaller proportion receive any compensation. Figure 18.1, adapted by the Office of Technology Assessment from J. R. Posner's work, depicts this experience.

Despite the inequities and even injustices of the tort system for handling medical malpractice, it has persisted, with only the piecemeal changes described ear-

## FIGURE 18.1.  MEDICAL INJURIES, NEGLIGENT CONDUCT, AND MALPRACTICE CLAIMS.

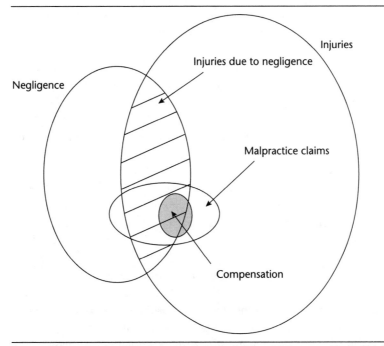

*Source:* Office of Technology Assessment, *Impact of Legal Reforms on Medical Malpractice Costs,* OTA–BP–H–19 (Washington, D.C.: U.S. Government Printing Office, October 1993), p. 9; adapted from J. R. Posner, "Trends in Medical Malpractice Insurance, 1970–1985," *Law and Contemporary Problems* 49, 2 (Spring 1986): 37.

lier, because, as consumer advocates point out, it is "often the only practical means available to patients for exposing, punishing, and deterring substandard medical practice."[67]

Various alternatives have been proposed, however, and the four main types are summarized briefly here: alternative dispute resolution (ADR), which includes conciliation, mediation, and arbitration; enterprise liability; no-fault insurance, which includes medical adversity insurance and *neo no-fault* insurance; and the Model Medical Accident Compensation Act, patterned after the workers' compensation system.

## Alternative Dispute Resolution

ADR is a nonjudicial process that includes conciliation (bringing the parties together), mediation (bringing the parties together and suggesting possible solutions), and arbitration (holding a hearing at which the parties present their cases and an award is made). The most important of these is arbitration, which may be voluntary or mandatory, binding or nonbinding, and an independent proceeding or related to a court case.

Arguments urged in favor of arbitration are: it resolves claims quickly, it reduces costs, it provides greater access for small claims, and it reduces the burden on the courts.

Arguments urged against arbitration are: it may favor providers if a provider is a member of the arbitration panel, it may not compensate the injured person adequately, it may reduce the provider's incentive to lower the incidence of malpractice because the private arbitration process avoids the stigma of a court suit, agreements to arbitrate may not be fully understood by the patient and thus may give an unfair advantage to the provider, and the informality of arbitration hearings may violate the due process rights of the parties.[68]

Experience with alternative dispute resolution is still limited. The courts have encouraged its use. Some state statutes provide for binding irrevocable arbitration agreements in medical malpractice cases, or as in California, private agreements may provide for arbitration. In 1981, authorities in the field pointed out that arbitration has the advantages of accommodating all types of cases; of offering various arbitration arrangements; and of being expeditious, economical, and generally acceptable, so that it should be considered "not alone as a procedural alternative to litigation, but as a substantive contribution to resolution of medical issues."[69] In the 1990s, as new strategies are being adopted for conflict resolution in many fields, alternative dispute resolution of medical liability may have a resurgence.

## Enterprise Liability

Related to alternative dispute resolution is the concept of enterprise liability, which allows patients, providers, and health care institutions to enter into a contract placing all liability for physician actions on the health care institution.

Arguments urged for contracting for enterprise liability are: it encourages health care institutions to strengthen their quality control measures, it reduces the cost of liability insurance and improves the physician-patient relationship by eliminating the threat of suit, it reduces the need for defensive medicine, it promotes early and more certain awards, and it reduces insurers' administrative costs by reducing the number of individual policies and claims.

Arguments urged against contracting for enterprise liability are: it does not cover all patients, the courts may look unfavorably on the contracts as an unfair limitation on the tort rights of patients, and consumers are not sufficiently informed or sufficiently powerful to protect their interests in contract negotiations.[70]

Enterprise liability may be a realistic possibility because of its compatibility with managed competition.[71] Even in the absence of managed competition, enterprise liability may gain acceptance because 80 percent of malpractice claims arise from hospital care, and the hospital would be the enterprise responsible for this care. HMOs that employ physicians directly are legally responsible for actions of their staff physicians. Hospitals are similarly responsible for care provided by interns and residents. *Darling* v. *Charleston Community Memorial Hospital* established the legal obligation of the hospital for the quality of care it provides.[72]

The growth of integrated health care delivery systems in which an organizational unit bears the insurance risk and also provides clinical services has fueled new support for replacing the current system of medical malpractice liability with a system of enterprise medical liability.[73] The arguments advanced for enterprise liability are as follows.[74] The current system suffers from the well-known deficiencies of failing to compensate many injured patients and failing to deter negligence. Moreover, certain practices of malpractice insurers, such as not basing premiums on individual experience but rather on location and specialty, minimize incentives for quality improvement.[75] The organizational unit that is ultimately responsible for efficient health care should also bear financial liability for malpractice so that it can include the cost of patient harm in its calculations. In addition, placing liability for malpractice in the high policy-making level of the organizational unit will tend to decrease defensive medicine, which has been estimated to cost about 8 percent of diagnostic procedures.[76] Imposing liability at the high level of the organizational unit may also promote equity by encouraging policies that benefit the many with cost-effective procedures rather than the few with expensive procedures.[77] It can also be argued that imposing liability on health plans follows from a capitated payment system, since health plans must bear the cost of future medical care for the present payment, and enterprise liability would require plans to incorporate the cost of malpractice awards in their calculations. Health plans are in a position to reduce the incidence of malpractice through organizational and managerial strategies, and an integrated delivery system may have the capacity to arrange for sharing liability among different units in a health plan network.

Proponents of enterprise liability contend that such a system will promote quality by improving relations between health plans and health care professionals, by promoting teamwork, and by relieving physicians to some extent of the extremely negative experience of malpractice suits.

Despite the apparent cogency of these arguments, many questions are unanswered. Will enterprise liability be feasible in the absence of comprehensive health care reform? Which enterprise should be responsible—the health plan or the hospital or other enterprise directly involved in delivery of health care?[78] What inequities will result from the operation of different health plans? In a mixed health care system—part managed care and part traditional practice—how will malpractice liability be handled fairly? Despite the theoretical appeal of many of the arguments for enterprise medical liability, can such a system realistically be implemented? Can it withstand legal challenge? Will it prejudice the injured patient by shifting liability to a powerful and invisible defendant?

## No-Fault Compensation

The essence of the no-fault approach is that it is a compensation system that eliminates proof of negligence as a basis for the collection of damages. As Grad points out, a no-fault system would recognize the fact that the risk of medical injury is inherent in modern medicine and would provide compensation for all such injuries, without regard to negligence.[79]

In 1976–77, the California Medical Association and the California Hospital Association sponsored the Medical Insurance Feasibility Study in California to determine the economic feasibility of a pure no-fault system. This study is important for showing that adverse outcomes of medical care, although numerous, are finite and can be identified. The study found that 82 percent of adverse outcomes were class I type adverse outcomes involving complications of treatment, including giving drugs to patients. Class II adverse outcomes—the effects of incomplete or delayed diagnosis or treatment—accounted for only 15 percent of adverse outcomes.[80] Most existing no-fault systems in the world cover only class I adverse outcomes and not class II outcomes. It is therefore suggested that since class I type injuries account for 82 percent of total adverse outcomes, a no-fault system applicable to that 82 percent might be worthwhile, leaving class II outcomes in a residual fault-based liability system.[81]

Arguments urged for a no-fault insurance system are: it would provide compensation to a greater number of injured persons, it would provide compensation more promptly, it would avoid the substantial cost of proving negligence, it would provide similar compensation to patients with similar injuries, and it would provide incentives for improving the quality of care by defining the causes of untoward outcomes and means of avoiding them and by basing insurance premiums on each provider's experience rating.

Arguments urged against a no-fault insurance system are: it may cost more than the current system because more people will be compensated; although the question of negligence would be eliminated, the question of causation would remain; it would require work to define the compensable events and the compensation schedule; it would cover only economic damages, not pain and suffering, although the compensation schedule might reflect some elements of pain and suffering; it would remove a deterrent to substandard care; it may cause some providers to refuse to accept high-risk patients; and it may be complex in resolving claims involving multiple providers.[82]

Next we turn to two forms of limited no-fault insurance: medical adversity insurance and neo no-fault insurance.

• *Medical adversity insurance.* In 1973, Havighurst and Tancredi proposed a no-fault approach that they called "medical adversity insurance."[83] The proposal provided for identifying those injuries that deserve compensation, called *designated compensable events.* The proposal aimed to improve the quality of care by defining categories of untoward outcomes and means for avoiding them. Although this system has not been implemented, benefits claimed for it are the impact on the quality of medical care (it would provide a listing, specialty by specialty, of potential adverse effects of various procedures), administrative savings derived by avoiding court suits, and reduction of emotional stress and stigma for all parties.[84]

• *Neo no-fault insurance.* Another variation on the no-fault system is neo no-fault.[85] The essence of this proposal is to encourage early out-of-court settlement for the actual economic losses and use the money that would have been spent on litigation and pain and suffering to pay for adequate injury compensation. This proposal differs from pure no-fault because the tort system is retained as an alternative.[86]

Under this proposal, a provider facing a malpractice claim would have the option of offering the claimant, within 180 days after the claim is filed, periodic payments or a lump sum approved by the court as compensation for economic losses including medical expenses, rehabilitation, and wage losses not covered by other insurance. Certain disincentives to sue would prevail: recovery would be allowed only for wanton misconduct; the standard of proof required would be higher—not the usual standard in civil cases of preponderance of the evidence but rather proof by clear and convincing evidence; limitation of noneconomic damages; and a penalty on the plaintiff of having to pay the defendant's costs if the claimant is awarded less than the noneconomic loss offered by the defendant.

The advantage of this proposal is that it provides prompt payment for economic losses in return for giving up the right to sue. But in egregious cases with great pain and suffering, the claimant would be permitted to bring a tort action.

• *Examples of U.S. No-Fault Systems.* Three examples of limited no-fault systems exist in the United States.

In 1986, Congress enacted the National Childhood Vaccine Injury Act of 1986, providing for a no-fault compensation system for children injured as a result of side effects of immunization against childhood diseases. The legislation was designed to encourage vaccine manufacturers to increase their production of vaccines, which had declined dangerously because of the industry's fear of malpractice suits. Compensation is payable by the federal government on the basis of strict liability, that is, without regard to fault or negligence by the manufacturer or the administering physician.[87]

Two states—Virginia and Florida—have enacted no-fault compensation systems for birth-related neurological injuries. The Virginia Birth-Related Neurological Injury Compensation Act of 1987 was designed to make liability insurance for obstetrician-gynecologists affordable and available by taking claims for certain catastrophically injured newborns out of the tort system and thus to provide compensation more quickly and to increase access to obstetrical care.[88]

Compensation is awarded only for those infants who meet a narrow statutory definition of injury to the spinal cord or brain, caused by a deprivation of oxygen or mechanical injury in the course of labor, delivery, or resuscitation in the immediate postdelivery period in a hospital, that rendered the infant permanently "motorically disabled" and developmentally or cognitively disabled such that assistance in all activities of daily living is required, and that was not caused by congenital or genetic factors, degenerative neurological disease, or maternal substance abuse. The injury must have been caused by a physician participating in the program or at a participating hospital.

The program is funded by an annual assessment of $250 per licensed physician, voluntary assessments of $5,000 per participating physician, and $50 per delivery for participating hospitals, not to exceed $150,000 in any twelve-month period.[89]

The procedure is as follows. The claimant files a claim with the Workers' Compensation Commission and serves a petition on the fund that administers the program and determines whether the claim falls within the definition of the statute.

If the fund finds that the injury is compensable, the Workers' Compensation Board issues an order without a hearing and sends the case to a medical review panel of three qualified and impartial physicians, which makes a recommendation to the commission as to whether the case is covered by the act. If the fund does not determine that the case falls within the definition, then the commission holds a hearing at which the panel's recommendation is given considerable but not determinative weight.[90] Awards are made according to statutory provisions.

The plaintiff has no option of an alternative remedy if the delivery was performed by a participating hospital, but final appeal may be made to the Virginia Court of Appeals. By the end of 1992, only four claims had been filed under this program.

The Florida Birth-Related Neurological Injury Compensation Act was passed in 1988 and is similar to that of Virginia but differs in several respects. The claim must be filed within five years instead of ten, and it is not required that the infant need assistance in all activities. A hospital is protected from liability only if the delivery is done by a participating physician, so hospitals either require their physicians to participate or pay the physician's assessment. Thus, about 90 percent of obstetricians in Florida participate.[91]

• *Experience with no-fault insurance in other countries.* Three countries have adopted systems of no-fault compensation for personal injury—New Zealand, Sweden, and Finland.

Since 1974, New Zealand has had a comprehensive system of compensation for all personal injuries whether they occur at work, on the highway, in the home, in the hospital, or anywhere else. The scheme was introduced because of different results for people with equal problems and equal needs, because many people received no compensation for injuries, and because extravagant and drawn-out adversary techniques reduced compensation to claimants.[92]

The intent of the scheme is to compensate all instances of physical or mental harm caused by accident, while excluding those arising from illness or old age. The scope of the scheme is broad but excluded are the effects of a cardiovascular or cerebrovascular episode unless it is work related and the result of undue strain or unless the episode results from an injury by accident, and also any physical or mental damage caused exclusively by disease, infection, or the aging process.[93]

Administered by a nonprofit autonomous governmental organization, the Accident Compensation Corporation, the New Zealand program, as of 1989, provided compensation for total disability, in periodic payments, at a level of 80 percent of earnings up to a ceiling of $976 per week (NZ$1 = US$0.62 as of February 15, 1989). Proportionate adjustments are made for partial disability. The benefit level is fixed at 80 percent in order to create an incentive for rehabilitation.

Payments are made for disability, adjusted for inflation, until age sixty-five, when pensions take over.

In addition to payments for loss of earnings, reasonable costs of medical and dental treatment are covered as well as reasonable costs of transport to the doctor or hospital for initial treatment and for further rehabilitative treatment, reasonable costs of rehabilitation and retraining assistance, payment for reasonable cost of necessary constant personal attention of the injured person following the accident, lump sum for permanent physical disability, lump sum for pain and suffering, lump sum to dependent spouse and dependent children, and other benefits.[94]

The program is financed by contributions from employers and employees and the self-employed, together with payments from owners of motor vehicles (in 1989, NZ$100 a year for a private car!) and a small supplement from general taxation.

The New Zealand physician or surgeon in 1989 paid a levy based on income at the rate of 1.45 percent, or NZ$920 up to the maximum leviable income of NZ$63,458 (now raised to NZ$104,000, with the annual levy raised to NZ$2,600). These payments cover the physician for personal incapacity and also provide a complete release from all risk of claims for damages from others.[95]

The New Zealand system has enjoyed wide public support for the fifteen years that it has been in operation. New Zealand has not experienced the growth in defensive medicine or the harm to the doctor-patient relationship associated with malpractice suits. As for the effect on the quality of medical practice, the Right Honourable Sir Owen Woodhouse, who is largely responsible for the introduction and promotion of the New Zealand compensation system, states, "It is a strange argument that physicians need to be made fearful of court actions in order to maintain those professional standards upon which their whole livelihood will depend. Certainly there are no signs in New Zealand that medical standards have deteriorated in the 15 years during which the comprehensive scheme has been operating."[96]

On January 1, 1975, Sweden introduced a voluntary patient insurance scheme administered by a consortium of insurers headed by Scandia Life. The scheme is funded and paid by the county councils on a per capita basis, costing about $1.76 (in U.S. dollars) per year. Injured patients may elect to bring an action in tort or may receive compensation under the patient compensation program without having to prove fault.[97] The program was not enacted by the Swedish government but is the result of an agreement between the Federation of County Councils and a consortium of Swedish insurers. Although the program is generally described as no-fault, it is not strictly so because error underlies most payments. "Such an error, however, does not have to be proved negligent; error may be assumed where the outcome is unusual."[98]

In January 1978, Sweden introduced a pharmaceutical scheme, which is also a voluntary, nonstatutory system covering injuries from vaccination and blood products. Impelled by the threat of legislation, the drug industry pays for the program, with premiums based on each company's market share.

Five types of injury are covered under the Swedish compensation system: treatments, timing and accuracy of diagnosis, accidents, infections, and injuries caused by diagnostic treatments. To be compensated, an individual must have reported sick for a minimum of fourteen days or been hospitalized for at least ten days, have suffered permanent injury, or have died. Compensation is paid for loss of income and for medical care, with indemnities for pain and suffering and permanent disfigurement.

The philosophy of the Swedish system is based on the principles of tort law in that injuries, complications, or undesired results that were unavoidable consequences of the illness or necessary treatment are not covered. Compensation is paid whether or not the error of judgment or clinical practice was negligent, and therefore doctors and nurses are willing to admit errors and encourage patients to file claims.[99]

The claims process is simple, inexpensive, and easy to administer. The patient has the right to take an appeal to a claims panel that meets for a day about twelve times a year. If the claims panel rejects the appeal, the patient's final resort is to submit his claim to arbitration.

Finland has introduced comprehensive pharmaceutical and treatment injury insurance modeled after the Swedish system. The Patient Injury Act of 1986 provides payments for loss of earnings, loss of amenities, and pain and suffering. Ninety-three percent of all medical care is provided by the state. Compensation is payable for any injury that has arisen from examination, treatment, or any similar action or neglect of the same; that has been caused by an infection connected with examination or treatment; or that has been caused by accident connected with examination or treatment, occurring during ambulance transport, or resulting from a defect in medical equipment.

The scheme is financed through insurance that doctors and other health providers must obtain. The Patient Insurance Association issues policies and handles claims and settlements. Failure to carry insurance makes the uninsured provider liable for ten times the normal premium. If a provider is uninsured, the Patient Insurance Association pays the patient and then collects the increased premium.[100]

In Finland, the Patient Injury Act of 1986 has eliminated the need to prove negligence entirely. In Sweden, negligence need be proved only if the injured person elects to sue in tort instead of seeking compensation through the patient insurance program. But the damages paid under the insurance program are the same as those recoverable in tort, so there is little incentive to sue.[101]

## Model Medical Accident Compensation Act

Finally, we turn to the proposal for a system of medical accident compensation that applies the principles of workers' compensation to medical injury compensation.[102] In the belief that administrative or agency compensation is "both theoretically and realistically the ultimate solution for the medical professional liability dilemma,"[103] Halley and colleagues have advanced a model statute authored by Bryce B. Moore, former director of the Kansas workers' compensation program, and supported by extensive research by the Midwest Institute for Health Care and Law.

Like workers' compensation, the Model Medical Accident Compensation Act involves a trade-off; it provides benefits to a larger number of injured individuals than are compensated currently in exchange for restricting the tort system. The administrative process is designed to provide prompt, limited, and certain compensation for an increased number of injured individuals, avoiding the delay, costs, and uncertainties of court procedures. A greater proportion of the premium dollar would go to the injured person than occurs under the adversarial process. Attorneys may represent claimants and providers in the administrative process.

Definition of the medical injury or compensable event is not through a schedule of compensable events but rather through review of individual cases, applying the standard of reasonable care. Proof of negligence is not required, but the concept of medical error or *fault* (defined as responsibility for an outcome) is retained to distinguish compensable events from progression of the disease or unavoidable consequences of treatment. Administrative determination by the Medical Accident Compensation Board replaces adversarial tort litigation and the jury. The determination of compensable events is made by the Medical Accident Compensation Board, assisted by an expert review panel.

Payment of compensation claims is guaranteed through requirements that health care providers carry insurance and through a Recovery Guarantee Fund. Three methods of funding are provided: purchase of an insurance policy by an individual provider, provider self-insurance (usually for an institution), and membership in a group-funded self-insurance pool (a less expensive method than individual purchase of insurance).

The Recovery Guarantee Fund is established in the state treasury to assure payment of compensation in the event a provider is uninsured or unable to pay the benefits under the act. Payments from the fund are not expected to be large, since health care providers will generally carry the required insurance, just as most employers carry the appropriate workers' compensation insurance.

Benefits are based on economic loss with equivalent compensation for claimants without ascertainable earnings, such as housewives, homemakers, retired persons, and children. Benefits include those for medical care and rehabilitation and for temporary and permanent personal disability, death benefits, and burial expenses. The calculation of permanent personal injury benefits is based on the highest of three percentages—the percentage loss of the claimant's earning ability, the percentage overall reduction in the claimant's health level, and the percentage functional disability to the body as a whole.

The cost of an administrative system is an important concern because of the anticipated increase in the number of compensated injuries. These increased payments may be offset by the greater efficiency of the system and by cost controls built into the system, such as maximum limits on liability, a two-year statute of limitations on filing a claim, credit for duplicate payments (no windfall to the claimant from collateral sources), and limitation on attorneys' fees.

The act provides for appeal to the courts from a decision of the Board. As in workers' compensation, appeals are based on the record of proceedings before the board. The courts have jurisdiction to determine whether the board has made a correct finding under the act.

Most importantly, built into the model act are provisions to promote an acceptable quality of health care. Separate from the compensation provisions are provisions for strengthened state agencies providing surveillance of medical practice, institutional review procedures, and other peer review mechanisms. Quality assurance is linked to the data collection functions of the board, which are connected to state and national data banks.

# Medical Malpractice Reform in the U.S. Context

The many proposals for changes in the tort system of handling medical malpractice liability break down into three main types: piecemeal reforms or tinkering with the tort system, no-fault compensation systems, and an administrative program of compensation modeled on the workers' compensation system.

Twenty years' experience with piecemeal reforms has made only minor improvements in the tort system that fails to compensate many injured persons, pays only 25 percent to 40 percent of total premium cost to injured persons, and is fraught with delays, high costs, and inequities among injured persons suffering from the same or similar injuries. Careful evaluations of the effects of these piecemeal reforms have confirmed their minimal benefits. The recurrence in the 1980s of the medical malpractice insurance crisis of the 1970s attests to the need for an alternative approach.

No-fault compensation systems are currently operating in the federal vaccine compensation program and in two states for compensation for birth-related neurological injuries. Examples of the no-fault approach exist in automobile insurance. While the compensable event is clearly defined in automobile accidents, definition of potentially compensable medical events requires more work. The Medical Insurance Feasibility Study, sponsored by the California Medical Association and the California Hospital Association in the late 1970s, showed that it is possible to define potentially compensable events and that a no-fault system of medical injury compensation is feasible.[104] From a policy point of view, the well-documented report of the New York State Special Advisory Panel on Medical Malpractice in 1976 strongly recommended a compensation system that does not pay damages for injuries caused by malpractice but rather provides compensation for bad medical results.[105]

The experience of New Zealand, Sweden, and Finland with their differing no-fault systems of medical injury compensation shows the rationality, equity, and public acceptance of no-fault systems. These countries, however, have much more all-encompassing systems of health insurance and social security benefits than the United States.

Despite the soundness of the no-fault approach and the appeal of neo no-fault in retaining the option of a suit in tort, political realities seem to militate against adoption of this alternative. Objections to the no-fault approach have been detailed earlier, but the principal countervailing force lies in the power of the special interests that would be affected by adopting this approach—mainly the insurance companies and the trial lawyers.

In view of these realities, a feasible and rational alternative is the Model Medical Accident Compensation Act, which designs an administrative system for reasonable and rapid compensation for medical injuries patterned after the workers' compensation program. While workers' compensation may be in need of some modernization itself, such as increased benefits and strengthened rehabilitation provisions, no one would dream of ever returning to the tort system for redress of occupational injuries and diseases. Administrative law is increasingly the means in the United States for handling technical problems requiring expertise and prompt resolution. It provides an appropriate vehicle for the solution of the problem of medical injury compensation. Extensive research and investigation have explored the economic, constitutional, and medical features of such a system, and precedents exist in other administrative law programs.

Regardless of when and how medical malpractice liability reform should be undertaken, the fundamental issue is quality of care. While no system of medical care can eliminate all adverse outcomes (a certain number of which are inevitable in high-technology medicine) and no system can eliminate all bad actors and all substandard performance, strategies can be adopted to monitor and continually improve the quality of care. The Model Medical Accident Compensation Act contains provisions on data collection and surveillance of care that can strengthen current protections of the quality of care.

The enactment of national health insurance assuring universal coverage of the total population might reduce the propensity to sue, since all medical care, including that needed because of adverse outcomes of earlier care, would be covered. Patient anger with the health care system—a necessary ingredient for a lawsuit—would be reduced by universal coverage.[106] Malpractice suits may also be restrained by the introduction of quality control measures by health maintenance organizations and third-party administrators (such as Kaiser Permanente's Report Card on Quality of Care) that will strengthen the existing quality system of state licensure, disciplinary actions, and peer review processes.

In 1986, an authority on medical malpractice called the current system not a compensation system but a liability system, pointing out that our current system fails as a compensation system, offers little evidence of any deterrent effects, and imposes costs of liability coverage and administration that are too high.[107] More than a decade later, when health care reform is still on the national agenda, the climate of opinion may indeed be favorable for rationalizing our handling of medical injury compensation by adopting an administrative system that is more equitable and less costly than the tort system.

## Notes

1. Paul Starr, *The Logic of Health Care Reform: Why and How the President's Plan Will Work* (Knoxville, TN: Whittle Books in association with Penguin Books, 1994), p. 20; and Office of Technology Assessment, *Impact of Legal Reforms on Medical Malpractice Costs,* OTA–BP–H–19 (Washington, D.C.: U.S. Government Printing Office, October 1993).

2. Henry J. Aaron, *Serious and Unstable Condition: Financing America's Health Care* (Washington, D.C.: Brookings Institution, 1991). The Office of Technology Assessment states that "most defensive medicine is not of zero benefit." See, also, Office of Technology Assessment, *Defensive Medicine and Medical Malpractice,* OTA–H–602 (Washington, D.C.: U.S. Government Printing Office, July 1994).

3. Starr, *The Logic of Health Care Reform,* p. 20.

4. Office of Technology Assessment, *Defensive Medicine and Medical Malpractice,* p. 1.

5. Aaron, *Serious and Unstable Condition,* p. 48.

6. William J. Curran and George B. Moseley III, "The Malpractice Experience of Health Maintenance Organizations," *Northwestern University Law Review* 70, 1(1975): D, pp. 68–89.

7. Elaine Lu, "The Potential Effect of Managed Competition in Health Care on Provider Liability and Patient Autonomy," *Harvard Journal on Legislation* 30, 2 (Summer 1993): 519–552, p. 533; and Rex O'Neal, "Safe Harbor for Health Care Cost Containment," *Stanford Law Review* 43 (1986): 399–443, pp. 410–421.

8. Office of Technology Assessment, *Impact of Legal Reforms on Medical Malpractice Costs,* p. 19.

9. Recent data from the Physicians Insurers Association of America (PIAA) indicate that claims against office-based practitioners are rising. Presentation by Thomas E. Kirchmeier to the American Society of Healthcare Risk Management, Chicago, October 25, 1993, cited by William M. Sage, Kathleen E. Hastings, and Robert A. Berenson, "Enterprise Liability for Medical Malpractice and Health Care Quality Improvement," *American Journal of Law & Medicine* 20, 1 & 2 (1994): 1–28, p. 12, n. 62.

10. Sage, Hastings, and Berenson, "Enterprise Liability," p. 12.

11. Kenneth S. Abraham and Paul S. Weiler, "Enterprise Medical Liability and the Choice of the Responsible Enterprise," *American Journal of Law & Medicine* 20, 1 & 2 (1994): 29–36, p. 32.

12. Office of Technology Assessment, *Impact of Legal Reforms on Medical Malpractice Costs;* and U.S. General Accounting Office, *Medical Malpractice: No Agreement on the Problems or Solutions,* Report to Congressional Requesters, GAO/HRD 86–50 (Washington, D.C.: U.S. General Accounting Office, January 1986).

13. Patricia Munch Danzon, *The Frequency and Severity of Medical Malpractice Claims,* R–2870–ICJ/HCFA (Santa Monica, Calif.: Institute for Civil Justice, RAND, 1982), p. 1.

14. Patricia M. Danzon, *Medical Malpractice: Theory, Evidence, and Public Policy* (Cambridge, Mass.: Harvard University Press, 1985); and Peter D. Jacobson, "Medical Malpractice and the Tort System," *Journal of the American Medical Association* 262, 23 (December 15, 1989): 3320–3327.

15. Danzon, *Medical Malpractice,* p. 2.

16. Frank P. Grad, "Medical Malpractice and Its Implications for Public Health," in *Legal Aspects of Health Policy: Issues and Trends,* eds. Ruth Roemer and George McKray (Westport, Conn.: Greenwood Press, 1980), p. 398.

17. Danzon, *Medical Malpractice,* p. 85.

18. M. Martin Halley, "Tort Law Impact on Health Care," in *Medical Malpractice Solutions: Systems and Proposals for Injury Compensation,* eds. M. Martin Halley, Robert J. Fowks, E. Calvin Bigler, and David L. Ryan (Springfield, Ill.: Thomas, 1989), pp. 21–32; p. 21. (Hereinafter *Medical Malpractice Solutions.*)

19. Danzon, *Medical Malpractice,* p. 85.

20. E. Calvin Bigler, "Medical Professional Liability in the United States," in *Medical Malpractice Solutions,* pp. 33–46; p. 36.

21. Danzon, *Medical Malpractice,* p. 59.

22. Danzon, *The Frequency and Severity of Medical Malpractice Claims,* p. 36.

23. Margo L. Rosenbach and Ashley G. Stone, "Malpractice Insurance Costs and Physician Practice, 1981–1986," *Health Affairs* (Winter 1990): 176–185, p. 177.

24. Danzon, *Medical Malpractice,* p. 1.

25. Grad, "Medical Malpractice and Its Implications for Public Health," pp. 397–433 (see p. 415); and Danzon, *The Frequency and Severity of Medical Malpractice Claims,* p. 30.

26. Danzon, *The Frequency and Severity of Medical Malpractice Claims,* p. 36; and Jacobson, "Medical Malpractice and the Tort System," p. 3323.

27. Bigler, "Medical Professional Liability in the United States," p. 35.

28. U.S. General Accounting Office, *Medical Malpractice,* p. 67.

29. Halley, "Tort Law Impact on Health Care," p. 22.

30. Grad, "Medical Malpractice and Its Implications for Public Health," p. 403.

31. M. Martin Halley, "Tort Reform: The Response to Crisis," in *Medical Malpractice Solutions,* pp. 63–78 (see p. 64).

32. U.S. General Accounting Office, *Medical Malpractice,* p. 78.

33. Sylvia Law and Steven Polan, *Pain and Profit: The Politics of Malpractice* (New York: Harper-Collins, 1978), p. 84.

34. Patricia Munch Danzon, *Contingent Fees for Personal Injury Litigation* (Santa Monica, Calif.: U.S. Department of Health, Education, and Welfare and RAND, June 1980), p. vii. This work was prepared for the Health Care Financing Administration.

35. Danzon, *Medical Malpractice,* p. 187.

36. Office of Technology Assessment, *Impact of Legal Reforms on Medical Malpractice Costs,* p. 29.

37. *Roa* v. *Lodi Medical Group,* 37 Cal. 3d 920, 211 Cal. Rptr. 77, 695 P. 2d 164 (1985).

38. Halley, "Tort Reform: The Response to Crisis," p. 71.

39. Office of Technology Assessment, *Impact of Legal Reforms on Medical Malpractice Costs,* p. 285.

40. Danzon, *Medical Malpractice,* p. 199; and Office of Technology Assessment, *Impact of Legal Reforms on Medical Malpractice Costs,* p. 29.

41. Danzon, *Medical Malpractice,* p. 184.

42. Office of Technology Assessment, *Impact of Legal Reforms on Medical Malpractice Costs,* p. 31

43. U.S. General Accounting Office, *Medical Malpractice,* p. 81.

44. In incorporating into state law twenty practice guidelines for four specialties (anesthesiology, emergency medicine, obstetrics and gynecology, and radiology), the Maine legislature sought to resolve malpractice claims by eliminating the need to establish the standard of practice. Legislators hoped to control health care costs by reducing the incentive to perform unnecessary tests and procedures. See U.S. General Accounting Office, *Medical Malpractice: Maine's Use of Practice Guidelines to Reduce Costs,* GAO/HRD–94–80 (Washington, D.C.: U.S. General Accounting Office, October 1993).

45. Office of Technology Assessment, *Impact of Legal Reforms on Medical Malpractice Costs,* p. 33.

46. Office of Technology Assessment, *Impact of Legal Reforms on Medical Malpractice Costs,* p. 30.

47. Halley, "Tort Reform: The Response to Crisis," p. 72.

48. Office of Technology Assessment, *Impact of Legal Reforms on Medical Malpractice Costs,* p. 37; and Halley, "Tort Reform: The Response to Crisis," pp. 68–69.

49. Office of Technology Assessment, *Impact of Legal Reforms on Medical Malpractice Costs,* pp. 33–34; and Halley, "Tort Reform: The Response to Crisis," p. 66.

50. Halley, "Tort Reform: The Response to Crisis," p. 68.

51. Office of Technology Assessment, *Impact of Legal Reforms on Medical Malpractice Costs,* p. 36.

52. Office of Technology Assessment, *Impact of Legal Reforms on Medical Malpractice Costs,* p. 36.

53. Office of Technology Assessment, *Impact of Legal Reforms on Medical Malpractice Costs,* p. 35.

54. Halley, "Tort Reform: The Response to Crisis," pp. 71–72.

55. Halley, "Tort Reform: The Response to Crisis," p. 72.

56. Halley, "Tort Reform: The Response to Crisis," p. 70; and Office of Technology Assessment, *Impact of Legal Reforms on Medical Malpractice Costs,* p. 37.

57. Office of Technology Assessment, *Impact of Legal Reforms on Medical Malpractice Costs,* pp. 57–75. The six studies analyzed are E. K. Adams and S. Zuckerman, "Variation in the Growth and Incidence of Medical Malpractice Claims," *Journal of Health, Politics, Policy, and Law* 9, 3 (Fall 1984): 475–488; D. K. Barker, "The Effects of Tort Reform on Medical Malpractice Insurance Markets: An Empirical Analysis," *Journal of Health, Politics, Policy, and Law* 17, 1 (Spring 1992): 143–161; G. Blackmon and R. Zeckhauser, "State Tort Reform Legislation: Assessing Our Control of Risks," in *Tort Law and the Public Interest,* ed. Peter H. Schuck (New York: Norton, 1991); P. M. Danzon, "The Frequency and Severity of Medical Malpractice Claims: New Evidence," *Law and Contemporary Problems* 49, 2 (Spring 1986): 57–84; F. A. Sloan, P. M. Mergenhagen, and R. R. Bovbjerg, "Effects of Tort Reforms on the Value of Closed Medical Malpractice Claims: A Microanalysis," *Journal of Health, Politics, Policy, and Law* 14, 4 (Winter 1989): 663–689; and S. Zuckerman, R. R. Bovbjerg, and F. Sloan, "Effects of Tort Reforms and Other Factors on Medical Malpractice Insurance Premiums," *Inquiry* 27, 2 (Summer 1990): 167–182.

58. Office of Technology Assessment, *Impact of Legal Reforms on Medical Malpractice Costs*, pp. 72–73.

59. Office of Technology Assessment, *Defensive Medicine and Medical Malpractice*, pp. 75–93.

60. Halley, "Tort Reform: The Response to Crisis," p. 77.

61. Halley, "Tort Reform: The Response to Crisis," p. 77; and Sylvia A. Law. "A Consumer Perspective on Medical Malpractice," *Law and Contemporary Problems* 49, 2 (1986): 306–320, p. 315.

62. Halley, "Tort Reform: The Response to Crisis," p. 77.

63. State of New York, *Report of the Special Advisory Panel on Medical Malpractice*, New York City, January 1976; cited and discussed in Grad, "Medical Malpractice and Its Implications for Public Health," p. 431, n. 97.

64. Danzon, *Medical Malpractice*, p. 186.

65. Danzon, *Medical Malpractice*, p. 4.

66. Harvard Medical Practice Study, *Patients, Doctors, and Lawyers: Medical Injury, Malpractice Litigation, and Patient Compensation in New York: A Report of the Harvard Medical Practice Study to the State of New York* (Cambridge, Mass.: President and Fellows of Harvard College, 1990); New York State Health Department, *Medical Practice Study, Executive Summary* (Albany: New York State Health Department, 1990); and Howard W. Hiatt, Benjamin A. Barnes, Troyen A. Brennan, et al., "A Study of Medical Injury and Medical Malpractice," Special Report, *New England Journal of Medicine* 321, 7 (August 17, 1989): 480–484.

67. Law and Polan, *Pain and Profit*, p. 155.

68. U.S. General Accounting Office, *Medical Malpractice*, p. 46; and Robert J. Fowks, "Arbitration," in *Medical Malpractice Solutions*, pp. 79–89 (see p. 81).

69. Irving Ladimer, Joel C. Solomon, and Michael Mulvill, "Experience in Medical Malpractice Arbitration," *Journal of Legal Medicine* 2 (1981): 433–470 (see p. 452).

70. Clark C. Havighurst, "Malpractice Reform: Getting There by Private Vehicle," in *Medical Malpractice Solutions*, pp. 115–127.

71. Office of Technology Assessment, *Impact of Legal Reforms on Medical Malpractice Costs*, p. 45.

72. *Darling* v. *Charleston Community Memorial Hospital*, 33 Ill. 2d 326, 211 N.E. 2d 253 (1965).

73. Sage, Hastings, and Berenson, "Enterprise Liability"; and Abraham and Weiler, "Enterprise Medical Liability and the Choice of the Responsible Enterprise."

74. These arguments are drawn from Sage, Hastings, and Berenson, "Enterprise Liability."

75. Sage, Hastings, and Berenson, "Enterprise Liability," p. 3, citing Danzon, *Medical Malpractice*, p. 130; and Lori L. Darling, "The Applicability of Experience Rating to Medical Malpractice Insurance," *Case Western Reserve Law Review* 38 (1987–88): 255, 261–65.

76. Office of Technology Assessment, *Defensive Medicine and Medical Malpractice*, OTA–H–602 (Washington, D.C.: U.S. Government Printing Office, July 1994), pp. 1, 6. See, also, Sage, Hastings, and Berenson, "Enterprise Liability," p. 9, citing a 1992 study by Lewin-VHI, Inc., estimating that malpractice reform might save between $25 billion and $76 billion in unnecessary tests and procedures over a five-year period. For the study itself, see Robert Rubin and D. Mendelsohn, *Estimating the Costs of Defensive Medicine*, Lewin-VHI, Inc., October 21, 1992.

77. Sage, Hastings, and Berenson, "Enterprise Liability," p. 9.

78. Abraham and Weiler, "Enterprise Medical Liability."

79. Grad, "Medical Malpractice and Its Implications for Public Health," pp. 409–410.

80. Don Harper Mills, "The Case for and Against Pure No-Fault," in *Medical Malpractice Solutions*, pp. 143–157. For the original study, which was sponsored by the California Medical

Association and the California Hospital Association, see Don Harper Mills (ed.), *Report on the Medical Insurance Feasibility Study* (San Francisco: Sutter, 1977).

81. Mills, "The Case for and Against Pure No-Fault," p. 146.

82. Office of Technology Assessment, *Impact of Legal Reforms on Medical Malpractice Costs,* pp. 42–43; and Danzon, *Medical Malpractice,* pp. 213–217.

83. Clark C. Havighurst and Laurence R. Tancredi, "'Medical Adversity Insurance'—a No-Fault Approach to Medical Malpractice and Quality Assurance," *Insurance Law Journal* no. 13 (February 1974): 69–100.

84. Laurence R. Tancredi, "Designated Compensable Events," in *Medical Malpractice Solutions,* pp. 103–114.

85. Jeffrey O'Connell, "Neo No-Fault Remedies for Medical Injuries: Coordinated Statutory and Contractual Alternatives," *Law and Contemporary Problems* 49, 2 (1986): 125–141.

86. Jeffrey O'Connell, "Neo No-Fault: Settling for Economic Losses," in *Medical Malpractice Solutions,* pp. 91–101 (see p. 96).

87. National Childhood Vaccine Injury Act, P.L. No. 99–660, sec. 311, 100 Stat. 3755 (1986); and Frank P. Grad, *The Public Health Law Manual,* 2d ed. (Washington, D.C.: American Public Health Association, 1990).

88. Virginia Birth-Related Neurological Injury Compensation Act of 1987, Va. Code Ann., sec. 38.2–5000–5021 (1993); and Institute of Medicine, Division of Health Promotion and Disease Prevention, Committee to Study Medical Professional Liability and the Delivery of Obstetrical Care, *Medical Professional Liability and the Delivery of Obstetrical Care,* vol. 1 (Washington, D.C.: National Academy Press, 1989); and Institute of Medicine, Division of Health Promotion and Disease Prevention, Committee to Study Medical Professional Liability and the Delivery of Obstetrical Care, *Medical Professional Liability and the Delivery of Obstetrical Care;* vol. 2: *An Interdisciplinary Review,* eds. Victoria P. Rostow and Roger J. Bulger (Washington, D.C.: National Academy Press, 1989).

89. Institute of Medicine, *Medical Professional Liability and the Delivery of Obstetrical Care,* p. 137.

90. Office of Technology Assessment, *Impact of Legal Reforms on Medical Malpractice Costs,* pp. 43–44.

91. Florida Birth-Related Neurological Injury Compensation Act of 1988, Fla. Stat., sec. 766. 303–315 (1994); and Office of Technology Assessment, *Impact of Legal Reforms on Medical Malpractice Costs,* p. 44.

92. Sir Owen Woodhouse, "The New Zealand Experience," in *Medical Malpractice Solutions,* pp. 171–183.

93. Woodhouse, "The New Zealand Experience," p. 180.

94. U.S. General Accounting Office, *Medical Malpractice,* p. 156.

95. Woodhouse, "The New Zealand Experience," pp. 178–179.

96. Woodhouse, "The New Zealand Experience," p. 179.

97. Diana Brahams, "The Swedish and Finnish Patient Insurance Schemes," in *Medical Malpractice Solutions,* pp. 185–201; and U.S. General Accounting Office, *Medical Malpractice,* p. 167.

98. Brahams, "The Swedish and Finnish Patient Insurance Schemes," p. 186.

99. Brahams, "The Swedish and Finnish Patient Insurance Schemes," pp. 187–188.

100. Brahams, "The Swedish and Finnish Patient Insurance Schemes," pp. 196–197. See, also, Paula Kokkonen, "No-Fault Liability and Patient Insurance: The Finnish Patient Injury Law of 1986," *International Digest of Health Legislation* 40, 1 (1989): 241–246.

101. Brahams, "The Swedish and Finnish Patient Insurance Schemes," p. 200.

102. This section is based on part four, "Replacing Tort: A Model Medical Accident Compensation System" (chapters fifteen through eighteen) of *Medical Malpractice Solutions.* The editors of that work describe these chapters as follows: "Chapter 15 discusses the theory, development, framework, and claims procedure of this model administrative, standard-of-care-based system, which applies workers' compensation principles to health care injuries. Chapter 16 identifies substantive provisions, including the compensable event, the types of benefits payable, funding, and cost controls. The conclusions of Chapter 17 indicate the basic economic feasibility of the Model Medical Accident Compensation System by assuming different scenarios for analysis and projections. In Chapter 18 the state and federal constitutional legal problems are analyzed, especially as to due process and equal protection, indicating constitutionality of the Model Act."

103. Halley, Fowks, Bigler, and Ryan, "A Model Medical Accident Compensation Act, Part I," in *Medical Malpractice Solutions,* p. 206.

104. Mills, "The Case for and Against Pure No-Fault," in *Medical Malpractice Solutions,* pp. 143–157.

105. Grad, "Medical Malpractice and Its Implications for Public Health," p. 410, n. 97.

106. Louise Lander, *Defective Medicine: Risk, Anger, and the Malpractice Crisis* (New York: Farrar, Straus & Giroux, 1978).

107. Randall R. Bovbjerg, "Medical Malpractice on Trial: Quality of Care Is the Important Standard," *Law and Contemporary Problems* 49 (1986): 321–347.

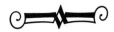

CHAPTER NINETEEN

# ETHICAL ISSUES IN PUBLIC HEALTH AND HEALTH SERVICES

Pauline Vaillancourt Rosenau and Ruth Roemer

The cardinal principles of medical ethics[1]—autonomy, beneficence, and justice—apply in public health ethics but in somewhat altered form. Personal autonomy and respect for autonomy are guiding principles of public health practice as of medical practice. In medical ethics, the concern is with the privacy, individual liberty, freedom of choice, and self-control of the individual. From this principle flows the doctrine of informed consent. In public health ethics, autonomy, the right of privacy, and freedom of action are recognized insofar as they do not result in harm to others. Thus, from a public health perspective, autonomy may be subordinated to the welfare of others or of society as a whole.

Beneficence, which includes doing no harm, promoting the welfare of others, and doing good, is a principle of medical ethics. In the public health context, beneficence is the overall goal of public health policy and practice. It must be interpreted broadly in light of societal needs, rather than narrowly in terms of individual rights.

Justice—whether defined as equality of opportunity, equity of access, or equity in benefits—is the core of public health. Serving the total population, public health is concerned with equity among various social groups, with protecting vulnerable populations, with compensating persons for disadvantages in health and health care, and with surveillance of the total health care system. As expressed in William H. Foege's now classic phrase, "Public health is social justice."[2]

This chapter concerns public health ethics as distinguished from medical ethics. Of course, some overlap exists between public health ethics and medical ethics, but public health ethics, like public health itself, applies generally to issues affecting populations, whereas medical ethics, like medicine itself, applies to individuals. Public health involves a perspective that is population-based, a view of conditions and problems that gives preeminence to the needs of the whole society rather than exclusively to the interests of single individuals.

Public health ethics evokes a number of dilemmas, many of which may be resolved in several ways depending on one's standards and values, that is, one's normative choices. Ours are indicated. Data and evidence are relevant to the normative choices involved in public health ethics. We refer the reader to health services research wherever appropriate.

In order to illustrate the concept of public health ethics, we raise several general questions to be considered in different contexts:[3]

- What tensions exist between protection of the public health and protection of individual rights?
- How should scarce resources be allocated and used?
- What should be the balance between expenditures and quality of life in cases of chronic and terminal illness?
- What are appropriate limits on the use of expensive medical technology?
- What obligations do health care insurers and health care providers have to meet the "right to know" of patients as consumers?
- What responsibility exists for the young to finance health care for older persons?
- What obligation exists for government to protect the most vulnerable sectors of society?

We cannot provide a clear, definitive answer that is universally applicable to any of these questions. Context and circumstances sometimes require qualifying even the most straightforward response. In some cases, differences among groups and individuals may be so great and conditions in society may be so diverse and complex that no single answer to a question is possible. In other instances, a balance grounded in a public health point of view is viable. Sometimes there is no ethical conflict at all because one solution is optimal for all concerned: for the individual, the practitioner, the payer, and society. For example, few practitioners would want to perform an expensive, painful, medical act that was without benefit and might do damage. Few patients would demand it, and even fewer payers would reimburse for it. A likely societal consensus would suggest that public health would be better served if scarce health resources were used for better purposes.[4] But in other circumstances, competition for resources would pose a dilemma, as between providing a new and effective but expensive drug of help to only a few persons on the one hand and use of a less expensive but less effective drug for a larger number of persons on the other. Such a dilemma was posed for the Medicaid program in 1988 when an expensive heart medicine became available that was only slightly more effective than a much less expensive product. In fact, drug formularies are based on the resolution of such problems.

Even in the absence of agreement on ethical assumptions and facing diversity and complexity that prohibit easy compromises, we suggest mechanisms for resolving the ethical dilemmas in health care that do exist. We explore these in the conclusion.

And a word of caution: space is short and our topic complex. We cannot explore every dimension of every relevant topic to the satisfaction of all readers. We offer here, instead, an introduction with a goal to awaken readers—be they practitioners, researchers, students, patients, or consumers—to the ethical dimension of public health. We hope to remind them of the ethical assumptions that underlie their own public health care choices. This chapter, then, is limited to considering selected ethical issues in public health and the provision of personal health services. We shall examine our topic by components of the health system: development of health resources, economic support, organization of services, management of services, delivery of care, and assurance of the quality of care.[5]

# Overarching Public Health Principles

We argue that the following are the general assumptions of a public health ethic:

- Provision of care on the basis of health need without regard to race, religion, gender, sexual orientation, or ability to pay
- Equity in distribution of resources, giving due regard to vulnerable groups in the population—ethnic minorities, migrants, children, pregnant women, the poor, the handicapped, and others
- Respect for human rights, including the right to autonomy, privacy, liberty, health, and well-being, keeping in mind social justice considerations

## Ethical Issues in the Development of Resources

When we talk about the development of *resources,* we mean health personnel, facilities, drugs and equipment, and knowledge. The choices among the kinds of personnel trained, the facilities made available, and the commodities produced are not neutral. The production and acquisition of each of these involve ethical assumptions, and they in turn have public health consequences.

The numbers and kinds of personnel required and their distribution are critical to public health. We need to have an adequate supply of personnel and facilities for a given population in order to meet the ethical requirements of providing health care without discrimination or bias. The proper balance of primary care physicians and specialists is essential to the ethical value of beneficence so as to maximize health status.[6] The ethical imperative of justice requires special measures to protect the economically disadvantaged, such as primary care physicians working in health centers. The imperfect free market mechanisms employed in the United States to date have resulted in far too many specialists relative to generalists. Canada has achieved some balance, but this has involved closely controlling medical school enrollments and residency programs.

At the same time, the ethical principle of autonomy urges that resource development also be diverse enough to permit consumers some choice of providers and facilities. Absence of choice is a form of coercion. It also reflects an inadequate supply. But it results, as well, from the absence of a range of personnel. Patients should have some, though not unlimited, freedom to choose the type of care they prefer. Midwives, chiropractors, and other effective and proven practitioners should be available if health resources permit it without sacrificing other ethical considerations. The ethical principle of autonomy here might conflict with that of equity, which would limit general access to specialists in the interest of a better distribution of health care access to the whole population. The need for ample public health personnel is another ethical priority, necessary for all individuals to live in a healthful, disease-free environment.

Physician assistants and nurses are needed, and they may serve an expanded role, substituting for primary care providers in some instances to alleviate the shortage of primary care physicians especially in underserved areas.[7] But too great a reliance on these providers might diminish quality of care, particularly with respect to differential diagnosis, when they are required to substitute entirely for physicians.[8] The point of service is also a significant consideration. For example, more effective and expanded health care and dental care for children could be achieved by employing the school as a geographical point for monitoring and providing selected services.[9]

Health personnel are not passive commodities, and freedom of individual career choices may conflict with public health needs. Here autonomy of the individual must be balanced with social justice and beneficence. In the past, the individual's decision to become a medical specialist took precedence over society's need for more generalists. A public health ethic appeals to the social justice involved and considers the impact on the population. A balance between individual choice and society's needs is being achieved today by restructuring financial compensation for primary care providers.

Similarly, in the United States an individual medical provider's free choice as to where to practice medicine has resulted in underserved areas, which makes ways to develop and train health personnel for rural and central city areas a public health priority.[10] Progress has been made in the complex problem of providing rural health clinics, but more needs to be done.[11] For example, one option is to increase funds for the National Health Service Corps (NHSC).[12] When needs and preferences of the NHSC doctors and their families are taken into consideration, they remain at their posts longer and have better morale.[13]

Similar ethical public health dilemmas are confronted with respect to health facilities. From a public health point of view, the need for equitable access to quality institutions and for fair distribution of health care facilities takes priority over an individual real estate developer's ends or the preferences of for-profit hospital owners. Providing a range of facilities to maximize choice would suggest the need for both public and private hospitals, community clinics and health centers, inpatient and outpatient mental health facilities, and long-term care facilities and hospices. The financial crisis facing public hospitals throughout the nation poses an ethical problem of major proportions.[14] At stake is the survival of facilities that provide an enormous volume of care for the poor, that train large numbers of physicians and other health personnel, and that provide specialized services— trauma centers, burn units, and so on—for the total urban and rural populations they serve.

Research serves a public health purpose, too. For example, research has advanced medical technology, and its benefits in new and improved products should be accessible to all members of society. Public health ethics also focuses on the importance of research in assessing health system performance, including equity of access and medical outcomes.[15] Only if what works and is medically effective can be distinguished from what does not and is medically ineffective, will public health interests be best served. Health care resources need to be used wisely and not wasted. Health services research can help assure this goal.

Research is central to the development of public health resources. Equity mandates a fair distribution of research resources among the various diseases that affect the public's health because research is costly, resources are limited, and choices have to be made. Research needs both basic and applied orientation to assure quality.[16] There is a need for research on matters that have been neglected in the past, as has been recognized in the field of women's health.[17] Correction of other gross inequities in the allocation of research funds is urgent. Recent reports indicate that younger scientists are not sufficiently consulted in the peer review process, and they do not receive their share of research funds. Ethical implications involving privacy, informed consent, and equity affect targeted research grants for AIDS, breast cancer, and other special diseases. The legal and ethical issues in the human genome project involve matters of such broad scope—wide use of genetic screening, information control, privacy, and possible manipulation of human characteristics—that Annas has called for "taking ethics seriously."[18] The orphan drug law, through tax exemption, focuses enormous resources on diseases that affect a very few individuals.[19] This law may be an instance where society assumes that beneficence takes precedence over equity and social justice. The apparent exaggerations in pricing and profitability have led to regulatory efforts to limit abuse.[20] By contrast, in some instances, discoveries made while researching diseases that affect only a few individuals, as occur in basic research, can lead to findings that benefit broader populations.

Conduct of biomedical research involving human subjects is governed by federal law in the United States. Ethical issues are handled by ethics advisory boards convened to advise the Department of Health and Human Services on the ethics of biomedical or behavioral research projects and by institutional review boards of research institutions seeking funding of research proposals. Both kinds of board are charged with responsibility for reviewing clinical research proposals and for assuring that the legal and ethical rights of human subjects are protected.[21] Among the principal concerns of these boards is the need to assure the autonomy of subjects by requiring fully informed and unencumbered consent by patients competent to give such consent. The boards are also concerned with protection of the privacy of human subjects and the confidentiality of their relation to the project. An important legal and ethical duty of researchers, in the event that a randomized clinical trial proves beneficial to health, is to terminate the trial immediately and make the benefits available to the control group and to the treated group alike.

While the ethical principles that should govern biomedical research involving human subjects are a high priority, criticism has been leveled at the operation of some institutional review boards as lacking objectivity and as being overly identified with the interests of the researcher and the institution.[22] Recommendations to correct this defect include appointing patient and consumer advocates to review boards along with physicians and others affiliated with the institution and in addition to the sole lawyer who is generally a member of the review board, having advocates involved early in the drawing up of protocols for the research, having third parties interview patients after they have given their consent to make sure that they understood the research and their choices, requiring the institution to include research in its quality assurance monitoring, and establishing a national human experimentation board to oversee the four thousand institutional review boards currently operating in the country.[23]

Correction of fraud in science and the rights of subjects are important ethical considerations in developing knowledge. Ethical conflict between the role of the physician as caregiver and as researcher is not uncommon inasmuch as what is good for the patient is not always what is good for the research project. Certainly, in some instances, society stands to benefit at the expense of the research subject, but respect for the basic worth of the individual means that an individual has a right to be informed before agreeing to participate in an experiment. Only when consent is informed, clear, and freely given can altruism for the sake of advancing science and humanity be authentic. Still, exceptions to informed consent are sometimes justified. For example, the need for medically trained emergency personnel permits a convincing case to be made for using deceased patients to teach resuscitation procedures. There is "no risk to the dead person, and families could not realistically be expected to discuss consent at such a difficult time."[24]

Policy makers concerned with the development of resources for health care thus confront tensions between protection of public health and protection of the rights of individual patients and providers. They face issues concerning the allocation of scarce resources and the use of expensive medical technology. We trust that in resolving these issues their decisions are guided by the principles of autonomy, beneficence, and justice as applied to the health of populations.

## Ethical Issues in Economic Support

Nowhere is the public health ethical perspective clearer than on issues of economic support. Personal autonomy and respect for privacy remain essential, as does beneficence. But a public health orientation suggests that the welfare of society merits a close regard for justice. It is imperative that everyone in the population have equitable access to health care services with dignity, so as not to discourage necessary use of such services, and in most cases this means universal health insurance coverage. Lack of insurance makes for poorer medical outcomes even though individuals without health insurance do receive care in hospital emergency rooms.[25] From a public health perspective, financial barriers to essential health care are inappropriate. If each and every human being is to develop to his or her full potential, to participate fully as a productive citizen in our democratic society, then preventive health services and the alleviation of pain and suffering due to health conditions that can be effectively treated must be provided without financial barriers. Removing economic barriers to health services will not mean that the difference in health status between rich and poor will disappear. But it is a necessary, if not a sufficient, condition for this goal.

From a public health point of view, the economic resources to support health services should be fair and equitable. Any individual's contribution should be progressive, based on ability to pay. While some individual contribution, no matter how small, is appropriate as a gesture of commitment to the larger community, it is also ethically fitting for the nation to take responsibility for a portion of the cost. The exact proportion may vary across nation and time, depending on the country's wealth and the public priority attributed to health services.[26]

Similarly, justice and equity suggest the importance of the ethical principle of social solidarity in any number of forms.[27] Social insurance by definition means that there is wisdom in assigning responsibility for payment by those who are young and working to support the health care of children and older people no longer completely independent. A public health orientation suggests that social solidarity forward and backward in time, across generations, is ethically persuasive. Those in the most productive stages of the life cycle today were once dependent children and are likely, one day, to be dependent older persons. Institutions such as Social Security and Medicare play a moral role in a democracy. They were established to attain common aims and are fair in that they follow agreed-upon rules.[28] The alternatives to social solidarity between the young and the elderly are simply unacceptable. As members of a society made up of overlapping communities, our lives are intricately linked together. No man or woman is an island; not even the most wealthy or most independent can exist alone. The social pact that binds us to live in peace together requires cooperation of such a fundamental nature that we could not travel by car (assuming respect for traffic signals) to the grocery store to purchase food (or assume it safe for consumption) without appealing to social solidarity. These lessons apply to health care as well.

In 1983, the President's Commission for the Study of Ethical Problems in Medicine and Biomedical and Behavioral Research made, as its first and principal recommendation on ethics in medicine, the assertion that society has an obligation to assure equitable access to health care for all its citizens.[29] Equitable access, the commission said, requires that all citizens be able to secure an adequate level of care without excessive burdens. Implementation of this principle as an ethical imperative is even more urgent twelve years later, as increasing numbers of people, of whom one-fourth are children, become uninsured.

## Ethical Issues in Organization of Services

The principal ethical imperative in organization of health services is that services be organized and distributed in accordance with health needs. This ethical principle is illustrated by the issues of geographical and cultural access.

A system of health care to be fair and just must minimize geographical inequities in the distribution of care. Rural areas are underserved and also inner cities. Any number of solutions have been proposed and tried in an effort to bring better access in health services to underserved areas, be they rural areas or inner cities. These include mandating a period of service for medical graduates as a condition of licensure, loan forgiveness and expansion of the National Health Service Corps, rural preceptorships, providing economic incentives for establishing practice in rural areas, and employment of physician assistants and nurse practitioners.[30] Telemedicine may provide the best available medical consultants to rural areas in the near future,[31] but the technology involves initial start-up costs that are not trivial.

Similarly, the principles of autonomy and beneficence require health services to be culturally relevant to the populations they are designed to serve.[32] This means that medical care professionals need to be able to communicate in the language of those they serve and to understand the cultural preferences of those for whom they seek to provide care.[33] The probability of success is enhanced if needed health professionals are from the same cultural background as those they serve. This suggests that schools of medicine, nursing, dentistry, and public health should intensify their efforts to reach out and extend educational and training opportunities to qualified and interested members of such populations. To carry out such programs, however, these schools must have the economic resources required to provide fellowships and teaching assistant positions.

The development of various forms of managed care—health maintenance organizations, prepaid group practices, preferred provider organizations, and independent practice associations—raises a different set of ethical questions. As experienced in the United States in recent years, managed care is designed more to minimize costs than to assure that health care is efficient and effective. If managed care ends up constraining costs by depriving individuals of needed medical attention (reducing medically appropriate access to specialists, for example), then it violates the ethical principle of beneficence because such management interferes with doing good for the patient. For example, if managed care is employed as a cost containment scheme for Medicaid and Medicare without regard to quality of care, it risks increasing inequity. It could even contribute to a two-tiered health care system in which those who can avoid various forms of managed care by paying privately for their personal health services will obtain a higher quality of care.

The advantages of managed care are clear: team practice, emphasis on primary care, generous use of diagnostic and therapeutic outpatient services, and prudent use of hospitalization, all contributing to cost containment. At the same time, managed care systems have the disadvantage of restricted choice of provider, run the risk of underservicing, and may achieve cost containment through cost shifting.[34]

The ethical issues in managed care are illustrated most sharply by the question of who decides what is medically necessary—the physician or others, such as the health plan, the insurer, the employer, or the state legislature.[35] This question is not unique to managed care; it has also arisen with respect to insurance companies and Medicaid.[36] On one hand, the physician has a legal and ethical duty to provide the standard of care that a reasonable physician in the same or similar circumstances would provide. On the other hand, insurers have traditionally specified what is covered or not covered as medically necessary in insurance contracts. The courts have reached different results in such cases, depending on the facts of the case, the character of the treatment sought (whether generally accepted or experimental), and the interpretation of medical necessity.[37]

As more and more integrated health care delivery systems are formed, as more mergers of managed care organizations occur, as pressures for cost containment persist, ethical issues concerning conflicts of interest, quality of care choices, restraints on expenditures, and patients' rights will attain increasing importance. The principles of autonomy, beneficence, and justice will be severely tested in the resolution of the ethical problems facing a complex, corporate health care system.

If medicine is practiced for profit, as seems to be the case today and for the near future in the United States, then the ethical dilemma between patients' interests and profits will be a continuing problem. Sometimes the two can both be served, but it is unlikely to be the case in all instances. That both consumers and employers are concerned about quality of care is clear from Paul Ellwood's statement expressing disappointment in the evolution of HMOs because "they tend to place too much emphasis on saving money and not enough on improving quality—and we now have the technical skill to do that."[38]

## Ethical Issues in Management of Health Services

Management involves planning, administration, regulation, and legislation. The style of management depends on the values and norms of the population. Planning involves determining the population health needs (with surveys and research, for example) and then assuring that programs are in place to provide these services. A public health perspective suggests that planning is appropriate to the extent that it provides efficient, appropriate health care (beneficence) to all who seek it (equity and justice). Planning may avoid waste and contribute to the rational use of health services. But it is also important that planning not be so invasive as to be coercive and deny the individual any say in his or her health care unless such intervention is necessary to protect public health interests. The ethical principle of autonomy preserves the right of the individual to refuse care, to determine his or her own destiny, especially when the welfare of others is not involved. A balance between individual autonomy and public health intervention that will provide benefit to the society is not easy to achieve. But in some cases the resolution of such dilemmas is clear, as with mandatory immunization programs. Equity and beneficence demand that the social burdens and benefits of living in a disease-free environment be shared. Therefore, for example, immunization requirements should cover all those potentially affected.

Health administration has ethical consequences that may be overlooked because they appear ethically neutral: organization, staffing, budgeting, supervision, consultation, procurement, logistics, records and reporting, coordination, and evaluation.[39] But all these activities involve ethical choices. The importance of privacy in record keeping, for example, raises, once again, the necessity to balance the ethical principles of autonomy and individual rights with social justice and the protection of society.[40]

The distribution of scarce health resources is another subject of debate. The principle of first come first served may at first seem equitable. But it also incorporates the "rule of rescue" whereby a few lives are saved at great cost, and this policy results in the invisible loss of many more lives. The cost-benefit or cost-effectiveness analysis of health economics attempts to apply hard data to administrative decisions. This approach, however, does not escape ethical dilemmas because the act of assigning numbers to years of life, for example, itself is value laden. If administrative allocation is determined on the basis of the number of years of life saved, then the younger are favored over the older, which may or may not be equitable. If one factors into such an analysis the idea of quality years of life, other normative assumptions must be made as to how important quality is and what constitutes quality. Some efforts have been made to assign a dollar value to a year of life as a tool for administering health resources. But here, too, we encounter worrisome normative problems. Does not ability to pay deform such calculations?[41]

Crucial to management of health services are legal tools—legislation, regulations, and sometimes litigation—necessary for fair administration of programs. Legislation and regulations are essential for authorizing health programs; they also serve to remedy inequities and to introduce innovations in a health service system. Effective legislation depends on a sound scientific base, and ethical questions are especially troubling when the scientific evidence is uncertain.

For example, in a landmark decision in 1976, the Court of Appeals for the District of Columbia upheld a regulation of the Environmental Protection Agency restricting the amount of lead additives in gasoline based largely on epidemiological evidence.[42] An analysis of this case and of the scope of judicial review of the regulatory action of an agency charged by Congress with regulating substances harmful to health underlines the dilemma the court faced:

the need of judges trained in the law, not in science, to evaluate the scientific and epidemiological evidence on which the regulatory agency based its ruling.[43] The majority of the court based its upholding of the agency's decision on its own review of the evidence. By contrast, Judge David Bazelon urged an alternative approach: "In cases of great technological complexity, the best way for courts to guard against unreasonable or erroneous administrative decisions is not for the judges themselves to scrutinize the technical merits of each decision. Rather, it is to establish a decision making process that assures a reasoned decision that can be held up to the scrutiny of the scientific community and the public."[44]

Coping with conflicting scientific evidence is a persistent ethical dilemma, as reflected by a 1993 decision of the U.S. Supreme Court involving the question of how widely accepted a scientific process or theory must be before it qualifies as admissible evidence in a lawsuit. The case involved the issue of whether a drug prescribed for nausea during pregnancy, Bendectin, causes birth defects. Rejecting the test of "general acceptance" of scientific evidence as the absolute prerequisite for admissibility, as applied in the past, the court ruled that trial judges serve as gatekeepers to ensure that pertinent scientific evidence is not only relevant but reliable. The court also suggested various factors that might bear on such determinations.[45]

Epidemiological evidence, which is the core of public health, is increasingly recognized as helpful in legal suits—a significant advance for the determination of ethical issues in cases where the scientific evidence is uncertain.[46] Of course, it should be noted that a court's or an agency's refusal to act because of uncertain scientific evidence is in itself a decision with ethical implications.

Enactment of legislation and issuance of regulations are important for management of a just health care system, but these strategies are useless if they are not enforced. For example, state legislation has long banned the sale of cigarettes to minors, but only recently have efforts been made to enforce these statutes rigorously through publicity, stings (arranged purchases by minors), penalties on sellers, threats of license revocation, and bans on cigarette sales from vending machines.[47] A novel case of enforcement involves a Baltimore ordinance prohibiting billboards promoting cigarettes in areas where children live, play, and go to school, enacted in order to enforce the minors' access law banning tobacco sales to minors.[48]

Thus, management of health services involves issues of allocating scarce resources, evaluating scientific evidence, measuring quality of life, and imposing mandates by legislation and regulations. Although a seemingly neutral function, management of health services must rely on principles of autonomy, beneficence, and justice in its decision-making process.

## Ethical Issues in Delivery of Care

Delivery of health services, the actual provision of health care services, is the end point of all the other dimensions discussed above. The ethical considerations of only a few of the many issues pertinent to delivery of care are discussed here.

Resource allocation in a time of cost containment inevitably involves rationing. While at first blush, rationing by ability to pay may appear natural, neutral, and inevitable, the ethical dimensions for delivery of care may be overlooked. If ability to pay is recognized as a form of rationing, the question of its justice is immediately apparent. The Oregon Medicaid program is another example. It is equitable by design and is grounded in good part in the efficacy of the medical procedure in question, thus respecting the principle of ethical beneficence. It is structured to extend benefits to a wider population of poor people than would be entitled to care under Medicaid. The plan does not qualify as equitable and fair, however, because it does not apply to the whole population of Oregon but only to the poor. In addition, it reduces the level of services to some persons who used to be on Medicaid, in order to widen the pool of beneficiaries. This also presents significant ethical problems.[49]

Rationing medical care is not always ethically dubious but rather may conform to a public health ethic. In some cases, too much medical care is counterproductive and may produce more harm than good. For example, Canada rations health care, pays one-third less per capita than the United States, and offers universal coverage; yet health status indicators do not suggest that Canadians suffer. In fact, on several performance indicators Canada surpasses the United States.[50] Because there is so little information about medical outcomes and the efficacy of many medical procedures, rationing would actually benefit patients if it discouraged unneeded and inappropriate treatment.

The rationing of organ transplants, similarly, is a matter of significant ethical debate. The number of organs available for transplant is less than the need. Rationing, therefore, must be used to determine who will be given a transplant. Employing tissue match makes medical sense and also seems ethically acceptable. But to the extent that ability to pay is a criterion, ethical conflict is inevitable. It may, in fact, go against scientific opinion and public health ethics if someone who can pay receives a transplant even though the tissue match is not so good as it would be for a patient who is also in need of a transplant but unable to pay the cost. Rationing on this basis seems ethically unfair and medically ill-advised.[51]

One solution would be to make more organs available through mandatory donation from fatal automobile accidents without explicit consent of individuals and families. A number of societies have adopted this policy because the public health interest of society and the seriousness of the consequences are so great for those in need of a transplant that it is possible to justify ignoring the individual autonomy (preferences) of the accident victim's friends and relatives. This has not been the case in the United States to date.[52]

Delivery of services raises conflict-of-interest questions for providers that are of substantial public health importance. Hospitals pressed by competitive forces strain to survive and in some cases do so only by less-than-honest cost shifting and even direct fraud. A recent survey of hospital bills finds that more than 99 percent included errors that favored the hospital.[53] Physicians who own or share ownership of laboratories and medical testing facilities have been found to refer patients to these facilities to a far greater extent than can be medically justified.[54] The public health ethic of beneficence is called into question by such unnecessary tests.

The practice of medical and public health screening presents serious ethical dilemmas. Screening for diseases for which there is no treatment is difficult to justify unless the information is explicitly desired by the patient for personal reasons such as life planning and reproduction, except in cases where the information can be used to postpone onset or prevent widespread population infection. In a similar case, screening without provision to treat those discovered to be in need of treatment is unethical. Public health providers need to be sure in advance that they can offer the health services required to provide care for those found to be affected. This is the ethical principle of beneficence and social justice.[55]

The tragic epidemic of HIV/AIDS has raised serious ethical questions concerning testing, reporting, and partner notification. The great weight of authority favors voluntary and confidential testing, so as to encourage persons to come forward for testing, counseling, and behavior change.[56] The majority of states require reporting of AIDS cases; only a few states require reporting of HIV+ status, and those have strong confidentiality protections in place.[57] Partner notification was at first generally disapproved on grounds of nonfeasibility and protection of privacy, but some states have enacted legislation permitting a physician to notify a partner of a patient's HIV+ status if the physician believes that the patient will not inform the partner.[58]

With the finding that administration of AZT during pregnancy to an HIV+ woman may protect the fetus, the question arises as to what extent pregnant women should be tested for HIV. Certainly, the option of voluntary confidential testing should be offered. Should anyone else be tested involuntarily? Some guidance for resolving ethical questions in this difficult sphere is presented by Stephen Joseph, the former commissioner of health for New York City, who states that the AIDS epidemic is a public health emergency involving extraordinary civil liberties issues—not a civil liberties emergency involving extraordinary public health issues.[59]

The field of reproductive health is a major public health concern affecting women in their reproductive years. Here the principles of autonomy, beneficence, and justice apply to the provision of contraceptive services, including long-acting means of contraception; abortion, including medical abortion made possible by the development of RU 486; and use of noncoital technologies for reproduction. The debate on these issues has been wide, abrasive, and divisive. Twenty-three years after abortion was legalized by the U.S. Supreme Court's decision in *Roe* v. *Wade*[60] protests against abortion clinics have escalated. Violence against clinics and murders of abortion providers threaten access to abortion services and put the legal right to choose to terminate an unwanted pregnancy in jeopardy. For presentation of various points of view on the moral and legal aspects of abortion and for selected judicial opinions in this field, the reader is referred to Beauchamp and Walters, *Contemporary Issues in Bioethics.*[61]

We state our position as strongly favoring the pro-choice point of view in order to assure the autonomy of women, beneficence for women and their families faced with unwanted pregnancy, and justice in society. In the highly charged debate on teenage pregnancy, we believe that social realities, the well-being of young women and their children, and the welfare of society mandate access to contraception and abortion and respect for the autonomy of young people. The ethics of parental consent and notification laws, which often stand as a barrier to abortions needed and wanted by adolescents, is highly questionable.[62]

Of the many important ethical issues in the delivery of health care not discussed here because of space limitations, three examples may be mentioned briefly.

- *The death debate* is generally considered a matter of medical ethics involving the patient, his or her family, and the physician. But this issue is also a matter of public health ethics because services at the end of life entail administrative and financial dimensions that are part of public health and management of health services.[63]

- *The mental health field's conflict* between the health needs and legal rights of patients, on one hand, and the need for protection of society, on the other, illustrates sharply the ethical problems facing providers of mental health services. This conflict has been addressed most prominently by reform of state mental hospital admission laws to make involuntary admission to a mental hospital initially a medical matter, with immediate and periodic judicial review as to the propriety of hospitalization, review in which a patient advocate participates.[64] The *Tarasoff* case presents another problem in the provision of mental health services: the duty of a psychiatrist or psychologist to warn an identified person of a patient's intent to kill the person, despite the rule of confidentiality governing medical and psychiatric practice. In both instances, a public health perspective favors protection of society over the legal rights of individuals.[65]

- *Records and statistics* are basic to public health strategies and effective delivery of preventive and curative services. The moral and legal imperative of privacy to protect an individual's medical record gives way to public health statutes requiring reporting of gunshot wounds, communicable diseases, child abuse, and AIDS.[66] More generally, the right of persons to keep their medical records confidential conflicts with the need of society for epidemiological information to monitor the incidence and prevalence of diseases in the community and to determine responses to this information. A common resolution of this problem is to make statistics available without identifying information.

Ethical problems in the delivery of services will surely increase in number and kind in a period of great change in the health service system as private fee-for-service solo practice is being replaced by new ways of financing and providing health care. The most prominent problem will be the question of who decides the appropriateness of services—the payer or the provider, the managed care plan or the physician—and what role the consumer will have in the new system that is evolving.

## Ethical Issues in Assuring Quality of Care

If a public health ethic requires fair and equitable distribution of medical care, then it is essential that waste and inefficiency be eliminated. Spending scarce resources on useless medical acts is a violation of a public health ethic. To reach this public health goal, knowledge about what is useful and medically efficacious is essential.

As strategies for evaluating the quality of health care have become increasingly important, the ethical dimensions of peer review, practice guidelines, and malpractice suits—all methods of quality assurance—have come to the fore. Established in 1972 to monitor hospital services under Medicare to assure that they were medically necessary and delivered in the most efficient manner, professional standards review organizations came under attack as overregulatory and too restrictive.[67] Congress ignored the criticism and in 1982 passed the Peer Review Improvement Act, which did not abolish outside review but consolidated the local peer review agencies, replaced them with statewide bodies, and increased their responsibility.[68] In 1986, Congress passed the Health Care Quality Improvement Act, which established national standards for peer review at the state and hospital levels for all practitioners regardless of source of payment.[69] The act also established a national data bank on the qualifications of physicians and provided immunity from suit for reviewing physicians acting in good faith.

The functions of peer review organizations (PROs) in reviewing the adequacy and quality of care necessarily involve some invasion of the patient's privacy and the physician's confidential relationship with the patient. Yet beneficence and justice in an ethical system of medical care mandate a process of control of the cost and quality of care. The work of PROs has been furthered by finding an accommodation between protection of privacy and confidentiality on one hand and necessary but limited disclosure on the other. Physicians whose work is being reviewed are afforded the right to a hearing at which the patient is not present, and patients are afforded the protection of outside review in accord with national standards.

Practice guidelines developed by professional associations, health maintenance organizations and other organized providers, third-party payers, and government agencies are designed to evaluate the appropriateness of procedures. Three states—Maine, Minnesota, and Vermont—have passed legislation permitting practice guidelines to be used as a defense in malpractice actions under certain circumstances.[70] Such a simplistic solution, however, avoids the question of fairness: whose guidelines should prevail in the face of multiple sets of guidelines issued by different bodies, and how should accommodation be made to evolving and changing standards of practice?[71]

Malpractice suits constitute one method of regulating the quality of care, although an erratic and expensive system. The subject is fully discussed in Chapter Eighteen. Here we raise only the ethical issue of the right of the injured patient to compensation for the injury and the need of society for a system of compensation that is more equitable and more efficient than the current system.

The various mechanisms for assuring quality of care all pose ethical issues. Peer review requires some invasion of privacy and confidentiality to provide surveillance of quality, although safeguards have been devised. Practice guidelines involve some interference with physician autonomy but in return provide protection for both the patient and the provider. Malpractice suits raise questions of equity, since many injured patients are not compensated. In the process of developing and improving strategies for quality control, the public health perspective justifies social intervention to protect the population.

## Mechanisms for Resolving Ethical Issues in Health Care

Even in the absence of agreement on ethical assumptions and in the face of diversity and complexity that prohibit easy compromise, mechanisms for resolving ethical dilemmas in public health do exist. Among these are ombudsmen, institutional review boards, ethics committees, standards set by professional associations, practice guidelines, financing mechanisms, and courts of law. Some of these mechanisms are voluntary. Others are mandated by law. None is perfect. Some, such as financing mechanisms, are particularly worrisome.

While ethics deals with values and morals, the law has been very much intertwined with ethical issues. In fact, the more that statutes, regulations, and court cases decide ethical issues, the narrower is the scope of ethical decision making by providers of health care.[72] For example, because the *Cruzan* case defines the conditions for terminating life support for persons in a persistent vegetative state (clear and cogent evidence of a prior statement by the patient when competent of desire not to be kept alive by artificial means in a persistent vegetative state), the scope of decision making by physicians and families is constrained.[73] Courts of law, therefore, are important mechanisms for resolving ethical issues.

The law deals with many substantive issues in numerous fields, including that of health care. It also has made important procedural contributions to resolving disputes by authorizing, establishing, and monitoring mechanisms or processes for handling claims and disputes. Such mechanisms are particularly useful for resolving ethical issues in health care because they are generally informal and flexible and often involve the participation of all the parties. Administrative mechanisms are much less expensive than litigation and in this respect are potentially more equitable.

Ombudsmen in health care institutions are a means of providing patient representation and advocacy. They may serve as channels for expression of ethical concerns of patients and their families.

Ethics committees in hospitals and managed care organizations operate to resolve ethical issues involving specific cases in the institution. They may be composed solely of the institution's staff, or they may include an ethicist specialized in handling such problems.

Institutional review boards, discussed earlier, are required to evaluate research proposals for their scientific and ethical integrity.

Practice guidelines, also discussed earlier, provide standards for ethical conduct and encourage professional behavior that conforms to procedural norms generally recognized by experts in the field.

Finally, financing mechanisms that provide incentives for certain procedures and practices have the economic power to encourage ethical conduct. At the same time, they may function to encourage the opposite behavior.[74]

As the health care system continues to deal with budget cuts, increasing numbers of uninsured persons, and the process of restructuring fee-for-service care into managed care and integrated delivery systems, ethical questions loom large. Perhaps their impact can be softened by imaginative and rational strategies to finance, organize, and deliver health care in accordance with the ethical principles of autonomy, beneficence, and justice.

Ethical issues in public health and health services management are likely to become increasingly complex in the future. New technology and advances in medical knowledge will challenge us and raise ethical dilemmas. These will need to be evaluated and applied in a public health context and submitted to a public health ethical analysis. Few of these developments are likely to be entirely new and without precedent, however. Current discussion such as that presented here may inform these new developments.

# Notes

1. Tom L. Beauchamp and James F. Childress, *Principles of Biomedical Ethics* (New York: Oxford University Press, 1989), chaps. 3, 4, and 5; and Tom L. Beauchamp and LeRoy Walters (eds.), *Contemporary Issues in Bioethics*, 4th ed. (Belmont, Calif.: Wadsworth, 1994).

2. William H. Foege, "Public Health: Moving from Debt to Legacy, 1986 Presidential Address," *American Journal of Public Health* 77 (1987): 1276–1277.

3. Another public health question is how threats to the environment should be reconciled with the need for employment. We acknowledge that issues in environmental control have an enormous impact on public health. Here, however, our focus is on the ethical issues in policy and management of personal health services. For a discussion of equity and environmental matters see Robert Paehlke and Pauline Vaillancourt Rosenau, "Environment/Equality: Tensions in North American Politics," *Policy Studies Journal* 21, 4 (1993): 672–686.

4. For some examples, see David Eddy, "Rationing Resources While Improving Quality," *Journal of the American Medical Association* 272 (1994): 818–820.

5. This outline is taken from Milton I. Roemer, *National Health Systems of the World;* vol. 1: *The Countries* (New York: Oxford University Press, 1991), pp. 33–80. Financial resources are treated later in this chapter, under "Ethical Issues in Economic Support."

6. Richard A. Cooper, "Seeking a Balanced Physician Workforce for the 21st Century," *JAMA* 272 (September 7, 1994): 680–687. Quality of care declines where specialists are not available. See J. Ayanian, P. J. Hauptman, E. Guadagnoli, E. Antman, C. Pashos, and B. McNeil, "Knowledge and Practices of Generalist and Specialist Physicians Regarding Drug Therapy for Acute Myocardial Infarction," *New England Journal of Medicine* (October 27, 1994): 1136.

7. State regulation has a significant impact on the success of such programs. See Edward Sekscenski, Stephanie Sansom, Carol Bazell, Marla Salmon, and Fitzhugh Mullan, "State Practice Environments and the Supply of Physician Assistants, Nurse Practitioners, and Certified Nurse-Midwives," *New England Journal of Medicine* (November 10, 1994): 1266.

8. Milton I. Roemer, "Primary Care and Physician Extenders in Affluent Countries," *International Journal of Health Services* 7, 4 (1977): 545–555.

9. U.S. General Accounting Office, *Health Care: School-Based Health Centers Can Expand Access for Children*, GAO/HEHS–95–35 (Washington, D.C.: U.S. General Accounting Office, December 1994). Also available on the Internet info@www.gao.gov).

10. Jill Braden, *Health Status and Access to Care of Rural and Urban Populations* (Rockville, Md.: U.S. Department of Health and Human Services, 1994); and David Helms, *Delivering Essential Health Care Services in Rural Areas* (Rockville, Md.: U.S. Department of Health and Human Services, 1991).

11. Lawrence A. Fogel and Cindy MacQuarrie, "Benefits and Operational Concerns of Rural Health Clinics," *Healthcare Financial Management* (November 1994): 40–46.

12. Leah Wolfe, "From the Congressional Office of Technology Assessment: The National Health Service Corps: Improving on Past Experience," *JAMA* 266 (November 27, 1991): 2808.

13. Donald Pathman, Thomas Konrad, and Thomas Ricketts, "The National Health Service Corps Experience for Rural Physicians in the Late 1980s," *JAMA* 272 (November 2, 1994): 1341.

14. Kevin Sack, "Public Hospitals Around Country Cut Basic Service," *New York Times* (August 20, 1995), p. A1.

15. The Joint Commission on Accreditation of Healthcare Organizations is going to provide consumers with information about provider performance or outcomes. The National Committee on Quality Assurance, a national agency located in Washington, D.C., will undertake similar activities. See Ron Winslow, "Accreditation Group to Publish Reports on Performance of Health Providers," *Wall Street Journal* (October 28, 1994), p. B7A.

16. Julius H. Comroe, Jr., and Robert D. Dripps, "Scientific Basis for the Support of Biomedical Science," *Science* 192 (1976): 105–111.

17. Chris Hafner-Eaton, "When the Phoenix Rises, Where Will She Go? The Women's Health Agenda," in *Health Care Reform in the Nineties*, ed. Pauline Vaillancourt Rosenau (Newbury Park, Calif.: Sage, 1994); Council on Ethical and Judicial Affairs, American Medical Association, "Gender Disparities in Clinical Decision Making," *JAMA* 266 (1991): 559–562; and U.S. Public Health Service, *Women's Health: Report of the Public Health Service Task Force on Women's Health Issues* (Washington, D.C.: U.S. Department of Health and Human Services, 1985).

18. George J. Annas, "Who's Afraid of the Human Genome?" *Hastings Center Report* 19 (July/August 1989): 19–21.

19. See Judith Wagner (guest ed.) *International Journal of Technology Assessment in Health Care on Orphan Technologies* 8, 4, special issue (1992): entire issue.

20. John M. Coster, "Recombinant Erythropoietin, Orphan Product with a Silver Spoon," *International Journal of Technology Assessment in Health Care* 8 (1992): 635, 644–646.

21. A new section, Protection of Human Subjects of Biomedical and Behavioral Research, was added to the Public Service Act, Title IV, Part 1; see U.S.C.A., vol. 42, secs. 289, 289a–1–6 (1995), C.F.R., vol. 21, part 56 (1995). Irving Ladimer and Roger W. Newman (eds.), *Clinical Investigation in Medicine: Legal, Ethical and Moral Aspects, an Anthology and Bibliography* (Boston: Law-Medicine Research Institute, Boston University, 1963).

22. George J. Annas, "Ethics Committees: From Ethical Comfort to Ethical Cover," *Hastings Center Report* (May/June 1991): 18–21. At the same time, U.S. institutional review boards object to studies carried out in Europe on the grounds that they are not adequately protective of subjects. See Peter A. Patriarca, "A Randomized Controlled Trial of Influenza Vaccine in the Elderly: Scientific Scrutiny and Ethical Responsibility," *JAMA* 272 (December 7, 1994): 1701.

23. Philip J. Hilts, "Conference Is Unable to Agree on Ethical Limits of Research: Psychiatric Experiment Helped Fuel Debate," *New York Times* (January 15, 1995), p. A12.

24. Jeffrey Burns, Frank Reardon, and Robert Truog, "Using Newly Deceased Patients to Teach Resuscitation Procedures," *New England Journal of Medicine* 331 (December 15, 1994): 1653. See, also, J. P. Orlowski, G. A. Kanoti, and J. J. Mehlman, "The Ethics of Using Newly Dead Patients for Teaching and Practicing Intubation Techniques," *New England Journal of Medicine* 319 (1988): 439–441.

25. J. S. Weissman and A. M. Epstein, *Falling Through the Safety Net: Insurance Status and Access to Health Care* (Baltimore, Md.: Johns Hopkins University Press, 1994); Paula A. Braverman,

Mylo Schaaf, Susan Egerter, Trude Bennett, and William Schecter, "Insurance-Related Differences in the Risk of Ruptured Appendix," *New England Journal of Medicine* (August 18, 1994): 444; Jennifer Haas, Steven Udvarhelyi, and Arnold Epstein, "The Effect of Health Coverage for Uninsured Pregnant Women on Maternal Health and the Use of Cesarean Section," *JAMA* 270, 1 (1993): 61–64.

26. Roemer, *National Health Systems of the World*, p. 67.

27. For an explanation of the Communitarian form of social solidarity see "The Responsive Communitarian Platform: Rights and Responsibilities: A Platform," *The Responsive Community* (Winter 1991/1992): 4–20. Robert Bellah, Richard Madsen, William Sullivan, Ann Swindler, and Steven Tipton take a similar view in *Habits of the Heart* (New York: HarperCollins, 1985). See, also, Meredith Minkler, "Intergenerational Equity: Divergent Perspectives," paper presented at the annual meeting of the American Public Health Association, Washington, D.C., November, 1994; and Meredith Minkler and Anne Robertson, "Generational Equity and Public Health Policy: A Critique of 'Age/Race War' Thinking," *Journal of Public Health Policy* 12, 3 (August 1991): 324–344.

28. Robert Bellah, Richard Madsen, William Sullivan, Ann Swindler, and Steven Tipton, *The Good Society* (New York: Knopf, 1991).

29. President's Commission for the Study of Ethical Problems in Medicine and Biomedical and Behavioral Research, Alexander M. Capron, Executive Director, *Securing Access to Health Care: The Ethical Implications of Differences in the Availability of Health Services*, vol. 3: Appendices (Washington, D.C.: The Commission, 1983).

30. Charles E. Lewis, Rashi Fein, and David Mechanic, *The Right to Health: The Problem of Access to Primary Medical Care* (New York: Wiley, 1976), pp. 43, 141–245.

31. Susan V. Wheeler, "TeleMedicine," *BioPhotonics* (Fall 1994): 34–40; and Ronald Smothers, "150 Miles Away, the Doctor Is Examining Your Tonsils," *New York Times* (September 16, 1992), p. C14.

32. Gerardo Marin and Barbara VanOss Marin, *Research with Hispanic Populations* (Newbury Park, Calif: Sage, 1991), chap. 3. See, for example: Mario Orlandi (ed.), *Cultural Competence for Evaluators* (Rockville, Md.: U.S. Department of Health and Human Services, 1992).

33. Jill Rafuse, "Multicultural Medicine," *Canadian Medical Association Journal* 148 (1993): 282–284; and John Maher, "Medical Education in a Multilingual and Multicultural World," *Medical Education* 27 (1993): 3–5.

34. Harold S. Lutz, *Health Maintenance Organizations: Dimensions of Performance* (New York: Wiley, 1981).

35. Wendy K. Mariner, "Patients' Rights After Health Care Reform: Who Decides What Is Medically Necessary?" *American Journal of Public Health* 84, 9 (September 1994): 1515–1519.

36. *Pinneke* v. *Preisser,* 623 F2d 546 (8th Cir. 1980); and *Bush* v. *Barham,* 625 F2d 1150 (5th Cir. 1980).

37. Mariner, "Patients' Rights After Health Care Reform," p. 1516.

38. Holcomb B. Noble, "Quality Is Focus for Health Plans," *New York Times* (July 3, 1995), pp. A1, A7. For discussion of problems in business ethics, see Jerry Cederblom and Charles J. Dougherty, *Ethics at Work* (Belmont, Calif.: Wadsworth, 1990); A. Pablo Iannone (ed.), *Contemporary Moral Controversies in Business* (New York: Oxford University Press, 1989); Michael D. Bayles, *Professional Ethics*, 2d ed. (Belmont, Calif.: Wadsworth, 1989); and Joan C. Callahan, *Ethical Issues in Professional Life* (New York: Oxford University Press, 1988).

39. Roemer, *National Health Systems of the World*, p. 68–70.

40. See, for example: *Whalen* v. *Roe,* 429 U.S. 589 (1977) upholding the constitutionality of a state law requiring that patients receiving legitimate prescriptions for drugs with an abuse

potential have their names, addresses, ages, and other information reported to the state department of health.

41. A. L. Hillman, J. M. Eisenberg, M. V. Pauly, et al., "Avoiding Bias in the Conduct and Reporting of Cost-Effectiveness Research Sponsored by Pharmaceutical Companies," *New England Journal of Medicine* 324 (May 9, 1991): 1362–1365.

42. *Ethyl Corporation v. Environmental Protection Agency,* 541 F2d 1 (D.C. Cir. 1976).

43. Laurens Silver, "An Agency Dilemma: Regulating to Protect the Public Health in Light of Scientific Uncertainty," in *Legal Aspects of Health Policy: Issues and Trends,* eds. Ruth Roemer and George McKray (Westport, Conn.: Greenwood Press, 1980), pp. 60–93.

44. Silver, "An Agency Dilemma," p. 81, quoting this passage from Judge Bazelon's concurring opinion in *International Harvester Company v. Ruckelshaus,* 478 F2d 615, 652 (D.C. Cir. 1973).

45. *Daubert v. Merrell Dow Pharmaceuticals, Inc.,* 509 U.S., 113 S. Ct. 2786, 125 L.Ed. 2d 469 (1993).

46. Harold M. Ginzburg, "Use and Misuse of Epidemiologic Data in the Courtroom: Defining the Limits of Inferential and Particularistic Evidence in Mass Tort Litigation," *American Journal of Law & Medicine* 22, 3 & 4 (1986): 423–439.

47. Ruth Roemer, *Legislative Action to Combat the World Tobacco Epidemic,* 2d ed. (Geneva, Switzerland: World Health Organization, 1993), pp. 117–126; Centers for Disease Control, *Reducing the Health Consequences of Smoking: 25 Years of Progress. A Report of the Surgeon General,* DHHS Pub. No. (CDC) 89–8411 (Rockville, Md.: U.S. Department of Health and Human Services, 1989), pp. 597–608.

48. Baltimore, Maryland, Ordinance No. 307 (1994), upheld in *Penn Advertising of Baltimore, Inc. v. Mayor of Baltimore,* 63 F3d 1318 (4th Cir. 1995), aff'g 862 F. Supp. 1402 (D.Md. 1994).

49. George J. Annas, *The Standard of Care: The Law of American Bioethics* (New York: Oxford University Press, 1993), pp. 211–213; and Sara Rosenbaum, "Mothers and Children Last: The Oregon Medicaid Experiment," *American Journal of Law and Medicine* 23, 1 & 2 (1992): 97–126.

50. U.S. General Accounting Office, *Canadian Health Insurance,* BAP/HRD–91–90 (Washington D.C.: U.S. General Accounting Office, June 1991), p. 16. Also available on the Internet (info@www.gao.gov).

51. Sale of organs is unethical as well as scientifically unsound as a means of rationing, yet it exists and persists. See Renee Fox and Judith Swazey, *Spare Parts, Organ Replacement in American Society* (New York: Oxford University Press, 1992); and U.S. General Accounting Office, *Organ Transplants: Increased Effort Needed to Boost Supply and Ensure Equitable Distribution of Organs,* GAO/HRD–93–56 (Washington D.C.: April 1993). Also available on the Internet (info@www.gao.gov).

52. L. Roels, Y. Vanrenterghem, M. Waer, et al., "Three Years of Experience with a 'Presumed Consent' Legislation in Belgium: Its Impact on Multiorgan Donation in Comparison with Other European Countries," *Transplantation Procedures* 23 (1991): 903–904; and Associated Press, "Bill Would Allow Automatic Donation," *American Medical News* (March 22–29, 1993), p. 10.

53. General Accounting Office estimate quoted in Elisabeth Rosenthal, "Confusion and Error Are Rife in Hospital Billing Practices," *New York Times* (January 27, 1993), p. C16. See, also, Peter Kerr, "Glossing Over Health Care Fraud," *New York Times* (April 5, 1992), p. F17; U.S. General Accounting Office, *Health Insurance: Remedies Needed to Reduce Losses from Fraud and Abuse—Testimony,* GAO/T–HRD–9308 (Washington D.C.: U.S. General Accounting Office, March 8, 1993). Alan Hillman, director of the Center for Health Policy at the University of Pennsylvania, suggests that hospital records are so deformed and manipulated

for billing and reimbursement purposes that they are no longer of any use for outcomes research—see quote in "New Frontier in Research: Mining Patient Records," *New York Times* (August 9, 1994), p. A11.

54. Bruce Hillman, G. Olson, P. Griffith, J. Sunshine, C. Joseph, S. Kennedy, W. Nelson, and Lee Bernhardt, "Physicians' Utilization and Charges for Outpatient Diagnostic Imaging in a Medicare Population," *JAMA* 268 (October 21, 1992): 2050–2054; Jean Mitchell and Elton Scott, "Physician Ownership of Physical Therapy Services: Effects on Charges, Utilization, Profits, and Service Characteristics," *JAMA* 268 (October 21, 1992): 2055–2059; Gina Kolata, "Pharmacists Help Drug Promotions: Pharmacists Paid by Companies to Recommend Their Drugs," *New York Times* (July 29, 1994), pp. A1, D2; Philip J. Hilts "F.D.A. Seeks Disclosures by Scientists: Financial Interests in Drugs Are at Issue," *New York Times* (September 24, 1994), p. A7; Roy Winslow, "Drug Company's PR Firm Made Offer to Pay for Editorial, Professor Says," *Wall Street Journal* (September 8, 1994), p. B12; and U.S. General Accounting Office, *Medicare: Referrals to Physician-Owned Imaging Facilities Warrant HCFA's Scrutiny*, GAO/HEHS–95–2 (Washington D.C.: U.S. General Accounting Office, October 1994).

55. Elizabeth Heitman and Pauline Vaillancourt Rosenau, "The New Gene Technology: Old Material in Fresh Guise or Tracking Unexplored Terrain?" paper presented at the annual meeting of the American Public Health Association, San Francisco, October 1993.

56. World Health Organization, *WHO Consultation on Testing and Counseling for HIV Infection*, WHO/GPA/NF/93.2 (Geneva, Switzerland: Global Programme on AIDS, World Health Organization, 1993); Martha A. Field, "Testing for AIDS: Uses and Abuses," *American Journal of Law & Medicine* 16, 1 & 2 (1990): 33–106; Sev S. Fluss and Dineke Zeegers, "AIDS, HIV, and Health Care Workers: Some International Perspectives," *Maryland Law Review* 48, 1 (1989): 77–92 (see pp. 84–87).

57. Ronald Bayer, "Public Health Policy and the AIDS Epidemic: An End to AIDS Exceptionalism," *New England Journal of Medicine* 324, 21 (May 23, 1991): 1500–1504.

58. See, for example, California Health and Safety Code, sec. 199.25 (1990) and the insightful analysis by Ronald Bayer, "HIV Prevention and the Two Faces of Partner Notification," *American Journal of Public Health* 82, 8 (August 1992): 1156–1164.

59. Stephen C. Joseph, *Dragon Within the Gates: The Once and Future AIDS Epidemic* (New York: Carroll & Graf, 1992), pp. 53–54.

60. *Roe* v. *Wade*, 410 U.S. 113 (1973).

61. Beauchamp and Walters, *Contemporary Issues in Bioethics*. See, also, Cynthia R. Daniels, *At Women's Expense: State Power and the Politics of Fetal Rights* (Cambridge, Mass.: Harvard University Press, 1993); and Michele McKeegan, *Abortion Politics: Mutiny in the Ranks of the Right* (New York: Free Press, 1992).

62. See *Abortion Denied: Shattering Young Women's Lives*, video produced by the Feminist Majority Foundation, 8105 W. 3rd Street, Los Angeles, CA 90048, 1990.

63. Anne A. Scitovsky, "Medical Care in the Last Twelve Months of Life: The Relation Between Age, Functional Status, and Medical Care Expenditures," *Milbank Quarterly* 66, 4 (1988): 640–660; Helena Temkin-Greener, Mark S. Meiners, Elizabeth A. Petty, and Jill S. Szydlowski, "The Use and Cost of Health Services Prior to Death: A Comparison of the Medicare-Only and the Medicare-Medicaid Elderly Populations," *Milbank Quarterly* 70, 4 (1992): 679–701. For an insightful analysis of how a society's cultural beliefs, concept of autonomy, and informed consent laws influence resource allocation at the end of life, see George J. Annas and Frances H. Miller, "The Empire of Death: How Culture and Eco-

nomics Affect Informed Consent in the U.S., the U.K., and Japan," *American Journal of Law & Medicine* 20, 4 (1994): 359–394.

64. See, for example, N.Y. Mental Hygiene Law, article 9, secs. 9.01–9.59 (1988 and Supp. 1995); and Special Committee to Study Commitment Procedures of the Association of the Bar of the City of New York in Cooperation with the Cornell Law School, *Mental Illness and Due Process, Report and Recommendations on Admission to Mental Hospitals Under New York Law* (Ithaca, N.Y.: Cornell University Press, 1962).

65. *Tarasoff* v. *Regents of the University of California*, 17 Cal. 3d 425, 551 P2d 334, 131 Cal. Rptr. 14 (1976).

66. Frank P. Grad, *The Public Health Law Manual*, 2d ed. (Washington, D.C.: American Public Health Association, 1990): 67–69.

67. For a thoughtful discussion of peer review organizations under the law as it existed in November 1979, see Stanton J. Price, "Health Systems Agencies and Peer Review Organizations: Experiments in Regulating the Delivery of Health Care," in *Legal Aspects of Health Policy*, eds. Ruth Roemer and George McKray (Westport, Conn.; Greenwood Press, 1980), pp. 359–385, see pp. 380ff.

68. U.S.C., vol. 42, sec. 1320c et seq.

69. U.S.C., vol. 42, sec. 11101 et seq.

70. Office of Technology Assessment, *Impact of Legal Reform on Medical Malpractice Costs*, OTA-BP-H-19 (Washington, D.C.: U.S. Government Printing Office, October 1993), p. 33.

71. For analysis of various aspects of practice guidelines, see Alexander Morgan Capron, "Practice Guidelines: How Good Are Medicine's New Recipes?" *Journal of Law, Medicine & Ethics* 23:1 (Spring 1995): 47–56; Christine W. Parker, "Practice Guidelines and Private Insurers," *Journal of Law, Medicine & Ethics* 23:1 (Spring 1995): 57–61; Robert L. Kane, "Creating Practice Guidelines: The Dangers of Over-Reliance on Expert Judgment," *Journal of Law, Medicine & Ethics* 23:1 (Spring 1995): 62–64; Mark V. Pauly, "Practice Guidelines: Can They Save Money? Should They?" *Journal of Law, Medicine & Ethics* 23:1 (Spring 1995): 65–74; and Jodi Halpern, "Can the Development of Practice Guidelines Safeguard Patient Values?" *Journal of Law, Medicine & Ethics* 23:1 (Spring 1995): 75–81.

72. Frank P. Grad, "Medical Ethics and the Law," *Annals of the American Academy of Political and Social Science* 437 (May 1978): 19–36, p. 19.

73. *Cruzan* v. *Missouri Department of Health*, 497 U.S. 261 (1990).

74. Annas, *The Standard of Care: The Law of American Bioethics;* and Rosenbaum, "Mothers and Children Last: The Oregon Medicaid Experiment."

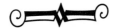

# NAME INDEX

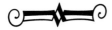

# SUBJECT INDEX